Psychiatric Case Studies for Advanced Practice

KATHLEEN M. PRENDERGAST, MSN, APN
Owner, Psychiatric Nurse Practitioner
Caldwell Mental Health Treatment Center
Psychiatric Nurse Practitioner
Counseling Center
Caldwell University
Caldwell, New Jersey
Psychiatric Consultant
Counseling and Psychological Services
Seton Hall University
South Orange, New Jersey

KASEY B. JACKMAN, PHD, RN, PMHNP-BC
Postdoctoral Research Fellow
Columbia University School of Nursing
New York, New York
Psychiatric Nurse Practitioner
Children's Crisis Intervention Service
St. Clare's Hospital
Boonton, New Jersey

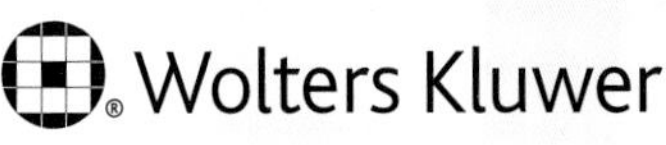

Philadelphia • Baltimore • New York • London
Buenos Aires • Hong Kong • Sydney • Tokyo

Acquisitions Editor: Nicole Dernoski
Editorial Coordinator: Lauren Pecarich
Production Project Manager: David Saltzberg
Design Coordinator: Theresa Mallon
Manufacturing Coordinator: Kathleen Brown
Marketing Manager: Linda Wetmore
Prepress Vendor: S4Carlisle Publishing Services

First Edition

9 8 7 6 5 4 3 2 1

Printed in China

Library of Congress Cataloging-in-Publication Data

Names: Prendergast, Kathleen M., editor. | Jackman, Kasey B., editor.
Title: Psychiatric case studies for advanced practice / [edited by] Kathleen M. Prendergast, Kasey B. Jackman.
Description: Philadelphia: Wolters Kluwer Health, [2019] | Includes bibliographical references and index.
Identifiers: LCCN 2018004181 | ISBN 9781496367822
Subjects: | MESH: Mental Disorders | Advanced Practice Nursing | Case Reports
Classification: LCC RC454 | NLM WM 40 | DDC 616.89—dc23
LC record available at https://lccn.loc.gov/2018004181

LWW.com

CCS0318

Psychiatric Case Studies for Advanced Practice

This book is dedicated to my husband, Mark, and children, Melissa, Matthew, Bryan, and David.

KATHLEEN M. PRENDERGAST

To Aleksey, Leo, and Dasha, my strongest allies and most steadfast supporters. And to my patients and students from whom I've learned so much.

KASEY B. JACKMAN

ACKNOWLEDGMENTS

I would like to acknowledge my psychiatric nurse instructors from The Mercer Hospital School of Nursing, Trenton, New Jersey: Mrs. Kearney, RN, and Delores Hunt, RN, BSN. Their influence has shaped my practice.

I would also like to express my appreciation to my former professor from Rutgers University, Marlene Rankin, PhD, APN, who was inspirational, and my former colleague, Dr. Adrian Coblentz, who was very supportive.

My acknowledgments would not be complete without a recognition of the contributions of my coauthor, Kasey B. Jackman, who agreed to coauthor this book despite many other commitments. Kasey's involvement definitely made this book, *Psychiatric Case Studies for Advanced Practice*, a much better resource, and for that I am appreciative.

Kathleen M. Prendergast

First, I would like to thank my coauthor, Kathleen M. Prendergast. Without her initiative and enthusiasm, this book would not exist. I am grateful for how much I have learned with her and from her throughout the process of writing and editing together.

I would also like to thank my professors and mentors at the Columbia University School of Nursing, for the excellent education I received there. Their dedication to patient care and the nursing profession inspires me to strive to be a better clinician, educator, and researcher.

Kasey B. Jackman

CONTENTS

SECTION II Adult Case Studies

SECTION III Older Adult Case Studies

LIST OF CONTRIBUTORS

Mary Askew, DNP, APN
Medical Director
Intensive Residential Treatment Services
Youth Consultation Service
Newark, New Jersey

Dorothy A. Borresen, PhD, MSN
Assistant Professor
Family Medicine and Community Health
Rutgers Robert Wood Johnson Medical School
New Brunswick, New Jersey

Jordon D. Bosse, MS, RN
PhD Candidate
College of Nursing
University of Massachusetts
Amherst, Massachusetts

Richard H. Broach, PMHNP-BC
Instructor
College of Nursing
Alverno College
Milwaukee, Wisconsin
Telepsychiatry Department
Waukesha Community Health Center
Waukesha, Wisconsin

Barbara Ann Caldwell, PhD, APN-BC
Professor
Advanced Nursing Practice Division
Rutgers University, School of Nursing
Newark, New Jersey

Laura Cannito, MSN, APN, PMHNP
Psychiatric Advanced Practice Nurse
Vanguard Medical Group
Verona, New Jersey

Krystyna de Jacq, PhD, RN, PMHNP-BC
Assistant Professor
Pace University
New York, New York

Suzanne Drake, PhD, APN
Clinician/Consultant
Private Practice
The Wellness Group of New Jersey, LLP
Edison, New Jersey

Valeria Dworkowitz, DNP
Psychiatric Advanced Practice Nurse
Innerspace Counseling, LLC
Old Bridge, New Jersey

Kelly Gardiner, PhD, PMHNP, CNS, BC
Psychiatric Mental Health Nurse Practitioner
ANCC Board Certified Adult Psychiatric Clinical Nurse Specialist
Public Health—Community Health and Education
Wales, Michigan

Brigitte Gordon, DNP
Assistant Professor
Nursing Graduate Program
Columbia University
New York, New York
Psychiatric Provider
Department of Psychiatry
Orange Regional Medical Center
Middletown, New York

Kasey B. Jackman, PhD, RN, PMHNP-BC
Postdoctoral Research Fellow
Columbia University School of Nursing
New York, New York
Psychiatric Nurse Practitioner
Children's Crisis Intervention Service
St. Clare's Hospital
Boonton, New Jersey

Christina E. Jacobs, MS, PMHNP-BC
Psychiatric Nurse Practitioner
Soho MD
New York, New York

Laura G. Leahy, DrNP, APRN, PMH-CNS/FNP, CARN-AP, FAANP
Advanced Senior Lecturer
School of Nursing
University of Pennsylvania
Philadelphia, Pennsylvania
Psychiatric & Addictions Advanced Practice Nurse
APRN-Owned Private Practice
APNSolutions, LLC
Sewell, New Jersey

Mellen Lovrin, DNP, APRN-BC
Faculty
Department of Nursing
Columbia University
New York, New York

Beth Maletz, DNP
Assistant Professor
Clinical Nursing
Columbia University
Nurse Practitioner
Pediatric Psychiatry
New York Presbyterian Hospital/Columbia University Medical Center
New York, New York

Kathleen M. Prendergast, MSN, APN
Owner, Psychiatric Nurse Practitioner
Caldwell Mental Health Treatment Center
Psychiatric Nurse Practitioner
Counseling Center
Caldwell University
Caldwell, New Jersey
Psychiatric Consultant
Counseling and Psychological Services
Seton Hall University
South Orange, New Jersey

Tara J. Richardson, MSN, PMHNP-BC
Psychiatric Mental Health Nurse Practitioner
New Alternatives for Children
New York, New York

Mary Santorelli, APRN, PMHNP (MSN)
Advanced Practice Nurse
Psychiatry
Atlantic Health System
Morristown Medical Center
Morristown, New Jersey
Overlook Medical Center
Summit, New Jersey

Barbara R. Sprung, DNP, RN, NPP, PMHNP-BC, Certified Family Therapist
Clinical Assistant Professor, Program Director
School of Nursing
Stony Break University
Stony Brook, New York

Robin H. Starr, MS, AGPCNP, PMHNP
Nurse Practitioner Specialist, Gerontology
MOFDAPS Comprehensive Behavioral Health Services
Myrtle Beach, South Carolina

Donna D. Templeton, APN
Psychiatric Nurse Practitioner
Adult Crisis Intervention Service
St. Clare's Hospital
Boonton, New Jersey

Robert White, DNP, FNP, PMHNP, APN, BC
Assistant Professor
Department of Nursing
Rowan University
Glassboro, New Jersey

Cathi Zillmann, NPP, CPNP
Nurse Practitioner
Clinical Preceptor
Department of Nursing
Stony Brook University
Stony Brook, NY

PREFACE

Psychiatric Case Studies for Advanced Practice was written to provide a resource for student nurse practitioners. As clinical educators for these graduate students, we were unable to find a case study resource for and by nurse practitioners that encompassed their future practice. In this book, we included patient cases from our own clinical practices, and we invited other experienced psychiatric nurse practitioners to contribute cases or composites of cases to provide examples from a greater diversity of patient populations and treatment settings. Becoming proficient as a psychiatric nurse diagnostician and practitioner is a complex process. This book is but one tool to help develop these skills.

Each case in this book describes the patient's clinical presentation and history with subsequent questions to guide the student through the process of arriving at a diagnosis using the *Diagnostic and Statistical Manual of Mental Disorders*, Fifth Edition (*DSM-5*). Questions to help the student identify treatment interventions are listed following the diagnosis.

Although this book was conceived with students in mind, many of the cases presented will be valuable for practitioners with various levels of experience. Common as well as complex cases are included from a variety of treatment settings and populations, such as university counseling centers, correctional facilities, homeless shelters, inpatient psychiatric units, hospital consultation and liaison services, geriatric facilities, telepsychiatry, and primary care. Newer diagnoses in the *DSM-5* such as gender dysphoria, binge-eating disorder, and autism spectrum disorder are included. The latest treatments for alcohol and opiate addiction and other conditions are reviewed.

While editing the book, we fine-tuned our own diagnostic skills and understanding of treatment options. We learned that the *DSM-5*, like earlier versions of the *DSM*, attempts to provide clear criteria for psychiatric diagnoses. However, as you will see with many of the cases, the diagnoses can only be identified as "other specified" or "unspecified," which indicates that specific diagnostic criteria are not met. This lack of specificity when diagnosing reflects the complexity and uniqueness of individuals and their life experiences and the difficulty in categorizing their presentations. Fortunately, psychiatric nurse practitioners, given their nursing background, provide care based on a broad understanding of behavior and can respond to individuals and their families with a holistic perspective.

We are extremely grateful to the expert psychiatric nurse practitioners who gave their time and effort to contribute cases for this book. Information that would identify the patients in the cases was deleted or altered to maintain the patients' anonymity.

Nurse practitioners may make treatment decisions that vary, and this is reflected in the cases presented in this book. For instance, the decision to obtain a baseline electrocardiogram before initiating psychostimulants in children may be made by one practitioner and not by another, on the basis of their assessment of existing risk factors as well as protocols specific to their practice setting. This inconsistency may be confusing to new practitioners, but they should be reminded to provide the best patient-centered treatment according to the latest evidence combined with their own clinical judgment.

Kathleen M. Prendergast and Kasey B. Jackman

ABOUT THE AUTHORS

KATHLEEN M. PRENDERGAST, MSN, RN, APN, PMHNP-BC

Kathleen's teaching positions have included Instructor in Clinical Nursing, Columbia University School of Nursing, New York and as a part-time lecturer for the Graduate Psychiatric Nurse Practitioner Program at Rutgers, The State University of New Jersey. She is the Psychiatric Consultant at Seton Hall University Counseling and Psychological Services and a Psychiatric APN at Caldwell University Counseling Center. She is the originator and moderator of The Psychiatric Nurse Practitioners Listserve, a national electronic forum for PMHNPs and students to collaborate regarding clinical issues. Kathleen is the president of the Society of Psychiatric Advanced Practice Nurses of New Jersey.

Kathleen has published in the *Journal of Psychosocial Nursing and Mental Health*. She has presented the topic "Post Traumatic Stress Disorder across the Life Span" at Morristown Memorial Medical Center Continuing Nursing Education Conference. She has been a speaker for the New Jersey Association of Mental Health and Addictions. She has also been a presenter for the Rutgers College of Nursing Update on Prescribing Controlled Dangerous Substances for Advanced Practice Nurses.

Kathleen graduated from The Mercer Hospital School of Nursing, Trenton, New Jersey, as a registered nurse and later from Rutgers College of Nursing with a master's degree in psychiatric nursing. She became ANCC Board–Certified adult psychiatric nurse practitioner in 2006. She is the owner and the psychiatric nurse practitioner at Caldwell Mental Health Center, Caldwell, New Jersey. Kathleen M. Prendergast is a Neuroscience Education Institute (NEI) Certified Master Psychopharmacologist.

KASEY B. JACKMAN, PhD, RN, PMHNP-BC

Dr. Jackman earned a PhD in nursing from the Columbia University School of Nursing Kasey has taught courses in the psychiatric-mental health nurse practitioner program at Columbia Nursing and precepted students in the clinical setting. Kasey's current clinical practice is with children and adolescents at an inpatient psychiatric hospital. Kasey is the co-founder and co-chair of the LGBTQIA Health and Health Disparities Research Interest Group of the Eastern Nursing Research Society. Kasey's research interests focus on the health of sexual and gender minority populations, with the goal of decreasing health disparities and promoting resilience. Prior to completing a bachelor's degree in nursing and a master's degree in psychiatric-mental health nursing, both at Columbia University, Kasey earned a bachelor's degree in sociology from Yale University.

LIST OF ABBREVIATIONS

AA	Alcoholics Anonymous
AACAP	American Academy of Child and Adolescent Psychiatry
ACE	Adverse Childhood Experiences
ACT	Acceptance and Commitment Therapy
ADDA	Attention Deficit Disorder Association
ADHD	Attention Deficit Hyperactivity Disorder
AIMS	Abnormal Involuntary Movement Scale
ANC	absolute neutrophil count
APA	American Psychiatric Association
ASRS	Adult ADHD Self-Report Scale
AH	auditory hallucinations
BDI	Beck Depression Inventory
BID	twice a day
BMI	body mass index
BPRS	Brief Psychiatric Rating Scale
C&S	culture and sensitivity
CBC	complete blood count
CBCL-AP	The Child Behavior Checklist–Attention Problem
CBT	cognitive behavioral therapy
CDSS	Calgary Depression Scale for Schizophrenia
CHADD	children and adults with ADHD
CMP	comprehensive metabolic panel
CPSS	Child PTSD Symptom Scale
CRS-R	Conners' Rating Scale–Revised
CY-BOCS	Children's Yale–Brown Obsessive-Compulsive Scale
DBD	disruptive behavior disorders
DBSA	Depression and Bipolar Support Alliance
DBT	dialectical behavioral therapy
DUI	driving under the influence
ECT	electroconvulsive therapy
EEG	electroencephalogram
EKG, ECG	electrocardiogram
EMDR	eye movement desensitization and reprocessing
EMS	emergency medical services
EOMI	extraocular movements intact
EPS	extrapyramidal symptoms
FDA	Food and Drug Administration
GED	general educational development

HAM-A	Hamilton Anxiety Scale
HAM-D	Hamilton Depression Scale
HEENT	Head, eyes, ears, nose, and throat
HS	hour of sleep
ICD	International Classification of Diseases and Related Health Problems
IOP	intensive outpatient program
IV	intravenous
LSAS	The Leibowitz Social Anxiety Scale
MDQ	Mood Disorder Questionnaire
MFQ	The Mood and Feelings Questionnaire
MMSE	Mini Mental State Examination
MoCA	Montreal Cognitive Assessment
MRI	magnetic resonance imaging
NAC	*N*-acetylcysteine
NAMI	National Alliance on Mental Illness
NICU	neonatal intensive care unit
NIMH	National Institute of Mental Health
NKDA	no known drug allergy
NPI-NH	Neuropsychiatric Inventory–Nursing Home Version
NSSI	nonsuicidal self-injury
ODD	oppositional defiant disorder
PANSS	Positive and Negative Syndrome Scale
PBA	pseudobulbar affect
PCIT	parent–child interaction therapy
PCL-C	PTSD CheckList–Civilian Version
PCP	primary care provider
PERRLA	pupils equal, round, reactive to light and accommodation
PFLAG	Parents, Families, and Friends of Lesbians, Gays, Bisexual, Transgender, and Queer
PHQ-9	Patient Health Questionnaire
PO	per os (by mouth)
PRN	as needed
QD	daily
RBC	red blood cells
ROS	review of systems
RPR	rapid plasma regain test to screen for syphilis
SADQ-C	The Severity of Alcohol Dependence Questionnaire
SAMHSA	Substance Abuse and Mental Health Services Administration
SAPAS	Standardised Assessment of Personality: Abbreviated Scale
SIB	self-injurious behavior
SITBI	Self-Injurious Thoughts and Behaviors Interview
SNAP-IV	Swanson, Nolan, and Pelham Questionnaire–fourth revision
SNRI	serotonin–norepinephrine reuptake inhibitor
SSRI	selective serotonin reuptake inhibitor

STI	sexually transmitted infection
T_3	triiodothyronine
T_4	thyroxine
TD	tardive dyskinesia
TF-CBT	trauma-focused cognitive behavioral therapy
TSH	thyroid-stimulating hormone
UA	urinalysis
VDRL	Venereal Disease Research Laboratory
VPA	valproic acid
WNL	within normal limits
Y-BOCS	Yale–Brown Obsessive-Compulsive Scale

INTRODUCTION

Psychiatric Case Studies for Advanced Practice provides student and new psychiatric nurse practitioners with child, adolescent, adult, and geriatric inpatient and outpatient psychiatric cases in order to enhance their skills. Since many of the more common mental health conditions are treated in primary care settings, some of the cases presented may provide a valuable up-to-date resource for family nurse practitioners as well. Experienced psychiatric nurse practitioners may also find this book valuable because it includes case studies about the diagnosis and treatment of complex cases and newer treatment modalities, such as telepsychiatry.

The cases are organized in sections by age group: child/adolescent, adult, and older adult. Although many psychiatric nurse practitioners treat all ages in their clinical practice, this format was chosen for easy reference.

The cases are presented in the standard format of chief complaint, history, mental status, diagnosis, differential diagnosis, and treatment plan. The template for the case studies is provided following this introduction.

The sections "Formulating the Diagnosis" and "Formulating the Treatment Strategy" are presented in each case study to help organize the information in a systematic manner. However, the holistic and integrative process of patient assessment and treatment planning, which is the hallmark of nursing, cannot be easily compartmentalized. Nonetheless, as a starting point, particularly for new practitioners, the sections delineate information gathering, analysis of the information, and help to identify how to proceed in a comprehensive manner. It should be noted, however, that assessing the patient and evaluating the response to treatment is an ongoing, dynamic process with the development of the therapeutic alliance as the core feature.

Only pertinent information is presented in order to make the cases readable and user-friendly. For instance, detailed risk assessments are not included in the cases unless specifically indicated by the patient's presentation. However, in clinical practice all findings, including negative findings, should be documented in a formal psychiatric evaluation. The importance of conducting a comprehensive risk assessment cannot be overstated. Several useful risk assessment tools can be accessed online at: https://www.integration.samhsa.gov/clinical-practice/Columbia_Suicide_Severity_Rating_Scale.pdf and http://www.forensic-psychiatry.no/violence_risk/v_risk_10_english.pdf.

Standard laboratory tests are not listed for each case to avoid repetition of information, but it should be understood that they are to be completed on initial assessment and as indicated thereafter. Standard testing provides baseline laboratory data and allows medical conditions that may contribute to psychiatric symptoms to be ruled out. Typically, routine tests would include a comprehensive metabolic panel, complete blood count with a differential, platelet count, thyroid-stimulating hormone, triiodothyronine (free T3), vitamin D-25 hydroxy, vitamin B_{12}, folic acid, VDRL, and routine urinalysis. For children under 12 years of age, a blood lead level would be standard. In some practice settings, routine pregnancy tests would also be indicated or when a patient is prescribed a medication that is potentially teratogenic. Weight, height, blood pressure, and heart rate should be obtained with each appointment and are not listed in the case studies unless findings are abnormal.

The rationale for each diagnosis is included following the diagnostic criteria from the *Diagnostic and Statistical Manual of Mental Disorder*, Fifth Edition (*DSM-5*). Specific screening tools, when applicable, are listed to help clarify the diagnosis. The treatment strategy and the rationale for the treatment utilizing evidence-based practice are presented. The Treatment Strategy section is divided into the following subheadings: Psychopharmacology, Diagnostic Tests, Referrals, Psychotherapy, Psychoeducation, and Treatment Guidelines. Safety measures and consultations are also described where indicated.

In the Psychopharmacology section the medications prescribed are listed along with the rationale. To identify medications that are Food and Drug Administration (FDA) approved for psychiatric diagnoses, the following link is provided: https://www.centerwatch.com/drug-information/fda-approved-drugs/therapeutic-area/17/psychiatry-psychology. However, many medications prescribed in the cases in this book are "off label" (i.e., prescribed in a manner not specifically approved by the FDA). The use of medications not specifically FDA approved to treat individual diagnoses is quite common and necessary in many instances. New practitioners in particular should consult with colleagues and the published literature regarding off-label use of medications.

Drug–drug interactions should be routinely checked before prescribing psychotropic medications. This can be accomplished with a variety of computerized applications. Drug–drug incompatibility is discussed in the case studies where relevant. For safe clinical practice, evaluation of risk regarding the interaction of medications, both psychotropic and nonpsychotropic medication, is standard practice. The nurse practitioner must also ask the patient about use of over-the-counter products and herbal remedies because these may contribute to additional interactions or side effects.

When prescribing controlled substances, an electronic database that provides prescription data on controlled dangerous substances (CDS) should be consulted to ensure safe prescribing practices. State-based electronic database systems vary, but they are becoming more common and should be utilized. It should be assumed that there is no electronic record of multiple providers of controlled medications or other dangerous practices in the cases presented in this book unless otherwise stated.

Psychopharmacologic and psychotherapeutic treatment provided by the same practitioner is ideal. However, in many instances, the norm is a split treatment model where medication and therapy are provided by two separate health care providers. In these cases, interprofessional collaboration is essential for optimal patient care. The patient must be asked to give written consent for the two providers to communicate regarding the patient's case. This interprofessional collaboration should take place on a regular basis. Even in this model, the nurse practitioner should be able to provide some form of brief psychotherapy and, if indicated, refer the patient for additional therapy. The type of psychotherapy recommended for each case (whether provided by the treating nurse practitioner or referred to another psychotherapist) is listed with the rationale. For more detailed information regarding types of psychotherapy, readers can refer to many of the valuable existing resources, such as Kathleen Wheeler's *Psychotherapy for the Advanced Practice Psychiatric Nurse.*

Education for the patient and family is included in the psychoeducation section. Understanding the diagnosis and treatment plan facilitates adherence to medication and therapy, and enhances the collaborative relationship with the practitioner. In addition, educating patients and their families about the treatment is important so that they can participate in the risk/benefit analysis and provide informed consent for medication.

Treatment guidelines are listed with each case when applicable. The guidelines, however, should not be a substitute for clinical judgment. They may inform the diagnosis and treatment, but because each case is unique, individual assessment and tailored treatment recommendations by the nurse practitioner are essential.

The section entitled Clinical Notes describes additional relevant information about aspects of the case. Expectations about the course of treatment or similar presentations are elucidated in this section.

The final section of the case studies, References/Recommended Readings, lists sources that support the diagnosis or treatment plan of the case or related cases.

TEMPLATE FOR CASE STUDIES

Following each heading are examples of what can be included in each section of a psychiatric evaluation, however, these lists are not exhaustive.

Identification: (Age, marital status, sex, occupation, language if other than English, ethnic background, religion, current living circumstances if pertinent; whether referred or brought by someone)

Chief Complaint: (Patient's own words in quotes)

History of Chief Complaint: (Chronological picture of the events that brought the patient to treatment, onset of current episode, precipitating factors)

Past Psychiatric History: (First episode of illness, types of treatments, hospitalizations, suicidal attempts, assaultive behavior, psychiatric medications)

Medical History: (Allergies, review of symptoms, any major medical illnesses, surgeries, head trauma, tumors, seizures, infectious diseases, sexually transmitted infections, autoimmune diseases, exposure to environmental hazards or toxins, hospitalizations, recent international travel; include current medications, appetite, sleep pattern, sexual behavior)

History of Drug or Alcohol Abuse: (Description of pattern of alcohol and/or drug [illicit or prescribed] abuse. Include any history of substance-related blackouts or seizures or any intravenous drug use.)

Family History: (Psychiatric illnesses, hospitalizations, substance abuse, home environment, relationships, include genogram when appropriate)

Personal History

Perinatal: (Perinatal exposure to alcohol or drugs, full-term birth, vaginal or C-section, breast or bottle-fed)

Childhood: (Developmental milestones, history of head banging, rocking, attachment history, separation anxiety, gender identity development, friendships, intellectual and motor skill, learning disabilities, nightmares, phobias, bedwetting, fire setting, cruelty to animals)

Adolescence: (School groups, activities, sports, sexual activity, self-esteem, body image)

Adulthood: (Education, employment, marital or relationship issues, cultural, religious, social, military, legal issues)

Trauma/Abuse History:
(Describe characteristics of exposure to trauma, such as violence, sexual abuse, military trauma in combat, medical trauma)

Mental Status Examination
Appearance: (Posture, clothing, grooming, attitude toward examiner)

Behavior and Psychomotor Activity: (Attitude toward examiner, Mannerisms, tics, stereotyped behavior, echopraxia, hyperactivity, gait)

Consciousness: (Alert, stuporous, lethargic, somnolent)

Orientation: (Person, place, time)

Memory: (Recent, e.g., "What is my name?" "What did you have for breakfast?"
Remote, e.g., "Name the last 3 presidents."
Immediate retention, e.g., Repeat 6 digits forward and backward, repeat 3 words 5 minutes later.)

Concentration and Attention: (Calculations, e.g., serial sevens, or spell "world" backward, or name 5 things that begin with F)

Visuospatial Ability: (Copy figure or draw a clock face)

Abstract Thought: (Similarities, proverbs)

Intellectual Functioning: (Vocabulary and general fund of knowledge)

Speech and Language: (Quantity, rate, dysprosody, spontaneity)

Perceptions: (Hallucinations, depersonalization, derealization, formication)

Thought Processes: (Flight of ideas, poverty of ideas, loose associations, logical, coherent, illogical perseveration, thought blocking, tangential, circumstantial, punning)

Thought Content: (Obsessions, compulsions, phobias, ideas of reference, ideas of influence, persecutory, grandiose, or bizarre delusions, worries, antisocial urges)

Suicidality or Homicidality: (Detailed risk assessment if indicated)

Mood: (Depressed, irritable, anxious, angry, expansive, euphoric, empty, guilty, hopeless, self-contemptuous, frightened, perplexed, labile)

Affect: (Congruent with mood, normal range, constricted, blunted, flat)

Impulse Control: (Difficulty controlling immediate reaction, e.g., blurting out answers to questions or inappropriate comments. Among children and adolescents may be evidenced by touching or grabbing objects in the room during the evaluation.)

Judgment/Insight/Reliability: (Judgment is evaluated by the patient's capacity to make appropriate decisions and come to sensible conclusions. Insight is evaluated by the degree of the patient's understanding about their illness. Reliability is the degree to which the patient is able to provide accurate information.)

Formulating the Diagnosis

Which diagnosis (or diagnoses) should be considered?

The diagnosis formed with the information provided in the clinical presentation and history is listed.

DSM-5 code (*ICD-10* code) diagnostic criteria

The diagnostic criteria from the *DSM-5* is listed for quick reference.

What is the rationale for the diagnosis?

The rationale describes the specific symptomatology that qualifies the clinical presentation to be identified as the *DSM-5* diagnosis, including diagnostic specifiers.

What test or tools should be considered to help identify the correct diagnosis?

Tools with a brief description are identified. Example: Beck Depression Inventory (BDI) to assess the severity of depressive symptoms.

What differential diagnosis (or diagnoses) should be considered?

The *DSM-5* code (*ICD-10* code) diagnosis is listed followed by the rationale for why it is a differential.

Formulating the Treatment Strategy

What treatment would you prescribe, and what is the rationale?

Evidence-based treatment and/or accepted practice for the diagnosis and clinical presentation is provided, supported by guidelines or references.

Safety measures required: (E.g., if inpatient, what are the observation orders, q 15 minutes, etc.)

Consultations with specialist if needed to coordinate treatment: (Obstetrician for pregnant patient, etc.)

Psychopharmacology: Medication with dose-instructions listed.

Describes the medication category, whether FDA approved for the diagnosis or if off label for specific target symptoms. Explanation is provided for the choice of this medication over other medications in the same category.

Diagnostic tests: Diagnostic tests that are specific to the case are described with the rationale.

Referrals: Referrals and rationale are listed (special types of psychotherapist, medical referrals, etc).

Type of psychotherapy: Type and rationale listed explaining why the therapy would apply to this case or diagnosis.

Psychoeducation: Pertinent information regarding medications or black box warnings.

Educational sites for information such as NIMH, CHADD, etc.

What standard guidelines would you use to treat or assess this patient? Guidelines to treat diagnosis are listed.

Clinical Note

Bullet points about relevant insight regarding this type of case or similar cases listed.

References/Recommended Readings

References to support rationale for treatment provided.

Readings that may inform diagnosis or treatment of the case or similar cases provided.

Appendix

Screening tool or information specific to the case is provided when applicable.

SECTION I

Child and Adolescent Case Studies

CASE 1

Preschooler with Emotional and Behavioral Difficulties

IDENTIFICATION: The patient is a 3-year, 4-month-old female who resides with her biologic mother and maternal grandmother, referred by her primary care provider for further evaluation.

CHIEF COMPLAINT: Mother states, "She has so many tantrums that I am completely overwhelmed."

HISTORY OF CHIEF COMPLAINT: Mother reports that the patient has always been a strong-willed child and has tested limits with adults since early toddlerhood. Mother reports, however, that the patient's angry and aggressive outbursts have worsened in recent weeks. Mother reports that the patient cries, yells, throws objects, refuses to follow directions to take a time-out, and hits and kicks her in the midst of these outbursts. Mother reports the main trigger is patient's being told "no," particularly in the context of breastfeeding. Mother reports patient remains reliant on being nursed by mother in order to fall asleep, have a bowel movement, and in times of distress. Mother reports patient has become increasingly demanding about breastfeeding, including pulling down mother's shirt and hitting mother when not permitted to breastfeed promptly.

Mother reports both patient and mother are currently experiencing sleep deprivation. Mother reports maternal grandmother does not enforce a consistent, developmentally appropriate bedtime, and frequently, the patient is still awake when the mother returns home late at night from work. Mother reports she and patient co-sleep, and patient wakes frequently throughout the night and requires breastfeeding in order to fall back asleep. On further discussion, it is evident neither patient nor mother is getting adequate quantity or quality of sleep.

Mother reports that current stressors include the patient's transition from a familiar family daycare setting to a new, center-based preschool program as well as witnessing the discord between the mother and maternal grandmother. Mother further reports that it has been challenging to balance her work schedule with caring for the patient and that the maternal grandmother has therefore taken on a larger caretaking role. Per mother, she and the maternal grandmother have differing styles of discipline; mother states, "She lets her do whatever she wants and there is no structure." Mother reports her goal is to establish clearer boundaries and limit setting with patient as well as improve their relationship.

PAST PSYCHIATRIC HISTORY: The patient has had no previous psychiatric evaluations or treatment.

MEDICAL HISTORY: Patient has a past medical history of anemia. Patient has chronic tonsillar hypertrophy and allergic rhinitis.

HISTORY OF DRUG OR ALCOHOL ABUSE: Not applicable because of patient's age.

FAMILY HISTORY: Mother reports she has had no contact with patient's biologic father since her pregnancy with the patient and that patient has never had any contact or visitation with father. Mother reports maternal grandmother has recently become more involved with patient out of necessity, because of financial limitations requiring their residing together and mother's work schedule. Mother reports patient is "very attached" to maternal grandmother, seeking her support and reassurance when upset. Mother further reports her belief that the patient intentionally pits mother and maternal grandmother against one another and seeks permission from maternal grandmother for things even after mother has said "no." Lastly, mother reports her own history of depression, for which she is currently not in treatment because of financial limitations.

PERSONAL HISTORY

Perinatal: Mother reports a healthy pregnancy and full-term, normal spontaneous vaginal delivery without complications.

Childhood: Mother reports patient's developmental milestones have all been within normal limits until this time, other than the emotional and behavioral difficulties described. Patient has attended a small, family daycare since age 2 and is currently transitioning to a center-based program. Per mother, patient makes friends easily and socializes appropriately for her age.

TRAUMA/ABUSE HISTORY: Denied.

MENTAL STATUS EXAMINATION

Appearance: Well groomed, dressed in casual clothing. Initially, withdrawn and avoidant with evaluator, but opens up and engages more appropriately as session progresses.

Behavior and psychomotor activity: Mildly intrusive at times; seeks frequent reassurance from mother and requests/demands breastfeeding multiple times during session; needs multiple prompts and has difficulty leaving the office at the end, including crying, yelling, and hitting mother.

Consciousness:	Alert.
Orientation:	Oriented to person, place, and time.
Memory:	Recent and distant memory observed as intact.
Concentration and attention:	Appropriate for age and developmental level.
Visuospatial ability:	Appropriate for age and developmental level.
Abstract thought:	N/A per developmental level.
Intellectual functioning:	Average to above average.
Speech and language:	English speaking, regular rate and rhythm, good articulation.
Perceptions:	None reported or observed.
Thought processes:	Circumstantial and concrete per developmental level.
Thought content:	Appropriate for developmental level; no abnormalities.
Suicidality or homicidality:	Denied.
Mood:	Irritable.
Affect:	Congruent with mood; full range.
Impulse control:	Impaired.
Judgment/Insight/Reliability:	Limited per developmental level.

FORMULATING THE DIAGNOSIS

Which diagnosis (or diagnoses) should be considered?

309.4 (F43.25) Adjustment Disorder with Mixed Disturbance of Emotions and Conduct

Diagnostic Criteria

A. The development of emotional or behavioral symptoms in response to an identifiable stressor(s) occurring within 3 months of the onset of the stressor(s).
B. These symptoms or behaviors are clinically significant, as evidenced by one or both of the following:
   1. Marked distress that is out of proportion to the severity or intensity of the stressor, taking into account the external context and the cultural factors that might influence symptom severity and presentation.
   2. Significant impairment in social, occupational, or other important areas of functioning.
C. The stress-related disturbance does not meet the criteria for another mental disorder and is not merely an exacerbation of a preexisting mental disorder.
D. The symptoms do not represent normal bereavement.
E. Once the stressor or its consequences have terminated, the symptoms do not persist for more than an additional 6 months.

Specify whether:

- **309.0 (F43.21) With depressed mood:** Low mood, tearfulness, or feelings of hopelessness are predominant.
- **309.24 (F43.22) With anxiety:** Nervousness, worry, jitteriness, or separation anxiety is predominant.
- **309.28 (F43.23) With mixed anxiety and depressed mood:** A combination of depression and anxiety is predominant.
- **309.3 (F43.24) With disturbance of conduct:** Disturbance of conduct is predominant.
- **309.4 (F43.25) With mixed disturbance of emotions and conduct:** Both emotional symptoms (eg, depression, anxiety) and disturbance of conduct are predominant.
- **309.9 (F43.20) Unspecified:** For maladaptive reactions that are not classifiable as one of the specific subtypes of adjustment disorder.

Specify if:

- **Acute:** If the disturbance lasts less than 6 months.
- **Persistent (chronic):** If the disturbance lasts for 6 months or longer.

(Reprinted with permission from the *Diagnostic and Statistical Manual of Mental Disorders*. 5th ed. Arlington, VA: American Psychiatric Publishing; 2013.)

What is the rationale for the diagnosis?

At this time, the patient's symptoms meet criteria for adjustment disorder with mixed disturbance of emotions and conduct. One stressor to which the patient is having difficulty adjusting is disrupted caregiving, as a result of mother's work schedule and maternal grandmother's increased role, as well as her transition from a familiar daycare setting to an unfamiliar one. In addition, the patient is likely responding to the increased conflict between her mother and maternal grandmother. The patient's emotional symptoms include irritability, crying, and difficulty self-soothing. The patient's behavioral symptoms include angry outbursts and aggression.

What test or tools should be considered to help identify the correct diagnosis?

Collateral information from the patient's teachers indicating her functioning in the school setting should also be obtained. The patient's symptoms should be monitored over time to determine whether she meets criteria for another mental disorder.

The Child Behavior Checklist for Ages 1.5 to 5 (CBCL/1.5-5) for parents and the Caregiver-Teacher Report Form for Ages 1.5 to 5 (C-TRF) for teachers are two standardized screening measures that should be administered to clarify symptoms and help identify the correct diagnosis.

What differential diagnosis (or diagnoses) should be considered?

313.81 (F91.3) Oppositional Defiant Disorder

At this time, this patient demonstrates some of the symptoms of the criteria for oppositional defiant disorder (ODD). However, her symptoms have been evident for less than 6 months, which is the time frame required for children younger than 5 years. If this patient's symptoms persist for 6 months or longer, a diagnosis of ODD can be considered and could help inform and guide treatment recommendations. However, caution should prevail when making this diagnosis because many of the behaviors associated with ODD occur normally during the preschool and later developmental periods. Therefore, the frequency and intensity must be carefully assessed to make sure that they are significantly elevated before making this diagnosis.

FORMULATING THE TREATMENT STRATEGY

What treatment would you prescribe and what is the rationale?

Psychopharmacology: Psychopharmacologic treatment is not indicated at this time.

Diagnostic Tests: None indicated. Refer to pediatrician for routine testing.

Referrals: The psychiatric nurse practitioner will refer the family for more intensive and comprehensive mental health services to include dyadic treatment for the patient and mother and individual treatment for the mother.

Type of Psychotherapy: Parent-Child Interactional Therapy (PCIT) is an appropriate modality for this family, given its dual emphases on the development of a secure attachment and the need for effective and consistent discipline. At the start of PCIT treatment, parents are coached to engage in child-directed play to improve the parent-child relationship and interactions. Parents are then coached in setting limits and the skills necessary to maintain an authoritative approach with their child. PCIT is a highly evidenced-based treatment with demonstrated mental health benefits for both children and parents. Separate individual treatment for the mother's clinical depression is also indicated.

Psychoeducation: Information regarding positive parenting and child development may be beneficial for the mother, including the importance of boundaries and structure to promote children's sense of safety and security. The mother may benefit from additional education regarding sleep requirements and the effects of chronic sleep deprivation in young children. Future efforts to include the grandmother in treatment may also promote the stability of the family system.

What standard guidelines would you use to treat or assess this patient?

The Practice Parameter for the Assessment and Treatment of Children and Adolescents With Oppositional Defiant Disorder (http://www.jaacap.com/article/S0890-8567(09)61969-9/pdf).

CLINICAL NOTE

- It is important to view the patient, particularly a child this young, in the context of her family system.
- The negative impacts of sleep deprivation on young children are important to address early in treatment. This may promote the effectiveness of further treatment interventions.

REFERENCES/RECOMMENDED READINGS

American Academy of Child and Adolescent Psychiatry. Practice parameter for the assessment and treatment of children and adolescents with oppositional defiant disorder. *J Am Acad Child Adolesc Psychiatry*. 2007;46:1.

American Academy of Pediatrics Supports Childhood Sleep Guidelines. https://www.aap.org/en-us/about-the-aap/aap-press-room/pages/American-Academy-of-Pediatrics-Supports-Childhood-Sleep-Guidelines.aspx. 2016. Accessed February 15, 2017.

American Psychiatric Association. *Diagnostic and Statistical Manual of Mental Disorders*. 5th ed. Arlington, VA: American Psychiatric Publishing; 2013.

ASEBA Preschool Assessments. http://www.aseba.org/preschool.html. Accessed January 27, 2017.

Parent-Child Interaction Therapy. http://www.pcit.org/. Accessed February 15, 2017.

CASE 2

In Foster Care and Very Active

IDENTIFICATION: The patient is a 6-year-old African American male accompanied by his foster mother and 7-year-old brother. Two months ago, the child was placed in foster care secondary to substantiated allegations of neglect by his biological parents and unsafe living conditions.

CHIEF COMPLAINT: "My foster son is like the energizer bunny. When he plays, he is too rough with other kids and talks about people being killed."

HISTORY OF CHIEF COMPLAINT: This boy was previously diagnosed with attention-deficit/hyperactivity disorder (ADHD). The school reports that he cannot stay seated, frequently calls out in class, is disorganized, cannot complete his assignments, and has been known to be disrespectful to adults. According to the foster mother, he is very impatient and impulsive, and he engages in repetitive play with violent themes. He was exposed to a chaotic upbringing marked by homelessness, exposure to violence, weapons in the home, and parental substance abuse and neglect. After giving birth, the boy's mother was homeless. The child, his brother, and mother lived on the streets and in multiple homeless shelters for about 2 years. When the child was around age 2, his mother was reunited with his father, who provided stable housing. In the home, the parents abused illicit drugs and were involved with holding weapons in the home. At age 3, the child was in the Head Start Program, and it was noted that he was demonstrating extreme hyperactivity, poor impulse control, and difficulty sustaining focus. Peer interactions were marked by aggression such as kicking and biting others. When told "no," he would have extreme temper tantrums, where he would cry, scream, and destroy property. Such behaviors resulted in being permanently expelled from the program. At age 4, he was evaluated and diagnosed with ADHD, combined type. Medication was not prescribed at that time.

When the child was 5 years old, he was attending a day care program, and his behavior was unmanageable. When he was pushed by a peer, the child became aggressive by destroying property and hitting his caregivers. The behaviors escalated to the point where mobile crisis was called. When mobile crisis arrived, the child was aggressive toward the screener and stated, "I wish I was dead." Consequently, the child was transported to the Emergency Room for a psychiatric evaluation. During the evaluation, the child stated, "I can't tell you what's going on at home, because I will be a bad boy and not get any Christmas presents." Upon evaluation, inpatient psychiatric hospitalization was deemed necessary. During that time, the child disclosed that a friend of his father held a gun to his head. The hospital notified child protective services, and an investigation revealed that the child had been neglected by parents and living conditions were unsafe.

HISTORY OF PSYCHIATRIC TREATMENT: The patient was admitted to child's crisis intervention services (CCIS) unit earlier this year for a 3-week stay and then discharged to a residential treatment program, where he stayed for 2 months until he was placed in his current foster home. Past psychiatric diagnoses include ADHD and rule out mood disorder. The child is prescribed methylphenidate ER 18 mg daily at 8 AM. It is noted in the records that he has responded well to the medication.

MEDICAL HISTORY: Allergies to medication, food, the environment, and/or latex are denied by the foster mother. Immunizations are up to date. The child has asthma, which is well managed with Proventil (Albuterol) prn. Foster mother denies any recent attacks. The child last saw a dentist 3 months ago, and there is no evidence of dental caries. Appetite can be excessive, and he attempts to hoard food in his bedroom. About 2 to 3 times a week, he has difficulties falling asleep and reports frequent nightmares.

Physical Examination (Obtained by Pediatrician 2 Days Earlier)

Height: 3′8″, weight: 65 lb, BMI: 23.9
Vital signs: B/P, 100/60; P, 78; R, 16; T, 98.4
General: Well-nourished 6-year-old male
HEENT: PERRLA, EOMI, vision is 20/20, and hearing acuity is unremarkable.
Neck: No masses
Pulmonary: No wheezing, rhonchi, or rales
Cardiac: S_1, S_2
Abdomen: No distension, bowel sounds × 4 quadrants, no masses or hernias
Lymph nodes: No swelling
Extremities: 2+ pulses bilaterally
Skin: No lesions or edema
Neuro: CN II-XII intact

FAMILY HISTORY: Prior to his most recent psychiatric hospitalization, the child resided with his biological mother (age 24), his father (age 26), and his 7-year-old brother. The parents never married. The biological father has not seen his children for the past 4 months. The biological father has a history of alcohol and drug abuse, unemployment, and physical abuse of the mother during pregnancy. The patient's biological parents separated during the pregnancy but reunited when the child was 2 years old. The biological mother has a history of substance use but has been clean for the past 8 months. She attends a 12-step program. When her son was hospitalized, she left his father and is currently renting a room. She works part-time in a bakery. The records indicate that the biological mother herself had been removed at the age of 6 from her mother's care because of her mother's substance abuse and had been in approximately 13 foster homes. The biological mother currently has biweekly supervised visits with the patient and his brother. According to the foster mother, the patient is happy after visits with his mother. There is a strong family history of substance abuse. Other family psychiatric history is unknown.

FAMILY GENOGRAM: All family members were born in the United States. No evidence of consanguinity (Figure 2.1).

PERSONAL HISTORY

Perinatal: The patient was born prematurely at 7 months. Weight at birth was approximately 4 lb and 15 oz, and he spent 1 month in the NICU. Records indicate that mother denied any substance abuse during pregnancy. The mother was physically abused by the biological father during her pregnancy. Referral materials indicate that earlier developmental milestones were met within normal time frames.

Childhood: At age 2, child protective services were involved with this family because of allegations of neglect; however, that case was closed. At age 5, child protective services assumed custody of the patient and his brother because the children were exposed to an unsafe environment and neglect. The parents were charged with endangering their children.

The child is a nonclassified first grade student who attends public school. According to a psychological evaluation conducted this year, the child has a full-scale intelligence quotient of 82 (low normal). "Lunch" is his favorite subject, and he reports not liking any other classes.

According to the child's foster mother, he demonstrates age-appropriate gross and fine motor skills. He is able to dress and undress, can tie his shoes, colors within the lines; he can balance on one foot, catch a tennis ball, and ride a bicycle with training wheels.

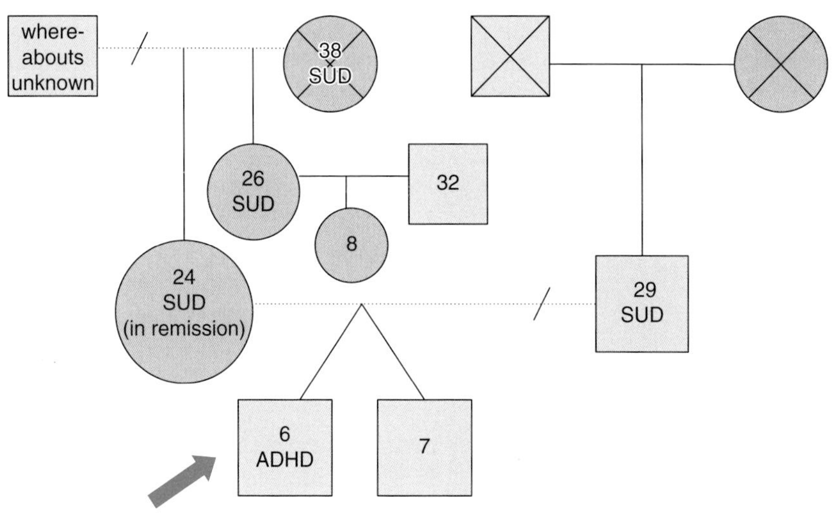

Key:

ADHD – Attention deficit hyperactivity disorder

SUD – Substance use disorder

-- Males

-- Females

Note: Arrow indicates the patient. Numbers indicate the family member's age.

Figure 2.1 Family genogram.

TRAUMA/ABUSE HISTORY: There is no documented history of physical and/or sexual abuse. Allegations of neglect were substantiated by child protective services.

MENTAL STATUS EXAMINATION

Appearance: The patient is a well-nourished 6-year-old, African American male who appears stated age. He is casually attired in a striped collared shirt, jeans, and sneakers, appropriate for age and weather. Hygiene and grooming are good.

Behavior: He separates easily from his foster mother and brother to come with interviewer. When he enters the office, he sits down in the chair, puts his hands on the desk and states, "Let's get to work." Initially, he stays seated with good posture, but after several minutes, he becomes hyperactive and cannot stay seated. Boundaries are poor, and he often grabs objects off the desk. He frequently interrupts. At one point during the interview, he picks up a doll, pretends to shoot it, and states, "We have to take care of the baby," and then he holds the doll in his arms.

Consciousness:	Alert.
Orientation:	Orients correctly to person, place, and time.
Memory:	Remote memory appears fair. He is able to repeat three objects immediately but not after 5 minutes.
Concentration:	When focused, he is able to sing the ABC's and count to 99. Otherwise, he has a very short attention span and is distracted.
Intelligence:	Intelligence appears to be average.
Speech and language:	Speech is spontaneous. At times, tone is loud. Rate is fast, and he talks excessively. He has a mild lisp and some age-appropriate articulation errors.
Thought processes/form:	Goal directed.
Thought content:	Auditory and/or visual hallucinations are denied. There is no evidence of psychosis.
Suicidal and/or homicidal ideations:	Cannot be elicited when questioned.
Mood:	"Happy."
Affect:	Constricted.
Impulse control:	Poor.
Judgment/Insight/Reliability:	He has some awareness but impaired judgment and impulse control. Fire play, stealing, animal cruelty, and/or self-injurious behaviors are denied.

Future aspirations:

When he grows up, he wants to be a "bus driver." When asked what his three wishes may be, he states:

1. "To go to Florida"
2. "To be with mommy"
3. "To have all the toys in the world"

FORMULATING THE DIAGNOSIS

What diagnosis should be considered?

309.81 (F43.10) Posttraumatic Stress Disorder

Posttraumatic Stress Disorder for Children 6 Years and Younger

A. In children 6 years and younger, exposure to actual or threatened death, serious injury, or sexual violence in one (or more) of the following ways:
   1. Directly experiencing the traumatic event(s).
   2. Witnessing, in person, the event(s) as it occurred to others, especially primary caregivers.
      - **Note:** Witnessing does not include events that are witnessed only in electronic media, television, movies, or pictures.
   3. Learning that the traumatic event(s) occurred to a parent or caregiving figure.

B. Presence of one (or more) of the following intrusion symptoms associated with the traumatic event(s), beginning after the traumatic event(s) occurred:
   1. Recurrent, involuntary, and intrusive distressing memories of the traumatic event(s).
      - **Note:** Spontaneous and intrusive memories may not necessarily appear distressing and may be expressed as play reenactment.
   2. Recurrent distressing dreams in which the content and/or affect of the dream is related to the traumatic event(s).
      - **Note:** It may not be possible to ascertain that the frightening content is related to the traumatic event.
   3. Dissociative reactions (eg, flashbacks) in which the child feels or acts as if the traumatic event(s) were recurring. (Such reactions may occur on a continuum, with the most extreme expression being a complete loss of awareness of present surroundings.) Such trauma-specific reenactment may occur in play.
   4. Intense or prolonged psychological distress at exposure to internal or external cues that symbolize or resemble an aspect of the traumatic event(s).
   5. Marked physiological reactions to reminders of the traumatic event(s).

C. One (or more) of the following symptoms, representing either persistent avoidance of stimuli associated with the traumatic event(s) or negative alterations in cognitions and mood associated with the traumatic event(s), must be present, beginning after the event(s) or worsening after the event(s):
   1. **Persistent avoidance of stimuli**
      - Avoidance of or efforts to avoid activities, places, or physical reminders that arouse recollections of the traumatic event(s).
      - Avoidance of or efforts to avoid people, conversations, or interpersonal situations that arouse recollections of the traumatic event(s).
   2. **Negative alterations in cognitions**
      - Substantially increased frequency of negative emotional states (eg, fear, guilt, sadness, shame, confusion).
      - Markedly diminished interest or participation in significant activities, including constriction of play.
      - Socially withdrawn behavior.
      - Persistent reduction in expression of positive emotions.

D. Alterations in arousal and reactivity associated with the traumatic event(s), beginning or worsening after the traumatic event(s) occurred, as evidenced by two (or more) of the following:
   1. Irritable behavior and angry outbursts (with little or no provocation) typically expressed as verbal or physical aggression toward people or objects (including extreme temper tantrums).
   2. Hypervigilance.
   3. Exaggerated startle response.
   4. Problems with concentration.
   5. Sleep disturbance (eg, difficulty falling or staying asleep or restless sleep).

E. The duration of the disturbance is more than 1 month.

F. The disturbance causes clinically significant distress or impairment in relationships with parents, siblings, peers, or other caregivers or with school behavior.

G. The disturbance is not attributable to the physiological effects of a substance (eg, medication or alcohol) or another medical condition.

(Reprinted with permission from the *Diagnostic and Statistical Manual of Mental Disorders*. 5th ed. Arlington, VA: American Psychiatric Publishing; 2013.)

What is your rationale for this diagnosis?

This child has experienced many life stressors, including homelessness, exposure to violence, guns and drugs, parental neglect, separation from his mother, and multiple out-of-home placements. When he was hospitalized, it was learned that he was threatened with a gun. This child feels easily threatened and demonstrates agitated and avoidant behaviors. During the evaluation, he reenacts the trauma, unprompted with a doll in the room. He has difficulty sleeping and frequent nightmares. Outbursts of anger are most likely secondary to hyperarousal. According to his foster mother, he has no friends, and he demonstrates a repetitive theme of violence during play.

What diagnosis should be considered?

314.01 (F90.2) Attention-Deficit/Hyperactivity Disorder, Combined Presentation

Diagnostic Criteria

A. A persistent pattern of inattention and/or hyperactivity-impulsivity that interferes with functioning or development, as characterized by (1) and/or (2):
   1. **Inattention:** Six (or more) of the following symptoms have persisted for at least 6 months to a degree that is inconsistent with developmental level and that negatively impacts directly on social and academic/occupational activities:
      - **Note:** The symptoms are not solely a manifestation of oppositional behavior, defiance, hostility, or failure to understand tasks or instructions. For older adolescents and adults (age 17 and older), at least five symptoms are required.
        a. Often fails to give close attention to details or makes careless mistakes in schoolwork, at work, or during other activities (eg, overlooks or misses details, work is inaccurate).
        b. Often has difficulty sustaining attention in tasks or play activities (eg, has difficulty remaining focused during lectures, conversations, or lengthy reading).
        c. Often does not seem to listen when spoken to directly (eg, mind seems elsewhere, even in the absence of any obvious distraction).
        d. Often does not follow through on instructions and fails to finish schoolwork, chores, or duties in the workplace (eg, starts tasks but quickly loses focus and is easily sidetracked).
        e. Often has difficulty organizing tasks and activities (eg, difficulty managing sequential tasks; difficulty keeping materials and belongings in order; messy, disorganized work; has poor time management; fails to meet deadlines).
        f. Often avoids, dislikes, or is reluctant to engage in tasks that require sustained mental effort (eg, schoolwork or homework; for older adolescents and adults, preparing reports, completing forms, reviewing lengthy papers).
        g. Often loses things necessary for tasks or activities (eg, school materials, pencils, books, tools, wallets, keys, paperwork, eyeglasses, mobile telephones).

h. Is often easily distracted by extraneous stimuli (for older adolescents and adults, may include unrelated thoughts).
i. Is often forgetful in daily activities (eg, doing chores, running errands; for older adolescents and adults, returning calls, paying bills, keeping appointments).

2. **Hyperactivity and impulsivity:** Six (or more) of the following symptoms have persisted for at least 6 months to a degree that is inconsistent with developmental level and that negatively impacts directly on social and academic/occupational activities:
   - **Note:** The symptoms are not solely a manifestation of oppositional behavior, defiance, hostility, or a failure to understand tasks or instructions. For older adolescents and adults (age 17 and older), at least five symptoms are required.

   a. Often fidgets with or taps hands or feet or squirms in seat.
   b. Often leaves seat in situations when remaining seated is expected (eg, leaves his or her place in the classroom, in the office or other workplace, or in other situations that require remaining in place).
   c. Often runs about or climbs in situations where it is inappropriate. (**Note:** In adolescents or adults, may be limited to feeling restless.)
   d. Often unable to play or engage in leisure activities quietly.
   e. Is often "on the go," acting as if "driven by a motor" (eg, is unable to be or uncomfortable being still for extended time, as in restaurants, meetings; may be experienced by others as being restless or difficult to keep up with).
   f. Often talks excessively.
   g. Often blurts out an answer before a question has been com pleted (eg, completes people's sentences; cannot wait for turn in conversation).
   h. Often has difficulty waiting his or her turn (eg, while waiting in line).
   i. Often interrupts or intrudes on others (eg, butts into conversations, games, or activities; may start using other people's things without asking or receiving permission; for adolescents and adults, may intrude into or take over what others are doing).

B. Several inattentive or hyperactive-impulsive symptoms were present before age 12.
C. Several inattentive or hyperactive-impulsive symptoms are present in two or more settings (eg, at home, school, or work; with friends or relatives; in other activities).
D. There is clear evidence that the symptoms interfere with, or reduce the quality of, social, academic, or occupational functioning.
E. The symptoms do not occur exclusively during the course of schizophrenia or another psychotic disorder and are not better explained

by another mental disorder (eg, mood disorder, anxiety disorder, dissociative disorder, personality disorder, substance intoxication or withdrawal).

Specify whether:

- **314.01 (F90.2) Combined presentation:** If both Criterion A1 (inattention) and Criterion A2 (hyperactivity-impulsivity) are met for the past 6 months.
- **314.00 (F90.0) Predominantly inattentive presentation:** If Criterion A1 (inattention) is met but Criterion A2 (hyperactivity-impulsivity) has not been met for the past 6 months.
- **314.01 (F90.1) Predominantly hyperactive/impulsive presentation:** If Criterion A2 (hyperactivity-impulsivity) is met and Criterion A1 (inattention) has not been met for the past 6 months.

Specify if:

- **In partial remission:** When full criteria were previously met; fewer than the full criteria have been met for the past 6 months; and the symptoms still result in impairment in social, academic, or occupational functioning.

Specify current severity:

- **Mild:** Few, if any, symptoms in excess of those required to make the diagnosis are present, and symptoms result in no more than minor impairments in social or occupational functioning.
- **Moderate:** Symptoms or functional impairment between "mild" and "severe" is present.
- **Severe:** Many symptoms in excess of those required to make the diagnosis, or several symptoms that are particularly severe, are present, or the symptoms result in marked impairment in social or occupational functioning.

(Reprinted with permission from the *Diagnostic and Statistical Manual of Mental Disorders*. 5th ed. Arlington, VA: American Psychiatric Publishing; 2013.)

What is your rationale for this diagnosis?

This child has a known diagnosis of ADHD—combined type. The clinical presentation supports this diagnosis.

What tests or tools should be considered to help identify the correct diagnosis?

Child PTSD Symptom Scale (CPSS)
Conners Rating Scale

What differential diagnosis should be considered?

313.81 (F91.3) Oppositional Defiant Disorder

Aspects of posttraumatic stress disorder (PTSD) can mimic oppositional defiant disorder, such as angry outbursts, being easily annoyed, not following rules, and easily losing temper. Children with PTSD are often defiant when told no because they need to maintain a sense of control.

315.8 (F88) Other Specified Neurodevelopmental Disorder

Neurodevelopmental disorder is associated with prenatal alcohol exposure. Prenatal alcohol exposure contributes to a range of effects on mental, cognitive, and behavioral functioning and frequently is misdiagnosed as ADHD. The mother was a known substance abuser but did deny using drugs/alcohol during the pregnancy.

296.99 (F34.8) Disruptive Mood Dysregulation Disorder

The symptoms of hyperarousal may mimic hypomania, irritability, and sleep difficulties. The reenactment of violent themes is similar to the aggressive and explosive behaviors that are commonly seen in children with mood disorders. Therefore, the diagnosis of Disruptive Mood Dysregulation Disorder should be considered. However, the patient does not exhibit the "temper outbursts" frequently enough to meet the criteria for this diagnosis.

FORMULATING THE TREATMENT STRATEGY

What treatment would you prescribe and what is the rationale?

Psychopharmacology

Continue methylphenidate ER 18 mg at 8 AM.

Start Intuniv 1 mg daily at 8 PM. This is a nonstimulant medication that is FDA indicated for ADHD. Guanfacine (a short-acting form of Intuniv) is commonly used off-label for children with PTSD because it is a selective α_2-adrenergic agent that has been known to decrease hyperarousal and improve sleep.

Diagnostic Tests: None.

Referrals: None.

Type of Psychotherapy

Trauma-Focused Cognitive Behavioral Therapy (TF-CBT)—This therapy helps with stress management skills, assists with verbalization of emotions and anger management, and can improve interpersonal skills. Compared with other types of therapy, TF-CBT provides the most empirical data to support symptom reduction. Weekly TF-CBT sessions should be preferably in the foster home. This child may feel safer and more relaxed in a home setting.

Eye Movement Desensitization Reprocessing (EMDR)—This type of therapy teaches self-awareness, helps identify stress in the body, and reprocesses the trauma so the past can be fully integrated into the present.

Alternative therapies that may be helpful include yoga, relaxation skills, and meditation.

Psychoeducation

Provide education about the impact of traumatic events in early life and the impact on development.

To promote positive behavioral changes, this child's environment should be predictable, safe, and nurturing.

Advise the foster mother that despite a child being reared in an abusive environment, most children have a strong loyalty to their biological parents, making attachments to other parental figures challenging.

The public school has a Child Study Team that can provide an Individualized Educational Plan that allows for special accommodations to make this child more successful.

The book *The Boy Who Was Raised as a Dog* is a good resource to help increase understanding of PTSD.

What guidelines would you use to treat or assess this patient?

American Academy of Child and Adolescent Psychiatry (AACAP) Practice Parameters for the Assessment and Treatment of Children and Adolescents with PTSD; AACAP Practice Parameters for the Assessment and Treatment of Children and Adolescents with ADHD.

CLINICAL NOTE

- Children younger than 6 years can rarely complete any type of screening tool. Screening tools should be completed by caregivers.
- Research on pharmacological agents for PTSD treatment in children is limited.
- In clinical practice, some children are known to become more aggressive on a stimulant, but there is no evidence in the literature to support this.

REFERENCES/RECOMMENDED READINGS

American Academy of Child and Adolescent Psychiatry. Practice parameters for the assessment and treatment of children and adolescents with attention deficit/hyperactivity disorder. *J Am Acad Child Adolesc Psychiatry*. 2007;46(7):894-921.

American Academy of Child and Adolescent Psychiatry. Practice parameters for the assessment and treatment of children and adolescents with posttraumatic stress disorder. *J Am Acad Child Adolesc Psychiatry.* 2010;49(4):414-430.

American Psychiatric Association. *Diagnostic and Statistical Manual of Mental Disorders.* 5th ed. Arlington, VA: American Psychiatric Publishing; 2013.

Barkley RA. *Taking Charge of ADHD: The Complete, Authoritative Guide for Parents.* 3rd ed. New York, NY: Guilford Publications; 2013.

Foa EB, Johnson KM, Feeny NC, Treadwell KR. The Child PTSD Symptom Scale: a preliminary examination of its psychometric properties. *J Clin Child Psychol.* 2001;30(3):376-384.

Perry BD, Szacavitz M. *The Boy Who Was Raised as a Dog.* New York, NY: Basic Books; 2006.

Stahl S. *Essential Psychopharmacology: The Prescriber's Guide.* New York, NY: Cambridge University Press; 2007.

William MK, Bowers R, Weston C, Jackson J. *Green's Child and Adolescent Clinical Psychopharmacology.* Philadelphia, PA: Lippincott Williams &Wilkins; 2014.

CASE 3

Aggression at a Young Age

IDENTIFICATION: The patient is a 6-year-old, white girl in the custody of child protective services, residing with a foster family. She is evaluated in a crisis unit at an inpatient psychiatric hospital.

CHIEF COMPLAINT: "I am fine."

HISTORY OF CHIEF COMPLAINT: The patient became very angry and aggressive toward her foster mother after being asked to turn off the television so that she could get ready for bed. She screamed and threw objects at her foster mother and then locked herself in the bathroom. When the foster mother opened the bathroom door, the patient threatened to kill the foster mother, and her foster siblings, and burn down the house. The foster mother called emergency services, and the police came to the house and transported the patient to the hospital emergency department.

PAST PSYCHIATRIC HISTORY: The patient was evaluated at the emergency department twice in the past for aggressive behavior. No prior psychiatric medication trials. In-home behavioral health services were instituted after the second emergency evaluation. No further details about the therapy are known at this time.

MEDICAL HISTORY: No known allergies. No acute or chronic medical conditions. Patient appears small for her age.

HISTORY OF DRUG OR ALCOHOL ABUSE: None.

FAMILY HISTORY: Patient's biologic mother and father have a history of substance use problems. Details are not known.

PERSONAL HISTORY

Perinatal: The patient has a possible history of intrauterine exposure to substances.

Childhood: Patient's biologic parents were charged with neglect 1 year ago. Patient and her younger sister (2 years younger) were left alone by the parents to feed themselves. Patient is reported to have cared for her younger sister by feeding her and changing her diapers.

She currently lives with her foster mother, her 4-year-old biologic sister, and 9-year-old foster sister (foster mother's biologic daughter). Foster mother works part-time in food services. Patient has trouble focusing at school and is frequently described by teachers as disruptive and distractible.

TRAUMA/ABUSE HISTORY: History of neglect by biologic parents.

MENTAL STATUS EXAMINATION

Appearance: Casual dress, fair grooming.

Behavior and psychomotor activity: Cooperative with assessment, somewhat hyperactive.

Consciousness:	Alert.
Orientation:	Oriented to person and place.
Memory:	Not formally assessed but appears to be average.
Concentration and attention:	Responded to questions in an age-appropriate manner.
Visuospatial ability:	Not assessed.
Abstract thought:	Concrete thought process.
Intellectual functioning:	Average, appropriate for age.
Speech and language:	Regular rate, rhythm, and volume.
Perceptions:	No evidence of perceptual disturbance.
Thought processes:	Concrete.

Thought content: No paranoia or grandiosity.

Suicidality or homicidality: Denied during this evaluation.

Mood: Euthymic.

Affect: Constricted.

Impulse control: Limited.

Judgment/Insight/Reliability: Poor/poor/poor.

FORMULATING THE DIAGNOSIS

Which diagnosis (or diagnoses) should be considered?

309.3 (F43.24) Adjustment Disorder, with Disturbance of Conduct

Diagnostic Criteria

A. The development of emotional or behavioral symptoms in response to an identifiable stressor(s) occurring within 3 months of the onset of the stressor(s).
B. These symptoms or behaviors are clinically significant, as evidenced by one or both of the following:
   1. Marked distress that is out of proportion to the severity or intensity of the stressor, taking into account the external context and the cultural factors that might influence symptom severity and presentation.
   2. Significant impairment in social, occupational, or other important areas of functioning.
C. The stress-related disturbance does not meet the criteria for another mental disorder and is not merely an exacerbation of a preexisting mental disorder.
D. The symptoms do not represent normal bereavement.
E. Once the stressor or its consequences have terminated, the symptoms do not persist for more than an additional 6 months.

Specify whether:

- **309.0 (F43.21) With depressed mood:** Low mood, tearfulness, or feelings of hopelessness are predominant.
- **309.24 (F43.22) With anxiety:** Nervousness, worry, jitteriness, or separation anxiety is predominant.
- **309.28 (F43.23) With mixed anxiety and depressed mood:** A combination of depression and anxiety is predominant.

- **309.3 (F43.24) With disturbance of conduct:** Disturbance of conduct is predominant.
- **309.4 (F43.25) With mixed disturbance of emotions and conduct:** Both emotional symptoms (eg, depression, anxiety) and disturbance of conduct are predominant.
- **309.9 (F43.20) Unspecified:** For maladaptive reactions that are not classifiable as one of the specific subtypes of adjustment disorder.

Specify if:

- **Acute:** If the disturbance lasts less than 6 months.
- **Persistent (chronic):** If the disturbance lasts for 6 months or longer.

(Reprinted with permission from the *Diagnostic and Statistical Manual of Mental Disorders*. 5th ed. Arlington, VA: American Psychiatric Publishing; 2013.)

What is the rationale for the diagnosis?

The patient appears to have developed behavioral symptoms since being placed with her new foster family 2 months ago. She has behavioral outbursts that are out of proportion to the current stressor and are causing impairment in her ability to live with her foster family. The disturbance does not meet the criteria for another diagnosis and is not an exacerbation of a previous disorder. The specifier "With disturbance of conduct" is chosen because her main symptoms are the behavioral outbursts. There are no reported mood problems, such as depression or anxiety, at this time.

What test or tools should be considered to help identify the correct diagnosis?

None.

What differential diagnosis (or diagnoses) should be considered?

312.34 (F63.81) Intermittent Explosive Disorder

The patient has episodes of aggressive behavior that are triggered by minor events, such as being asked to turn off the television or stop playing video games. They occur impulsively and without a tangible goal. However, the symptoms do not rise to the severity level of Intermittent Explosive Disorder and are more consistent with the criteria for an adjustment disorder diagnosis.

FORMULATING THE TREATMENT STRATEGY

What treatment would you prescribe and what is the rationale?

Psychopharmacology: No medications ordered. When the patient is followed in outpatient services after discharge, if nonpharmacologic treatments are not sufficient and the episodes persist, medications such as guanfacine or clonidine could be considered. Although these medications do not have an FDA-approved indication for impulsivity and aggression, they are frequently prescribed off-label for these symptoms.

Diagnostic Tests: Standard hospital admission laboratory work.

Referrals: Neuropsychologic evaluation for additional testing of several domains includes intellectual functioning, academic achievement, visuospatial processing, language processing, attention/concentration, verbal learning and memory, visual learning and memory, executive functions, speed of processing, sensory-perceptual functions, motor speed and strength, motivation, and personality assessment. This testing would help to identify any specific deficits that would guide treatment, particularly because this patient may have experienced in utero exposure to substances and/or may have unidentified learning disabilities.

Type of Psychotherapy: Family therapy to strengthen attachment between patient and foster mother. Consider referral for trauma-focused treatment for the patient.

Psychoeducation: Provide education to foster mother about the sequelae of early childhood neglect and maltreatment. Refer foster mother for parenting support group for parents/guardians of traumatized children.

What standard guidelines would you use to treat or assess this patient?

None.

CLINICAL NOTE

- Patients with early childhood abuse and/or neglect may develop reactive attachment disorder. Although this patient did not appear to meet criteria for this disorder when evaluated in the inpatient acute treatment setting, as the patient is followed in outpatient services, the potential for this should continue to be evaluated.

REFERENCES/RECOMMENDED READINGS

American Psychiatric Association. *Diagnostic and Statistical Manual of Mental Disorders*. 5th ed. Arlington, VA: American Psychiatric Publishing; 2013.

Gathright MM, Tyler LH. Disruptive Behaviors in Children and Adolescents. http://psychiatry.uams.edu/files/2015/02/disruptive.pdf. Accessed 2014.

McLaughlin KA, Greif Green J, Gruber MJ, Sampson NA, Zaslavsky AM, Kessler RC. Childhood adversities and first onset of psychiatric disorders in a national sample of US adolescents. *Arch Gen Psychiatry*. 2012;69(11):1151-1160.

CASE 4

Attention-Deficit/Hyperactivity Disorder and Low Frustration Tolerance

IDENTIFICATION: This patient is a 10-year-old biracial male who resides with his mother, father, and 7-year-old sister. He is being referred by his parents for behavioral issues at home.

CHIEF COMPLAINT: "I get angry too quickly."

HISTORY OF CHIEF COMPLAINT: This patient presents with feelings of low frustration tolerance, anxiousness, low self-esteem, and low concentration. The main concerns that prompted the patient's parents to seek treatment included the patient being very hostile toward his younger sister. They have reported unprecedented anger outbursts by the patient, which take the form of screaming and yelling at his sister, occasionally pushing her, and sometimes hitting walls. Anger outbursts have not resulted in any physical harm to others or destruction of property. He also occasionally displays this behavior toward his parents. Additionally, parents report that the patient has gotten into heated arguments with peers, often at the neighborhood basketball court, when he is angry. They report that this is very common, occurring 2 to 3 times weekly.

Patient was diagnosed with attention-deficit/hyperactivity disorder (ADHD) by a neurologist approximately 1 year ago. He is prescribed dexmethylphenidate XR 10 mg in the morning. Patient has not been followed up by the neurologist recently, so his dose of dexmethylphenidate has stayed the same for about 3 months. According to the parents, his teacher reported that his behavior has improved at school since taking dexmethylphenidate. Parents notice less hyperactivity at home. However, it was communicated that the patient is not motivated to go to school or complete his homework, and this often causes arguments at home. They state that although it has improved since starting on dexmethylphenidate, he still has a difficult time sitting down to complete his work. He has also presented with bullying issues at school and has shown low self-esteem and anxiety, as evidenced by patient continually asking, "Why do I have to go to therapy? Am I different? Am I stupid? Mental? Why do I have different homework than my friends? What if they make fun of me?" No significant anxiety has been reported in any situations aside from fear of judging by peers. Patient reports difficulty concentrating and has stated that he would like to work on not getting angry so quickly. His energy is high, and he sometimes has difficulty falling asleep in the evening; parents state that it takes about an hour after getting in bed before he can fall asleep. Symptoms are causing distress and impairment in functioning in his family, school, and social life.

PAST PSYCHIATRIC HISTORY: Patient was diagnosed with ADHD by a neurologist about 1 year ago. Patient has no past hospitalizations or other past mental health services.

MEDICAL HISTORY: No significant medical history reported. No known allergies. Average height and weight. No cardiac history.

HISTORY OF DRUG OR ALCOHOL ABUSE: Not reported.

FAMILY HISTORY: Parents deny significant family medical or psychiatric history. Family history of cardiac conditions is denied. Patient lives with his biologic parents and younger sister (7 years old). He is being raised by both parents. Patient's mother is Puerto Rican and father is Italian American. Maternal grandmother lives in Puerto Rico but is reported to visit often and stay in their home for long periods of time (the most recent time she stayed for >2 months). It is noted that his mother is Catholic, but religion has not been brought up as a significant factor.

PERSONAL HISTORY

Perinatal: Patient's mother denies use of alcohol or illicit substances during pregnancy.

Childhood: Patient is currently a fifth grade student at a public school. This is his first year at his current school, as it was reported that he was previously in a behavioral school. He receives services and extra help at school, although the exact type of services has not been explained. Patient reports that he gets "easier, different homework" than his same-grade classmates. He seems to be of average intelligence and appears able to process information appropriately for his age.

TRAUMA/ABUSE HISTORY: No physical/sexual/psychological abuse reported.

MENTAL STATUS EVALUATION

Appearance: A 10-year-old biracial male, average build and height for age. Athletic clothing. Normal gait and posture. Good hygiene.

Behavior and psychomotor activity: Cooperative/engaged. Good eye contact. Mildly distractible. Hyperactive at times.

Consciousness:	Alert.
Orientation:	Oriented to person, place, and time.
Memory:	Not formally assessed, but no issues with memory reported.
Concentration/Attention:	Low concentration in examination, reported impaired concentration at home and school.
Abstract thought:	Not formally assessed but appears average.
Intellectual functioning:	Average intelligence.
Speech and language:	English speaking. Normal in rate and volume.
Perceptions:	No abnormalities.
Thought processes:	Logical, coherent.
Thought content:	No auditory or visual hallucinations or delusions.
Suicidality or homicidality:	Denies.
Mood:	At time of initial evaluation, patient presents as anxious and shy.
Affect:	Congruent with mood.

Impulsivity: Not observed in initial evaluation; however, parents report issues with anger outbursts and impulsivity at home.

Judgment/Insight/Reliability: Good.

FORMULATING THE DIAGNOSIS

Which diagnosis (or diagnoses) should be considered?

314.01 (F90.2) Attention-Deficit/Hyperactivity Disorder, Combined Presentation, Mild

Diagnostic Criteria

A. A persistent pattern of inattention and/or hyperactivity-impulsivity that interferes with functioning or development, as characterized by (1) and/or (2):
   1. **Inattention:** Six (or more) of the following symptoms have persisted for at least 6 months to a degree that is inconsistent with developmental level and that negatively impacts directly on social and academic/occupational activities:
      - **Note:** The symptoms are not solely a manifestation of oppositional behavior, defiance, hostility, or failure to understand tasks or instructions. For older adolescents and adults (age 17 and older), at least five symptoms are required.
        a. Often fails to give close attention to details or makes careless mistakes in schoolwork, at work, or during other activities (eg, overlooks or misses details, work is inaccurate).
        b. Often has difficulty sustaining attention in tasks or play activities (eg, has difficulty remaining focused during lectures, conversations, or lengthy reading).
        c. Often does not seem to listen when spoken to directly (eg, mind seems elsewhere, even in the absence of any obvious distraction).
        d. Often does not follow through on instructions and fails to finish schoolwork, chores, or duties in the workplace (eg, starts tasks but quickly loses focus and is easily sidetracked).
        e. Often has difficulty organizing tasks and activities (eg, difficulty managing sequential tasks; difficulty keeping materials and belongings in order; messy, disorganized work; has poor time management; fails to meet deadlines).
        f. Often avoids, dislikes, or is reluctant to engage in tasks that require sustained mental effort (eg, schoolwork or homework; for older adolescents and adults, preparing reports, completing forms, reviewing lengthy papers).

g. Often loses things necessary for tasks or activities (eg, school materials, pencils, books, tools, wallets, keys, paperwork, eyeglasses, mobile telephones).
h. Is often easily distracted by extraneous stimuli (for older adolescents and adults, may include unrelated thoughts).
i. Is often forgetful in daily activities (eg, doing chores, running errands; for older adolescents and adults, returning calls, paying bills, keeping appointments).

2. **Hyperactivity and impulsivity:** Six (or more) of the following symptoms have persisted for at least 6 months to a degree that is inconsistent with developmental level and that negatively impacts directly on social and academic/occupational activities:
   - **Note:** The symptoms are not solely a manifestation of oppositional behavior, defiance, hostility, or a failure to understand tasks or instructions. For older adolescents and adults (age 17 and older), at least five symptoms are required.

   a. Often fidgets with or taps hands or feet or squirms in seat.
   b. Often leaves seat in situations when remaining seated is expected (eg, leaves his or her place in the classroom, in the office or other workplace, or in other situations that require remaining in place).
   c. Often runs about or climbs in situations where it is inappropriate. (**Note:** In adolescents or adults, may be limited to feeling restless.)
   d. Often unable to play or engage in leisure activities quietly.
   e. Is often "on the go," acting as if "driven by a motor" (eg, is unable to be or uncomfortable being still for extended time, as in restaurants, meetings; may be experienced by others as being restless or difficult to keep up with).
   f. Often talks excessively.
   g. Often blurts out an answer before a question has been completed (eg, completes people's sentences; cannot wait for turn in conversation).
   h. Often has difficulty waiting his or her turn (eg, while waiting in line).
   i. Often interrupts or intrudes on others (eg, butts into conversations, games, or activities; may start using other people's things without asking or receiving permission; for adolescents and adults, may intrude into or take over what others are doing).

B. Several inattentive or hyperactive–impulsive symptoms were present before age 12.

C. Several inattentive or hyperactive–impulsive symptoms are present in two or more settings (eg, at home, school, or work; with friends or relatives; in other activities).

D. There is clear evidence that the symptoms interfere with, or reduce the quality of, social, academic, or occupational functioning.
E. The symptoms do not occur exclusively during the course of schizophrenia or another psychotic disorder and are not better explained by another mental disorder (eg, mood disorder, anxiety disorder, dissociative disorder, personality disorder, substance intoxication or withdrawal).

Specify whether:

- **314.01 (F90.2) Combined presentation:** If both Criterion A1 (inattention) and Criterion A2 (hyperactivity-impulsivity) are met for the past 6 months.
- **314.00 (F90.0) Predominantly inattentive presentation:** If Criterion A1 (inattention) is met but Criterion A2 (hyperactivity-impulsivity) has not been met for the past 6 months.
- **314.01 (F90.1) Predominantly hyperactive/impulsive presentation:** If Criterion A2 (hyperactivity-impulsivity) is met and Criterion A1 (inattention) has not been met for the past 6 months.

Specify if:

- **In partial remission:** When full criteria were previously met; fewer than the full criteria have been met for the past 6 months; and the symptoms still result in impairment in social, academic, or occupational functioning.

Specify current severity:

- **Mild:** Few, if any, symptoms in excess of those required to make the diagnosis are present, and symptoms result in no more than minor impairments in social or occupational functioning.
- **Moderate:** Symptoms or functional impairment between "mild" and "severe" are present.
- **Severe:** Many symptoms in excess of those required to make the diagnosis, or several symptoms that are particularly severe, are present, or the symptoms result in marked impairment in social or occupational functioning.

(Reprinted with permission from the *Diagnostic and Statistical Manual of Mental Disorders*. 5th ed. Arlington, VA: American Psychiatric Publishing; 2013.)

What is the rationale for the diagnosis?

The patient's symptoms meet the criteria for ADHD. He has difficulty sustaining attention to tasks; for example, parents state he is normally unable to focus for the period of a half-hour television show. He fails to finish schoolwork or chores, as he is sidetracked easily, and has difficulty organizing his belongings. Parents report that he does not pay close attention to detail. He very much dislikes doing schoolwork or anything that requires a sustained mental effort. Parents report he is easily distracted and has difficulty following instructions. He also "squirms" and has a difficult time staying in his seat during class, per report from teacher. He talks excessively, is unable to wait his turn, and is uncomfortable being still for an extended period of time. His parents describe him as "restless." These symptoms have persisted for more than 6 months, are inconsistent with his developmental level, and negatively impact academic and social activities.

What test or tools should be considered to help identify the correct diagnosis?

NICHQ Vanderbilt Assessment scales for parents and teachers can be used to help identify the diagnosis of ADHD. These are available for free online. When diagnosing ADHD, it is essential to get information not only from parents but also from teachers.

Requesting previous psychiatric records from neurologist will be important to determine how ADHD diagnosis was reached and assess improvement from baseline.

What differential diagnosis (or diagnoses) should be considered?

312.89 (F91.8) Other Specified Disruptive, Impulse-Control, and Conduct Disorder

This category applies to presentations in which symptoms characteristic of a disruptive, impulse-control, and conduct disorder that cause clinically significant distress or impairment in social, occupational, or other important areas of functioning predominate but do not meet the full criteria for any of the disorders in the disruptive, impulse-control, and conduct disorders diagnostic class. The other specified disruptive, impulse-control, and conduct disorder category is used in situations in which the clinician chooses to communicate the specific reason that the presentation does not meet the criteria for any specific disruptive, impulse-control, and conduct disorder. This is done by recording "other specified disruptive, impulse-control, and conduct disorder" followed by the specific reason (eg, "recurrent behavioral outbursts of insufficient frequency").

Patient's impulsivity could be secondary to ADHD; however, it seems to be in excess of what is typically seen in ADHD. Patient's recurrent behavioral outbursts did not involve damage or destruction of property or physical assault, so patient does not meet full criteria for Intermittent Explosive Disorder at this time, resulting in a possible differential diagnosis of Other Specified Disruptive, Impulse-Control, or Conduct Disorder.

FORMULATING THE TREATMENT STRATEGY

What treatment would you prescribe and what is the rationale?

Psychopharmacology: Increase dexmethylphenidate XR to 15 mg daily in the morning. Dexmethylphenidate is a first-line drug for treatment of ADHD in children. It seems the patient's symptoms are not completely treated by 10 mg, so increasing the dosage may help.

Diagnostic Tests: Monitor height and weight on dexmethylphenidate because of risk of suppressed appetite. Blood pressure and heart rate will also be monitored. When prescribing stimulants, it is important to evaluate for family history and patient history of cardiac problems. Because cardiac problems in the patient and family were denied, no referral for cardiac evaluation or baseline electrocardiogram is necessary.

Referrals: Individual psychotherapy.

Type of Psychotherapy: Weekly psychotherapy should be initiated. Patient would be educated on strategies for impulse control and expressing anger appropriately. Cognitive behavioral therapy could be useful to target the ADHD and explosive symptoms. Relaxation techniques can also be taught to help manage anxiety. Patient is reported to have low self-esteem, so a strengths-based approach could be implemented.

Psychoeducation: Provide literature about ADHD from the National Institute of Mental Health (NIMH). Provide literature about dexmethylphenidate. Remind patient and parents about common side effects of dexmethylphenidate, such as suppressed appetite, insomnia, headache, irritability, overstimulation, tremor, dizziness, or exacerbation of tics.

What standard guidelines would you use to treat or assess this patient?

AACAP Practice parameter for the assessment and treatment of children and adolescents with attention-deficit/hyperactivity disorder.

CLINICAL NOTE

- Anxiety can be secondary to ADHD, because some people can feel anxious when they are not able to meet the demands of their environment. In this case, the patient experienced anxiety because he had different schoolwork than his classmates, which made him feel different than peers. However, it was not reported that he presents with significant anxiety in multiple situations, and he does not meet criteria for generalized anxiety disorder.

REFERENCES/RECOMMENDED READINGS

American Academy of Child and Adolescent Psychiatry. Practice parameters for the assessment and treatment of children and adolescents with attention deficit/hyperactivity disorder. *J Am Acad Child Adolesc Psychiatry*. 2007;46(7):894-921.

American Psychiatric Association. *Diagnostic and Statistical Manual of Mental Disorders.* 5th ed. Arlington, VA: American Psychiatric Publishing; 2013.

Stahl SM. *Stahl's Essential Psychopharmacology Prescriber's Guide*. 5th ed. San Diego, CA: Cambridge University Press; 2014.

CASE 5

Attention and Behavior Problems

IDENTIFICATION: The patient is a 12-year-old Hispanic female in the seventh grade, who is being referred by her parents for a psychiatric evaluation. Patient was seen at an outpatient mental health facility where Partial Hospitalization Programs and Intensive Outpatient Programs are offered.

CHIEF COMPLAINT: "I may be switched to a new school for my behavior."

HISTORY OF CHIEF COMPLIANT: The patient is being referred for behavioral issues in the school setting that have been occurring since approximately fifth grade.

A few days before the initial psychiatric evaluation, in school, the patient became angry and upset with a peer when she was asked to be quiet. She proceeded to call the peer a curse word and whispered under her breath, "I want to kill him." The patient was sent to the guidance office, where she was questioned about the comment; patient adamantly denied having any intention to hurt the other student and admitted she said it "out of anger." Patient was suspended from school because of her comment. The patient denies any access to a gun or lethal weapon and denies any suicidal/homicidal ideations, intent, or plan on initial evaluation. The patient is able to contract for safety. Parents deny that the patient has ever been violent toward another individual, yet she has made passive suicidal and homicidal statements. The patient threatened to "blow up the school" when she was being "bothered" by another peer during the fifth grade. The patient, in frustration, will also threaten to hurt herself. Parents state that patient "bottles up" feelings, does not articulate her feelings, and then becomes verbally aggressive. Patient has cursed at friends and has a history of friends telling her they do not want to be her friend anymore because of her behavior.

The patient displays signs and symptoms of low frustration tolerance, and she is quick to lose her temper, easily annoyed, angry almost daily, and sometimes blames others for her mistakes/misbehavior. Triggers for anger include primarily, as previously noted, being "annoyed" by others. Patient has no history of physical aggression toward animals or other individuals. Parents states that sometimes she engages in aggressive play and ruins her toys because of rough play. Patient denies either being bullied or bullying others. Patient has no history of fire setting, stealing, or running away. Parents state that when the patient gets into trouble at school, she lies and says nothing happened, and later in the day, the parents will receive a phone call from school informing them of her behavior that day. The patient essentially follows rules and requests from authority figures, yet will often need much redirection and reminding to stay on task and follow through. Patient does express remorse at her behavior, calling herself "stupid" for what she said, and does admit to regret of outbursts after they occur.

PAST PSYCHIATRIC HISTORY: The patient was diagnosed with attention-deficit/hyperactivity disorder (ADHD) in the third grade. Parents report that the patient experiences both inattentive and hyperactive symptoms. These symptoms are present in school and at home. However, despite significant symptoms of ADHD, she maintains essentially top grades in science, math, and language arts. The patient has had a 504 Plan since the third grade and an Individualized Education Plan as well. The patient was tried on methylphenidate extended release for ADHD. The trial was only 1 week long, because this medication significantly worsened tics.

Patient was diagnosed with generalized anxiety disorder in the fifth grade. However, she experiences anxiety mainly before a test or when demands are asked of her that she feels she cannot complete. She feels anxious when she has to complete homework. The patient was started on a selective serotonin reuptake inhibitor (SSRI, escitalopram 10 mg) in the fifth grade, and this, according to her parents, has helped her to worry less.

The patient was diagnosed with Tourette disorder (TD) last year by a neurologist. Physical tics began around 4 years of age, where she would experience eye twitches on and off. Patient also experienced a vocal tic, making a coughing sound. The patient currently has an exacerbation of twitches of her head and eyes when she feels more stressed; otherwise, the tics do not interfere with daily functioning. She is not medicated for TD.

The patient is currently taking escitalopram 10 mg daily, as previously noted, for anxiety and clonidine extended-release tablets 0.2 mg at bedtime for ADHD. The patient had a 2-month trial in the past with oxcarbazepine for mood stability; parents noted no change with this.

It is also important to note that the patient has a history of sleeping poorly. The patient is usually awake until midnight, still very active, and continues to be tired during the day. On a better night, the patient may sleep approximately 8 hours, if she is very tired.

The patient has no past psychiatric hospitalizations.

TRAUMA/ABUSE HISTORY: The patient denies any past or present physical, sexual, or emotional abuse of any kind.

MEDICAL HISTORY: No medical conditions reported. No known cardiac history. No past surgical history. The patient is of average height and weight.

HISTORY OF DRUG OR ALCOHOL ABUSE: Patient and parents deny any past or present use.

FAMILY HISTORY: Her parents were born in South America and speak English well. Her mother is a teacher and her father works in sales. The patient has been raised as a Catholic. The patient lives with her parents, who are married, her older brother (14 years old), and her older sister (16 years old).

Mother has a history of depression and anxiety and is currently taking an SSRI. Patient's brother, who is 2 years older, has ADHD as well. Father notes that on his side of the family, there is alcoholism and ADHD.

PERSONAL HISTORY

Perinatal: Mother denies any drug or alcohol use during pregnancy. Patient was born at 32 weeks, and the mother had placenta previa and was placed on bed rest for the remainder of her pregnancy. Maternal age was 31 years. Mother had a C-section because of prolonged labor. Patient was in the NICU for 1 week. Mother denies that the patient had any brain injuries or seizures in the past. Mother states the patient engaged in eye contact, smiled spontaneously, and had a happy disposition. Her first learned language was Spanish, which she speaks fluently with her parents, and she also speaks English fluently.

Childhood/Adolescence: Patient enjoys playing with her siblings, yet has had difficulty maintaining friendships because of her outbursts and poor impulse control. The patient is not engaged in any activities or sports outside of school. She denies being sexually active earlier or now.

MENTAL STATUS EXAMINATION

Appearance: Well groomed, normal gait and posture, appropriate for season.

Behavior and psychomotor activity: Head tics during assessment (most likely related to the patient being nervous). Psychomotor activity is normal, neither hyper- nor hypoactive.

Consciousness: Patient is alert.

Orientation: Oriented to person, place, and time.

Memory: Recent and remote memory intact.

Concentration and attention: Impaired.

Visuospatial ability: Not assessed.

Abstract thought: Not formally assessed but appears average.

Intellectual functioning: Average intelligence. Knowledge and awareness of events and past history are intact.

Speech and language: Slow, normal volume speech. Ability to name objects and repeat phrases is intact.

Perceptions: No abnormal perceptions apparent or reported. Patient denies any past or present hallucinations or delusions of any kind.

Thought process: Coherent.

Thought content: Patient's thought content appears to be negative, because she is worried about the future.

Suicidal/homicidal: Denies any current ideations, intent, or plan.

Mood: Euthymic.

Affect: Constricted.

Impulse control: Good during the interview.

Judgment: Impaired, poor.

Insight: Understands hospitalization.

Reliability: Fair.

FORMULATING THE DIAGNOSIS

Which diagnosis (or diagnoses) should be considered?

314.01 (F90.2) Attention-Deficit/Hyperactivity Disorder, Combined Presentation

Diagnostic Criteria

A. A persistent pattern of inattention and/or hyperactivity–impulsivity that interferes with functioning or development, as characterized by (1) and/or (2):
   1. **Inattention:** Six (or more) of the following symptoms have persisted for at least 6 months to a degree that is inconsistent with developmental level and that negatively impacts directly on social and academic/occupational activities:
      - **Note:** The symptoms are not solely a manifestation of oppositional behavior, defiance, hostility, or failure to understand tasks or instructions. For older adolescents and adults (age 17 and older), at least five symptoms are required.
        a. Often fails to give close attention to details or makes careless mistakes in schoolwork, at work, or during other activities (eg, overlooks or misses details, work is inaccurate).
        b. Often has difficulty sustaining attention in tasks or play activities (eg, has difficulty remaining focused during lectures, conversations, or lengthy reading).
        c. Often does not seem to listen when spoken to directly (eg, mind seems to be elsewhere, even in the absence of any obvious distraction).
        d. Often does not follow through on instructions and fails to finish schoolwork, chores, or duties in the workplace (eg, starts tasks but quickly loses focus and is easily sidetracked).
        e. Often has difficulty organizing tasks and activities (eg, difficulty managing sequential tasks; difficulty keeping materials and belongings in order; messy, disorganized work; has poor time management; fails to meet deadlines).
        f. Often avoids, dislikes, or is reluctant to engage in tasks that require sustained mental effort (eg, schoolwork or homework; for older adolescents and adults, preparing reports, completing forms, reviewing lengthy papers).
        g. Often loses things necessary for tasks or activities (eg, school materials, pencils, books, tools, wallets, keys, paperwork, eyeglasses, mobile telephones).
        h. Is often easily distracted by extraneous stimuli (for older adolescents and adults, may include unrelated thoughts).
        i. Is often forgetful in daily activities (eg, doing chores, running errands; for older adolescents and adults, returning calls, paying bills, keeping appointments).

2. **Hyperactivity and impulsivity:** Six (or more) of the following symptoms have persisted for at least 6 months to a degree that is inconsistent with developmental level and that negatively impacts directly on social and academic/occupational activities:
   - **Note:** The symptoms are not solely a manifestation of oppositional behavior, defiance, hostility, or a failure to understand tasks or instructions. For older adolescents and adults (age 17 and older), at least five symptoms are required.
     a. Often fidgets with or taps hands or feet or squirms in seat.
     b. Often leaves seat in situations when remaining seated is expected (eg, leaves his or her place in the classroom, in the office or other workplace, or in other situations that require remaining in place).
     c. Often runs about or climbs in situations where it is inappropriate. (**Note:** In adolescents or adults, may be limited to feeling restless.)
     d. Often unable to play or engage in leisure activities quietly.
     e. Is often "on the go," acting as if "driven by a motor" (eg, is unable to be or uncomfortable being still for extended time, as in restaurants, meetings; may be experienced by others as being restless or difficult to keep up with).
     f. Often talks excessively.
     g. Often blurts out an answer before a question has been completed (eg, completes people's sentences, cannot wait for turn in conversation).
     h. Often has difficulty waiting his or her turn (eg, while waiting in line).
     i. Often interrupts or intrudes on others (eg, butts into conversations, games, or activities; may start using other people's things without asking or receiving permission; for adolescents and adults, may intrude into or take over what others are doing).

B. Several inattentive or hyperactive–impulsive symptoms were present before age 12.

C. Several inattentive or hyperactive–impulsive symptoms are present in two or more settings (eg, at home, school, or work; with friends or relatives; in other activities).

D. There is clear evidence that the symptoms interfere with, or reduce the quality of, social, academic, or occupational functioning.

E. The symptoms do not occur exclusively during the course of schizophrenia or another psychotic disorder and are not better explained by another mental disorder (eg, mood disorder, anxiety disorder, dissociative disorder, personality disorder, substance intoxication or withdrawal).

Specify whether:

- **314.01 (F90.2) Combined presentation:** If both Criterion A1 (inattention) and Criterion A2 (hyperactivity–impulsivity) have been met for the past 6 months.
- **314.00 (F90.0) Predominantly inattentive presentation:** If Criterion A1 (inattention) is met but Criterion A2 (hyperactivity–impulsivity) has not been met for the past 6 months.
- **314.01 (F90.1) Predominantly hyperactive/impulsive presentation:** If Criterion A2 (hyperactivity–impulsivity) is met and Criterion A1 (inattention) has not been met for the past 6 months.

(Reprinted with permission from the *Diagnostic and Statistical Manual of Mental Disorders*. 5th ed. Arlington, VA: American Psychiatric Publishing; 2013.)

What is the rationale for the diagnosis?

The patient makes careless mistakes, has difficulty paying attention to detail, has difficulty sustaining attention and staying on task, often needs redirection and reminding to complete tasks or chores, feels overwhelmed and frustrated with homework, has difficulty organizing tasks, has very poor time management skills and overall concept of time, avoids and dislikes tasks that require sustained mental effort, feels more anxious when she is trying to stay organized and finish schoolwork, loses items necessary to complete tasks, is often easily distracted by extraneous stimuli, and often forgetful in daily activities. The patient also fidgets, leaves her seat, is often "on the go," talks excessively, has difficulty waiting her turn, and interrupts and intrudes on others. These symptoms are present in school and at home. Therefore, the patient meets criteria for ADHD, combined type.

Which diagnosis (or diagnoses) should be considered?

307.23 (F95.2) Tourette Disorder

Diagnostic Criteria

A. Both multiple motor and one or more vocal tics have been present at some time during the illness, although not necessarily concurrently.
B. The tics may wax and wane in frequency but have persisted for more than 1 year since first tic onset.
C. Onset is before age 18.
D. The disturbance is not attributable to the physiologic effects of a substance (eg, cocaine) or another medical condition (eg, Huntington disease, post-viral encephalitis).

(Reprinted with permission from the *Diagnostic and Statistical Manual of Mental Disorders*. 5th ed. Arlington, VA: American Psychiatric Publishing; 2013.)

What is the rationale for the diagnosis?

The patient exhibits both motor and vocal tics. The tics have persisted for more than 1 year. The onset occurred before the age of 18. The disturbance is not attributable to the effects of a substance or another medical condition. Therefore, this patient's symptoms meet the criteria for TD.

What test or tools should be considered to help identify the correct diagnosis?

The Child Behavior Checklist-Attention Problem (CBCL-AP)
Conner Rating Scale-Revised (CRS-R)
Connors Abbreviated Symptom Questionnaire (ASQ)
Disruptive Behavior Disorders (DBD) Rating Scale
DBD Structured Parent Interview

It is important to obtain information from both parents and teachers to have observations of patient's behavior throughout the day and throughout various activities, such as the patient's various teachers (if they change classes), babysitters, or other significant adults with whom they are in contact. The Vanderbilt Rating Scales, both parent and teacher versions, can be used to identify ADHD. The scales can be downloaded from http://www.nichq.org/childrens-health/adhd/resources/vanderbilt-assessment-scales

A majority of children with ADHD have at least one other Axis I psychiatric disorder, and the practitioner should inquire about symptoms of oppositional defiant disorder (ODD), conduct disorder (CD), depression, anxiety disorders, tic disorders, substance use disorders, and mania. Assessment scales such as The Child Behavior Checklist and the SNAP-IV may help identify these disorders.

What differential diagnosis (or diagnoses) should be considered?

As previously noted, it is important to assess for comorbidities that can occur with behavioral issues. Appropriate differential diagnoses would include ODD, CD, and/or impulse-control disorder. At the time of presentation, the patient's symptom did not meet full criteria for any of the *Diagnostic and Statistical Manual of Mental Disorders,* 5th ed. (*DSM-5*) disruptive, impulse-control, and conduct disorders (ie, ODD, intermittent explosive disorder, CD).

FORMULATING THE TREATMENT STRATEGY

What treatment would you prescribe and what is the rationale?

Psychopharmacology: Atomoxetine 40 mg in AM.

Atomoxetine was initiated to treat ADHD symptoms because this patient did not have a satisfactory response to clonidine extended release.

When the dose was increased, she became sedated, so the lower dose of 0.2 mg was resumed. When she was tried on methylphenidate extended-release tablets, her tics became more frequent, and she was not able to tolerate this side effect. Therefore, a trial of atomoxetine is indicated because it can be used to treat ADHD. First-line treatment for ADHD includes stimulants, atomoxetine, and guanfacine extended release. There is conflicting evidence about whether stimulant medications contribute to tics. It is important, as with any medication, to weigh risks and benefits; the parents of the patient in this case study specifically were unwilling to try another stimulant for her ADHD because of worsening tics in the past with a trial of methylphenidate extended-release tablets.

Atomoxetine is a selective norepinephrine reuptake inhibitor (SNRI). It works by increasing norepinephrine/noradrenaline and also possibly dopamine in the prefrontal cortex. The medication is FDA approved for ADHD in adults and children older than 6 years. Onset of action can occur as early as the first day of dosing; however, therapeutic actions may continue to improve for 8 to 12 weeks.

Continue escitalopram 10 mg daily. She has responded well to this medication for anxiety symptoms, so it will be continued.

Consider discussing a trial of a stimulant for this patient in the future with the parents. Although the patient's tics increased when tried on methylphenidate in the past, research has not established a clear causal relationship between stimulants and tics. It is known that tics occur more in patients with ADHD.

Diagnostic Tests: A comprehensive baseline bloodwork panel was ordered to establish safety before initiating medication.

A 12-lead electrocardiogram was ordered to establish a baseline. There are varying recommendations regarding screening for cardiac structural abnormalities without any known history. Because of the potential for undiagnosed cardiac abnormalities such as Wolf–Parkinson–White syndrome, hypertrophic cardiomyopathy, or prolonged QT syndrome and the potential for sudden death with atomoxetine, the testing was done.

It is recommended to monitor blood pressure and pulse when initiating treatment and until dosage increases are stabilized because atomoxetine has the potential for adverse effects on the cardiovascular system owing to its norepinephrine effects.

Referrals: The patient was admitted to the Partial Hospitalization Program, where she will be receiving individual, family, and group therapy.

The patient was receiving home schooling services via school and was being assisted with looking at options for therapeutic schools that will provide her with smaller classroom sizes and more individual attention to allow for increased success in the school setting.

Type of Psychotherapy: Behavioral parent training, behavioral classroom management, behavioral peer interventions, neurofeedback training, and organization interventions.

Psychoeducation: Atomoxetine carries a black box warning for increased risk of suicidality in children and adolescents with ADHD, especially during the first few months of treatment. Patients should be monitored closely for increasing suicidal thoughts or behaviors, clinical worsening, and/or unusual behavior.

Patient and parents may be referred to Children and Adults with Attention-Deficit/Hyperactivity Disorder (CHADD) (http://www.chadd.org) for further information and resources related to ADHD.

What standard guidelines would you use to treat or assess this patient?

The American Academy of Child & Adolescent Psychiatry Practice Parameter for ADHD (2007).

The American Academy of Pediatrics Clinical Practice Guideline for Children & Adolescents with ADHD (2011).

National Institute for Health and Care Excellence ADHD Pathway (2016).

CLINICAL NOTE

- Aggression is a frequent symptom of children with untreated or undertreated mental health conditions, including ADHD.
- Besides a morning dose, additional afternoon doses of atomoxetine may be needed to provide full daytime coverage of ADHD symptoms and maintain focus in the home setting as well as at school.
- After treating the ADHD appropriately, it is prudent to monitor for any remaining mood instability and/or behavioral issues that are unrelated to unmanaged ADHD and assess the need to administer psychotherapeutic and/or pharmacologic interventions.

REFERENCES/RECOMMENDED READINGS

American Psychiatric Association. *Diagnostic and Statistical Manual of Mental Disorders.* 5th ed. Arlington, VA: American Psychiatric Publishing; 2013.

Chang L, Wang M, Tsai P. Diagnostic accuracy of rating scales for attention-deficit/hyperactivity disorder: a meta-analysis. *Pediatrics*. 2015;137(3):e20152749.

Cohen SC, Mulqueen JM, Ferracioli-Oda E, et al. Meta-analysis: risk of tics associated with psychostimulant use in randomized placebo-controlled trials. *J Am Acad Child Adolesc Psychiatry.* 2015;54(9):728-736.

Evans S, Ownes J, Bunford N. Evidence-based psychosocial treatments for children and adolescents with attention-deficit/hyperactivity disorder. *J Clin Child Adolesc Psychol.* 2014;43(4):527-551.

Hamilton R, Gray C, Belanger A, et al. Cardiac risk assessment before the use of stimulant medications in children and youth: a joint position statement by the Canadian Paediatric Society, the Canadian Cardiovascular Society and the Canadian Academy of Child and Adolescent Psychiatry. *J Can Acad Child Adolesc Psychiatry.* 2009;18(4):349-355.

Kohn MR, Tsang TW, Clarke SD. Efficacy and safety of atomoxetine in the treatment of children and adolescents with attention deficit hyperactivity disorder. *Clin Med Insights Pediatr.* 2012;6:95-162.

Martin A, Scahill L, Kratochvil C. *Pediatric Psychopharmacology: Principles and Practice.* New York, NY: Oxford University Press; 2011.

Montoya A, Colom F, Ferrin M. Is psychoeducation for parents and teachers of children and adolescents with ADHD efficacious? A systematic literature review. *Eur Psychiatry.* 2011;26(3):166-175.

Posner J, Greenhill L. Attention-deficit/hyperactivity disorder. In: McVoy M, Findling RL, eds. *Clinical Manual of Child and Adolescent Psychopharmacology.* 2nd ed. Washington, DC: American Psychiatric Publishing; 2013:31-96.

Stahl SM. *The Prescriber's Guide.* 4th ed. New York, NY: Cambridge University; 2011.

CASE 6

Not Cooperating and Being Aggressive

IDENTIFICATION: The patient is a 12-year-old white male who is in seventh grade and lives with his parents and 7-year-old sister. Patient was referred to outpatient child and adolescent and family center.

CHIEF COMPLAINT: According to the mother, "My son's aggressive behavior is out of control."

HISTORY OF CHIEF COMPLAINT: The parents report that the patient has been a good student, receiving C and B grades over the past years, but in the last 6 months, his mood has been irritable and angry at home, and he has been having physical shoving matches with his sister that end in her crying and the patient being disciplined. He has been easily annoyed by anything his parents say to him, causing arguments with his parents and blaming them for annoying him. The teacher reports that he seems much more argumentative with her in Math class and at times disrupts the class. The Science teacher also reported one episode of being verbally aggressive with a student in his class last week.

PAST PSYCHIATRIC HISTORY: Mother reported that her son's behavior was somewhat a problem during his early kindergarten period. He did not like going to school, would protest, and then become aggressive with the other children, taking their toys, shoving and hitting them if they did not respond to his request. Mother indicated that during this time, the patient would be "mean" to the small dog that they adopted and kick the dog when he walked past him. Both had to be separated, and the father would become enraged and yell and scream to his son about what he was doing. He would sit in time-out for at least 15 minutes, which would work sometimes, and other times he would go back and try again to kick the dog. The pattern of behavior became so bad that the parents had to go for parent counseling to get their anger under control and learn how to manage their son. During the early years, the child was also evaluated by a child psychiatrist, who diagnosed the child with attention-deficit/hyperactivity disorder (ADHD) and recommended that he be started on a psychostimulant at the age of 7 years. At that time, the parents reported that they were fearful that he would become addicted and, anyway, according to his parents, he was doing better and getting good report cards, so no medication was started.

MEDICAL HISTORY: A history of tonsillectomy at 6 years from chronic streptococcal infections.

HISTORY OF DRUG OR ALCOHOL ABUSE: Denied.

FAMILY HISTORY: Mother reports that she married her husband 15 years ago after attending the same college. She works as high school math teacher in the local high school. Her husband is an engineer for a large aeronautical corporation and travels at least 5 days each month. They have a 7-year-old daughter who is in second grade and doing well. Mother reports that her mother has been treated for major depression and that the father's father is recovering from alcohol use. Both families are close and visit with each other on a weekly basis. They attend the Methodist Church each week, and both children attend weekly Bible class. The family is active in the community and does charitable work each month that includes the children.

PERSONAL HISTORY

Perinatal: The mother reported that she had attended prenatal care and that her son had weighed 8 lb and 1 oz at birth and had obtained his developmental milestone at the appropriate times.

Childhood: The one area in which the child was slow was his speech and articulation, for which he was sent for speech therapy at the age of 3, and it continued until he entered kindergarten. He had not attended nursery school and had trouble adjusting to kindergarten, where he was aggressive and had anger control problems. Because of the parent counseling that lasted about 6 months, both parents feel that they have been able to manage the patient's behavior well until 6 months ago when the aggression and irritability started out of nowhere. His grades in the elementary years were good, with Bs and Cs; he is active in sports and plays tennis each Saturday and also plays the piano with a local group of friends.

TRAUMA/ABUSE HISTORY: Child denied any abuse by parents but did report that he felt that one of the children at school was becoming more verbally aggressive toward him about his outside activities and making fun of him in front of other peers.

MENTAL STATUS EXAMINATION

Appearance: Well groomed. Short and thin for stated developmental age.

Behavior and psychomotor activity: Cooperative most of the time. Good eye contact with examiner. Had difficulty sitting, and fidgeted with a book he was reading and kept turning his head to look out of the window.

Consciousness:	Alert.
Orientation:	Oriented to time, place, and person.
Memory:	Intact.
Concentration and attention:	Because of his fidgeting, he was distracted by outside activity and needed to be redirected back to topic at hand.
Visuospatial ability:	Not assessed.
Abstract thought:	Intact and assessed by proverb.
Intellectual functioning:	Above average.
Speech and language:	Normal rate and volume with no problems with articulation.
Perceptions:	No abnormalities reported.
Thought processes:	Goal directed.
Thought content:	Concerned about why he needed to be here and angry at his parents for bringing him here. Denies any suicidal or homicidal ideation.
Mood:	Anxious and angry and reports that he can get very angry at times.
Affect:	Congruent with mood.
Impulse control:	Good and able to reflect on angry behavior without becoming agitated.

Judgment/Insight/Reliability: Was aware that his parents were trying to help in spite of his anger and able to understand that he was coming to see the nurse practitioner to get help for his anger problem.

FORMULATING THE DIAGNOSIS

Which diagnosis should be considered?

313.81 (F91.3) Oppositional Defiant Disorder, with Moderate Symptoms

A. A pattern of angry/irritable mood, argumentative/defiant behavior, or vindictiveness lasting at least 6 months as evidenced by at least four symptoms from any of the following categories and exhibited during interaction with at least one individual who is not a sibling.

Angry/Irritable Mood

1. Often loses temper
2. Is often touchy or easily annoyed
3. Is often angry and resentful

Argumentative/Defiant Behavior

4. Often argues with authority figures or, for children and adolescents, with adults
5. Often actively defies or refuses to comply with requests from authority figures or with rules
6. Often deliberately annoys others
7. Often blames others for his or her mistakes or misbehavior

Vindictiveness

8. Has been spiteful or vindictive at least twice within the past 6 months.

Note: The persistence and frequency of these behaviors should be used to distinguish a behavior that is within normal limits from a behavior that is symptomatic. For children younger than 5 years, the behavior should occur on most days for a period of at least 6 months unless otherwise noted (Criterion A8). For individuals 5 years or older, the behavior should occur at least once per week for at least 6 months unless otherwise noted (Criterion A8). Although these frequency criteria provide guidance on a minimal level of frequency to define symptoms, other factors should also be considered, such as whether the frequency and intensity of the behaviors are outside a range that is normative for the individual's developmental level, gender, and culture.

B. The disturbance in behavior is associated with distress in the individual or others in his or her immediate social context (eg, family, peer group, work colleagues), or it impacts negatively on social, educational, occupational, or other important areas of functioning.
C. The behaviors do not occur exclusively during the course of a psychotic, substance use, depressive, or bipolar disorder. Also, the criteria are not met for disruptive mood dysregulation disorder.

Specify current severity:

- **Mild:** Symptoms are confined to only one setting (eg, at home, at school, at work, with peers).
- **Moderate:** Some symptoms are present in at least two settings.
- **Severe:** Some symptoms are present in three or more settings.

(Reprinted with permission from the *Diagnostic and Statistical Manual of Mental Disorders*. 5th ed. Arlington, VA: American Psychiatric Publishing; 2013.)

What is your rationale for the diagnosis?

This patient has had aggressive behaviors in school and at home for over 6 months, with anger at parents and teachers, having arguments with teachers in both math and science class, blaming his teachers and parents for his angry and irritable behaviors, and being easily annoyed with teachers and parents, causing angry outbursts. Further, these behaviors have occurred at least once per week for the past 6 months. He meets criteria for moderate severity in displaying these behaviors in at least two settings. Therefore, he meets criteria for Oppositional Defiant Disorder (ODD) with moderate symptoms.

Which diagnosis should be considered?

314.01(F90.9) Unspecified Attention-Deficit/Hyperactivity Disorder

This category applies to presentations in which symptoms characteristic of ADHD that cause clinically significant distress or impairment in social, occupational, or other important areas of functioning predominate but do not meet the full criteria for ADHD or any of the disorders in the neurodevelopmental disorders diagnostic class. The unspecified ADHD category is used in situations in which the clinician chooses *not* to specify the reason that the criteria are not met for ADHD or for a specific neurodevelopmental disorder and includes presentations in which there is insufficient information to make a more specific diagnosis.

(Reprinted with permission from the *Diagnostic and Statistical Manual of Mental Disorders*. 5th ed. Arlington, VA: American Psychiatric Publishing; 2013.)

What is your rationale for the diagnosis?

The patient currently presents with hyperactivity (had difficulty sitting still and fidgeted) and distractibility (was distracted and kept looking out the window during the interview), which comprise some of the symptoms for the criteria for ADHD. In addition, this patient was evaluated for ADHD by a psychiatrist, who recommended starting a psychostimulant. So there is a likelihood that he has ADHD, but there is insufficient information to make a more specific diagnosis.

What tests or tools should be considered to help identify the correct diagnosis?

The Child Behavior Checklist (CBCL) parent and teacher forms should be used to screen for diverse areas of behavioral problems and used as a baseline for treatment planning.

Buss–Perry Aggression Questionnaire can be administered to evaluate the physical and verbal aggression, anger, and hostility. It can be used for children who are school age and older.

Vanderbilt ADHD Diagnostic Parent Rating Scale should be considered because the patient had already been diagnosed with ADHD, and it can be used to determine a baseline against which treatment progress can be measured.

What differential diagnosis should be considered?

296.99 (F34.81) Disruptive Mood Dysregulation Disorder may be considered, but the irritability or temper outburst needs to be present, on average, most of the day for three or more times per week over at least 1 year. The patient does not meet these criteria.

FORMULATING THE TREATMENT STRATEGY

What treatment would you prescribe and what is the rationale?

Consultation with School Counselor to explore patient's concerns about being bullied.

Psychopharmacology: Methylphenidate extended release formulation started at 18 mg/day in the morning can be increased by 18 mg each week with a maximum dosage of 72 mg/day. Methylphenidate is approved for ADHD and has been demonstrated to be effective in numerous controlled trials.

Diagnostic Tests: In addition to the routine laboratory tests, an electrocardiogram should be ordered to rule out any underlying cardiac comorbidity.

Regular monitoring of height and weight should be done at each visit to ensure consistent growth development given his current underweight status.

Referral: Hearing evaluation.

Psychotherapy: Recommend parent management training. It has been validated as a method to help parents better manage disruptive behavior and oppositional behaviors.

Psychoeducation: The parents should be provided with literature available from American Academy of Child and Adolescent Psychiatry (AACAP) on safety of psychostimulant use for ADHD and assisted with fears and anxiety about the use of medication.

Using a parent workbook to help improve parenting skills is also considered a supportive measure for families struggling with ODD.

What standard guidelines would you use to treat or assess this patient?

Practice guidelines from the AACAP for "Practice Parameter for the Assessment and Treatment of Children and Adolescents with Oppositional Defiant Disorder," which can be retrieved at http://www.jaacap.com/article/S0890-8567(09)61969-9/pdf.

CLINICAL NOTE

- With children and adolescents, a special issue relevant to the assessment is the child's involvement in bullying either as a victim or as a perpetrator. Such interactions may serve as an additional indicator that the child's functioning is impaired.

REFERENCES/RECOMMENDED READINGS

American Psychiatric Association. *Diagnostic and Statistical Manual of Mental Disorders*. 5th ed. Arlington, VA: American Psychiatric Publishing; 2013.

Martin A, Volkmar FR. *Lewis's Child and Adolescent Psychiatry*. Philadelphia, PA: Lippincott Williams & Wilkins; 2007.

Stahl SM. *Stahl's Essential Psychopharmacology*. New York, NY: Cambridge University Press; 2014.

CASE 7

Transgender Youth

IDENTIFICATION: The patient is a 14-year-old adopted African-American female-to-male transgender individual. The patient uses the name Joseph and masculine pronouns (he, him, his). He is evaluated in a child and adolescent inpatient crisis unit.

CHIEF COMPLAINT: "My parents don't understand me."

HISTORY OF CHIEF COMPLAINT: Patient came out as transgender on social media 2 years ago. At that time, he asked his parents and friends to call him Joseph and to refer to him using masculine pronouns (he, him, his). He wants to wear only boy's clothing, use the boy's bathroom at school, and participate in groups and activities for boys. Patient reports that his parents are not accepting of his transgender identity and that their lack of acceptance has contributed to increased anxiety, depression, and suicidal ideation. The patient told his outpatient therapist that he was planning to kill himself by running into oncoming traffic. The therapist contacted his parents, who brought him to the hospital for evaluation.

The patient reports engaging in self-injurious behavior by making superficial cuts to his forearms and occasionally to his breasts "because I hate them. I don't want them." Patient reports his last episode of self-injury was "two nights ago" when he used a razor to cut his left forearm.

He reports, "I can't seem to focus" and that he is in danger of failing two of his classes. He has been sleeping most afternoons after returning home from school. Patient reports feeling "very sad" for the past month. He states he has been eating more than usual and has gained 10 lb in the past month. He is currently prescribed fluoxetine 40 mg by his outpatient psychiatrist.

PAST PSYCHIATRIC HISTORY: The patient has been in outpatient therapy on and off since age 4 because of anxiety and issues with gender identity.

He had several trials of medications for attention-deficit/hyperactivity disorder (ADHD) as a young child. He is currently taking fluoxetine 40 mg with some effect on anxiety and depression. They had in-home family therapy for 6 months following a referral from the patient's school. This therapy ended 4 months ago. This is his first psychiatric hospitalization.

MEDICAL HISTORY: Exercise-induced asthma. Several superficial healing cuts observed on patient's left forearm.

HISTORY OF DRUG OR ALCOHOL ABUSE: Patient reports smoking about five cigarettes per day. He denies use of alcohol, marijuana, or other illicit substances. He denies use of any unprescribed hormones.

FAMILY HISTORY: Limited information available about patient's biologic family, but substance-abuse problems (specific substances unknown) were suspected in patient's biologic mother. Patient's adoptive mother has a history of depression.

PERSONAL HISTORY

Perinatal: Unknown because the patient is adopted.

Childhood: The patient was adopted at age 5 after having been in foster care since age 3 because of neglect and physical abuse by his biologic mother. No other children live in the home. The patient began to express cross-gender identity at age 12. He insisted on wearing boy's clothing and used the boys' bathroom at school even though the school did not permit this.

Adolescence: The patient expresses distress at developing secondary sex characteristics associated with females. He is currently binding his breasts to create the shape of a flatter chest. He reports intense dysphoria around the time of menstruation. He is attracted to girls and identifies as heterosexual.

TRAUMA/ABUSE HISTORY: Physical abuse and neglect by biologic mother from birth to age 3.

MENTAL STATUS EXAMINATION

Appearance: Short hair, dressed in masculine clothing, wearing eyeglasses.

Behavior and psychomotor activity: Restless, bouncing right leg throughout assessment.

Consciousness: Alert.

Orientation: Oriented to person, place, and time.

Memory: Not formally assessed but appears to be intact during this assessment.

Concentration and attention: Reports impaired concentration. Appears mildly distractible during assessment.

Visuospatial ability: Not assessed.

Abstract thought: Not assessed.

Intellectual functioning: Average.

Speech and language: Rapid, mildly pressured.

Perceptions: No evidence of perceptual disturbance.

Thought processes: Coherent, goal directed.

Thought content: No abnormalities.

Suicidality or homicidality: Suicidal ideation with plan to run into traffic. Uncertain intent.

Mood: "Down."

Affect: Congruent with mood, constricted.

Impulse control: Good during the assessment. His history of self-injurious behavior may be an indication of impulsivity.

Judgment/Insight/Reliability: Fair/Moderate/Moderate.

FORMULATING THE DIAGNOSIS

Which diagnosis (or diagnoses) should be considered?

296.23 (F32.2) Major Depressive Disorder, Severe, Single Episode Without Psychotic Features

Diagnostic Criteria

A. Five (or more) of the following symptoms have been present during the same 2-week period and represent a change from previous functioning;

at least one of the symptoms is either (1) depressed mood or (2) loss of interest or pleasure.

- **Note:** Do not include symptoms that are clearly attributable to another medical condition.
  1. Depressed mood most of the day, nearly every day, as indicated by either subjective report (eg, feels sad, empty, hopeless) or observation made by others (eg, appears tearful). (**Note:** In children and adolescents, can be irritable mood.)
  2. Markedly diminished interest or pleasure in all, or almost all, activities most of the day, nearly every day (as indicated by either subjective account or observation).
  3. Significant weight loss when not dieting or weight gain (eg, a change of more than 5% of body weight in a month) or decrease or increase in appetite nearly every day. (**Note:** In children, consider failure to make expected weight gain.)
  4. Insomnia or hypersomnia nearly every day.
  5. Psychomotor agitation or retardation nearly every day (observable by others, not merely subjective feelings of restlessness or being slowed down).
  6. Fatigue or loss of energy nearly every day.
  7. Feelings of worthlessness or excessive or inappropriate guilt (which may be delusional) nearly every day (not merely self-reproach or guilt about being sick).
  8. Diminished ability to think or concentrate, or indecisiveness, nearly every day (either by subjective account or as observed by others).
  9. Recurrent thoughts of death (not just fear of dying), recurrent suicidal ideation without a specific plan, or a suicide attempt or a specific plan for committing suicide.

B. The symptoms cause clinically significant distress or impairment in social, occupational, or other important areas of functioning.

C. The episode is not attributable to the physiologic effects of a substance or another medical condition.

Note: Criteria A–C represent a major depressive episode (MDE).

Note: Responses to a significant loss (eg, bereavement, financial ruin, losses from a natural disaster, a serious medical illness or disability) may include the feelings of intense sadness, rumination about the loss, insomnia, poor appetite, and weight loss noted in Criterion A, which may resemble a depressive episode. Although such symptoms may be understandable or considered appropriate to the loss, the presence of an MDE in addition to the normal response to a significant loss should also be carefully considered. This decision inevitably requires the exercise of clinical judgment based on the individual's history and the cultural norms for the expression of distress in the context of loss.

In distinguishing grief from an MDE, it is useful to consider that in grief the predominant affect is feelings of emptiness and loss, whereas in an MDE it is persistent depressed mood and the inability to anticipate happiness or pleasure.

The dysphoria in grief is likely to decrease in intensity over days to weeks and occurs in waves, the so-called pangs of grief. These waves tend to be associated with thoughts or reminders of the deceased. The depressed mood of an MDE is more persistent and not tied to specific thoughts or preoccupations. The pain of grief may be accompanied by positive emotions and humor that are uncharacteristic of the pervasive unhappiness and misery characteristic of MDE. The thought content associated with grief generally features a preoccupation with thoughts and memories of the deceased, rather than the self-critical or pessimistic ruminations seen in an MDE. In grief, self-esteem is generally preserved, whereas in an MDE feelings of worthlessness and self-loathing are common. If self-derogatory ideation is present in grief, it typically involves perceived failings vis-à-vis the deceased (eg, not visiting frequently enough, not telling the deceased how much he or she was loved). If a bereaved individual thinks about death and dying, such thoughts are generally focused on the deceased and possibly about "joining" the deceased, whereas in an MDE such thoughts are focused on ending one's own life because of feeling worthless, undeserving of life, or unable to cope with the pain of depression.

D. The occurrence of the MDE is not better explained by schizoaffective disorder, schizophrenia, schizophreniform disorder, delusional disorder, or other specified and unspecified schizophrenia spectrum and other psychotic disorders.
E. There has never been a manic episode or a hypomanic episode.
    - **Note:** This exclusion does not apply if all of the manic-like or hypomanic-like episodes are substance induced or are attributable to the physiologic effects of another medical condition.

(Reprinted with permission from the *Diagnostic and Statistical Manual of Mental Disorders*. 5th ed. Arlington, VA: American Psychiatric Publishing; 2013.)

What is the rationale for the diagnosis?

The patient meets criteria for major depressive disorder because of depressed mood over the past 2 weeks, along with loss of energy, decreased concentration, hypersomnia, hyperphagia, low self-esteem, and suicidal ideation. He denies symptoms of mania and psychosis. The symptoms are contributing to distress, as evidenced by his self-harm behavior, and the mood is not attributable to any other substance or medical condition.

Which diagnosis (or diagnoses) should be considered?

302.85 (F64.0) Gender Dysphoria in Adolescents and Adults

Diagnostic Criteria

A. A marked incongruence between one's experienced/expressed gender and assigned gender, of at least 6 months' duration, as manifested by at least two of the following:

1. A marked incongruence between one's experienced/expressed gender and primary and/or secondary sex characteristics (or in young adolescents, the anticipated secondary sex characteristics).
2. A strong desire to be rid of one's primary and/or secondary sex characteristics because of a marked incongruence with one's experienced/expressed gender (or in young adolescents, a desire to prevent the development of the anticipated secondary sex characteristics).
3. A strong desire for the primary and/or secondary sex characteristics of the other gender.
4. A strong desire to be of the other gender (or some alternative gender different from one's assigned gender).
5. A strong desire to be treated as the other gender (or some alternative gender different from one's assigned gender).
6. A strong conviction that one has the typical feelings and reactions of the other gender (or some alternative gender different from one's assigned gender).

B. The condition is associated with clinically significant distress or impairment in social, occupational, or other important areas of functioning.

(Reprinted with permission from the *Diagnostic and Statistical Manual of Mental Disorders*. 5th ed. Arlington, VA: American Psychiatric Publishing; 2013.)

What is the rationale for the diagnosis?

This patient meets criteria for gender dysphoria because he has expressed a cross-gender identity (female-to-male) for the past 2 years. He expressed a strong desire to be a male and to be treated as a boy. The patient exhibits at least two of the required diagnostic criteria and experiences significant distress in social functioning, and therefore meets criteria for this diagnosis.

What test or tools should be considered to help identify the correct diagnosis?

The Beck Depression Inventory (BDI)-II, the Patient Health Questionnaire (PHQ-9), or the Mood and Feelings Questionnaire (MFQ).

What differential diagnosis (or diagnoses) should be considered?

None.

FORMULATING THE TREATMENT STRATEGY

What treatment would you prescribe and what is the rationale?

Psychopharmacology: Increase fluoxetine to 50 mg. Fluoxetine is FDA approved for major depressive disorder for ages 8 to 18 years. He has experienced some benefit from fluoxetine but continues to experience depressive symptoms, so an increase in the medication is indicated.

Diagnostic Tests: Routine hospital admission laboratory tests (as described in the Introduction section).

Referrals: Cognitive behavioral therapy to address depressive symptoms. Supportive therapy to address gender-related stressors. Recommend that the patient attend a support group for transgender youth in order to increase peer support. The Trevor Project is a crisis intervention and suicide prevention hotline for lesbian, gay, bisexual, transgender, and queer/questioning youth (http://www.thetrevorproject.org/).

Refer the patient and family to resume family therapy. Talk to any potential referral sources before suggesting a provider to ensure that the provider is going to affirm the young person's gender. Refer the parents to local support groups for parents of transgender children, such as Parents, Families and Friends of Lesbians and Gays (PFLAG) for support groups and additional resources (www.pflag.org/transgender). If local parent groups do not exist, consider Internet-based resources. Transfamily.org has online discussion groups for parents, partners/spouses, and children of transgender people; they also have a discussion group specific for transgender youth. The Gender Spectrum (https://www.genderspectrum.org/) provides real-time online discussions and national phone calls for parents as well as a number of discussion boards.

Type of Psychotherapy: See above.

Psychoeducation: Provide education to parents that gender identity is not something that one chooses or that can be changed. Indeed, "conversion therapy" (therapy that attempts to change one's sexual orientation or gender identity) has been denounced as ineffective and harmful by many professional health care organizations as well as the federal government. Encourage parents to advocate for their transgender child in the school setting if needed.

Pamphlet: "Answers to Parents' Questions about Transgender People" can be accessed at www.pflagnyc.org/sites/pflagnyc/files/resources/pflag-nyc_trans_en.pdf.

Resource books for parents:

"The Transgender Child: A Handbook for Families and Professionals" by Stephanie Brill and Rachel Pepper

"The Transgender Teen: A Handbook for Parents and Professionals Supporting Transgender and Non-Binary Teens" by Stephanie Brill and Lisa Kenney

"Raising My Rainbow: Adventures in Raising a Fabulous, Gender Creative Son" by Lori Duron

What standard guidelines would you use to treat or assess this patient?

American Psychological Association. Guidelines for psychological practice with transgender and gender nonconforming people. *Am Psychol.* 2015;70(9):832.

CLINICAL NOTE

- Transgender individuals may experience misgendering (ie, being addressed as a gender other than the one they identify as) as a stressor that can worsen psychiatric symptoms. Providers and staff should use the name and gender pronouns of the patient's choice.
- Health care providers should be aware of nonbinary gender identities, meaning individuals who do not identify as either male or female but as another gender. Some people use identity terms such as "genderqueer" or "nonbinary," which indicates a gender identity outside of the binary options of male or female. Transgender people with nonbinary gender identities may use gender-neutral pronouns such as they, them, and theirs.

REFERENCES/RECOMMENDED READINGS

American Psychiatric Association. *Diagnostic and Statistical Manual of Mental Disorders.* 5th ed. Arlington, VA: American Psychiatric Publishing; 2013.

Bosse JD, Nesteby JA, Randall CE. Integrating sexual minority health issues into a health assessment class. *J Prof Nurs.* 2015;31(6):498-507.

Coleman E, Bockting W, Botzer M, et al. Standards of care for the health of transsexual, transgender, and gender-nonconforming people, version 7. *Int J Transgend.* 2012;14(4):165-232. doi:10.1080/15532739.2011.700873.

Hendricks ML, Testa RJ. A conceptual framework for clinical work with transgender and gender nonconforming clients: an adaptation of the Minority Stress Model. *Prof Psychol Res Pr.* 2012;43(5):460-467. doi:10.1037/a0029597.

Krieger I. *Helping Your Transgender Teen: A Guide for Parents.* New Haven, CT: Genderwise Press; 2011.

Olson J, Forbes C, Belzer M. Management of the transgender adolescent. *Arch Pediatr Adolesc Med.* 2011;165(2):171-176.

Substance Abuse and Mental Health Services Administration. *Ending Conversion Therapy: Supporting and Affirming LGBTQ Youth.* Rockville, MD: Substance Abuse and Mental Health Services Administration; 2015.

CASE 8

Self-Harm and Suicidality

IDENTIFICATION: The patient is a 16-year-old Hispanic female referred to the emergency department for evaluation by her school guidance counselor and subsequently referred for inpatient hospitalization.

CHIEF COMPLAINT: "I told my friend I was hurting myself."

HISTORY OF CHIEF COMPLAINT: The patient told her friend at school that she had been self-harming by making cuts on her left forearm and that she wanted to die. She states she cuts herself after arguments with her mother because it helps her to feel better. Her mother would not let her go out with her friends and expects her to help take care of the house and her younger siblings. Patient started to have suicidal thoughts about a month ago, and the thoughts have been increasing in intensity since then. She currently has a plan to overdose on over-the-counter sleep medication that her mother keeps at home. Patient reports difficulty focusing in school and recent loss of energy. She reports crying daily at home and denies history of symptoms of mania or hypomania.

PAST PSYCHIATRIC HISTORY: No previous psychiatric hospitalizations. Patient was in outpatient therapy about 6 months ago because of depression and anxiety. She stated that she had stopped going because insurance did not cover it anymore and her family could not afford to pay for it. No previous psychiatric medication trials.

MEDICAL HISTORY: No known allergies. No acute or chronic medication problems. Regular menses. Not using any birth control. Patient reports poor sleep and reduced appetite for the past month. Not intentionally restricting her diet. Height and weight are within normal limits. Superficial healing lacerations noted on left forearm.

HISTORY OF DRUG OR ALCOHOL ABUSE: Patient denied use of alcohol, marijuana, or other illicit substances.

FAMILY HISTORY: Patient's mother is from Ecuador and her father is from Puerto Rico. The patient was born in the United States. She lives at home with her mother and three younger siblings. The patient's father returned to Puerto Rico about 4 years ago, and she has minimal contact with him. Her mother works for a catering company. Patient's mother has a history of depression treated with fluoxetine. Maternal aunt and grandmother too may have depression. No reported psychiatric hospitalizations or family history of bipolar disorder.

PERSONAL HISTORY

Perinatal: Normal full-term vaginal birth. No known complications.

Childhood: No developmental delays or learning disorders.

Adolescence: The patient states she gets mostly As and Bs in her classes at school and does not require any special educational accommodations; however, her grades have declined significantly in the past month. She identifies as bisexual and denies any current intimate relationship. History of sexual activity with both male and female peers.

TRAUMA/ABUSE HISTORY: Patient denied.

MENTAL STATUS EXAMINATION

Appearance: Casual dress, adequate grooming and hygiene, bangs dyed blue.

Behavior and psychomotor activity: Normal gait, moderate eye contact.

Consciousness:	Alert.
Orientation:	Oriented to person, place, and time.
Memory:	Not formally tested but appeared intact during the assessment.
Concentration and attention:	Attention was intact during the assessment.
Visuospatial ability:	Not assessed.

Abstract thought:	Not formally assessed.
Intellectual functioning:	Good intellectual functioning and vocabulary.
Speech and language:	Quiet volume, low pressure, underproductive.
Perceptions:	No evidence of perceptual disturbance. Patient denied hallucinations.
Thought processes:	Logical, coherent.
Thought content:	Preoccupied with anger about having to take care of her siblings.
Suicidality or homicidality:	Suicidal ideation with plan to overdose on over-the-counter sleep medication, which she has access to at home. Patient reports uncertain intent to act on this plan.
Mood:	Depressed.
Affect:	Congruent with mood, constricted.
Impulse control:	Poor.
Judgment/Insight/Reliability:	Poor/Poor/Fair.

FORMULATING THE DIAGNOSIS

Which diagnosis (or diagnoses) should be considered?

296.23 (F32.2) Major Depressive Disorder, Single Episode, Severe

Diagnostic Criteria

A. Five (or more) of the following symptoms have been present during the same 2-week period and represent a change from previous functioning; at least one of the symptoms is either (1) depressed mood or (2) loss of interest or pleasure.
- **Note:** Do not include symptoms that are clearly attributable to another medical condition.
    1. Depressed mood most of the day, nearly every day, as indicated by either subjective report (eg, feels sad, empty, hopeless) or

observation made by others (eg, appears tearful). (**Note:** In children and adolescents, can be irritable mood.)
2. Markedly diminished interest or pleasure in all, or almost all, activities most of the day, nearly every day (as indicated by either subjective account or observation).
3. Significant weight loss when not dieting or weight gain (eg, a change of more than 5% of body weight in a month) or decrease or increase in appetite nearly every day. (**Note:** In children, consider failure to make expected weight gain.)
4. Insomnia or hypersomnia nearly every day.
5. Psychomotor agitation or retardation nearly every day (observable by others, not merely subjective feelings of restlessness or being slowed down).
6. Fatigue or loss of energy nearly every day.
7. Feelings of worthlessness or excessive or inappropriate guilt (which may be delusional) nearly every day (not merely self-reproach or guilt about being sick).
8. Diminished ability to think or concentrate, or indecisiveness, nearly every day (either by subjective account or as observed by others).
9. Recurrent thoughts of death (not just fear of dying), recurrent suicidal ideation without a specific plan, or a suicide attempt or a specific plan for committing suicide.

B. The symptoms cause clinically significant distress or impairment in social, occupational, or other important areas of functioning.
C. The episode is not attributable to the physiologic effects of a substance or another medical condition.

Note: Criteria A–C represent a major depressive episode (MDE).

Note: Responses to a significant loss (eg, bereavement, financial ruin, losses from a natural disaster, a serious medical illness or disability) may include the feelings of intense sadness, rumination about the loss, insomnia, poor appetite, and weight loss noted in Criterion A, which may resemble a depressive episode. Although such symptoms may be understandable or considered appropriate to the loss, the presence of the MDE in addition to the normal response to a significant loss should also be carefully considered. This decision inevitably requires the exercise of clinical judgment based on the individual's history and the cultural norms for the expression of distress in the context of loss.

In distinguishing grief from an MDE, it is useful to consider that in grief the predominant affect is feelings of emptiness and loss, whereas in an MDE, it is persistent depressed mood and the inability to anticipate happiness or pleasure. The dysphoria in grief is likely to decrease in intensity over days to weeks and occurs in waves, the so-called pangs of grief. These waves tend to be associated with thoughts or reminders of the deceased. The depressed mood of an MDE is more persistent and not tied to specific thoughts or preoccupations. The pain of grief may be accompanied by positive emotions and humor that are uncharacteristic of the pervasive unhappiness and misery characteristic of an MDE. The thought content associated with grief generally features a preoccupation with thoughts and memories of the deceased, rather than the self-critical or pessimistic ruminations seen in an MDE. In grief, self-esteem is generally preserved, whereas in an MDE, feelings of worthlessness and self-loathing are common. If self-derogatory ideation is present in grief, it typically involves perceived failings vis-à-vis the deceased (eg, not visiting frequently enough, not telling the deceased how much he or she was loved). If a bereaved individual thinks about death and dying, such thoughts are generally focused on the deceased and possibly about "joining" the deceased, whereas in an MDE, such thoughts are focused on ending one's own life because of feeling worthless, undeserving of life, or unable to cope with the pain of depression.

D. The occurrence of the MDE is not better explained by schizoaffective disorder, schizophrenia, schizophreniform disorder, delusional disorder, or other specified and unspecified schizophrenia spectrum and other psychotic disorders.
E. There has never been a manic episode or a hypomanic episode.
   - **Note:** This exclusion does not apply if all of the manic-like or hypomanic-like episodes are substance induced or are attributable to the physiologic effects of another medical condition.

(Reprinted with permission from the *Diagnostic and Statistical Manual of Mental Disorders*. 5th ed. Arlington, VA: American Psychiatric Publishing; 2013.)

What is the rationale for the diagnosis?

The patient's symptoms include depressed mood, loss of appetite, insomnia, loss of energy, diminished ability to concentrate, and recurrent thoughts of suicide. Therefore, she reports more than five symptoms required for diagnosis of a major depressive disorder. They have contributed to clinically significant distress and impairment of her academic functioning. Her symptoms are not attributable to physiologic effects of a substance or to another medical condition. In addition, the symptoms are not caused by other schizophrenic or psychotic disorders. Her symptoms have never included a manic or hypomanic episode.

Which condition should be considered?

There is no current *Diagnostic and Statistical Manual of Mental Disorders*, 5th ed. (*DSM-5*) code for Nonsuicidal Self-Injury (NSSI). It is listed in the section for Conditions for Further Study: Nonsuicidal Self-Injury in *DSM-5*.

Proposed Criteria

A. In the last year, the individual has, on 5 or more days, engaged in intentional self-inflicted damage to the surface of his or her body of a sort likely to induce bleeding, bruising, or pain (eg, cutting, burning, stabbing, hitting, excessive rubbing), with the expectation that the injury will lead to only minor or moderate physical harm (ie, there is no suicidal intent).
   - **Note:** The absence of suicidal intent has either been stated by the individual or can be inferred by the individual's repeated engagement in a behavior that the individual knows, or has learned, is not likely to result in death.

B. The individual engages in the self-injurious behavior with one or more of the following expectations:
   1. To obtain relief from a negative feeling or cognitive state.
   2. To resolve an interpersonal difficulty.
   3. To induce a positive feeling state.
      - **Note:** The desired relief or response is experienced during or shortly after the self-injury, and the individual may display patterns of behavior suggesting a dependence on repeatedly engaging in it.

C. The intentional self-injury is associated with at least one of the following:
   1. Interpersonal difficulties or negative feelings or thoughts, such as depression, anxiety, tension, anger, generalized distress, or self-criticism, occurring in the period immediately before the self-injurious act.
   2. Before engaging in the act, a period of preoccupation with the intended behavior that is difficult to control.
   3. Thinking about self-injury that occurs frequently, even when it is not acted upon.

D. The behavior is not socially sanctioned (eg, body piercing, tattooing, part of a religious or cultural ritual) and is not restricted to picking a scab or nail biting.

E. The behavior or its consequences cause clinically significant distress or interference in interpersonal, academic, or other important areas of functioning.

F. The behavior does not occur exclusively during psychotic episodes, delirium, substance intoxication, or substance withdrawal. In individuals with a neurodevelopmental disorder, the behavior is not part of a pattern of repetitive stereotypies. The behavior is not better explained by another mental disorder or medical condition (eg, psychotic disorder, autism spectrum disorder, intellectual disability, Lesch–Nyhan syndrome, stereotypic movement disorder with self-injury, trichotillomania [hair-pulling disorder], excoriation [skin-picking] disorder).

(Reprinted with permission from the *Diagnostic and Statistical Manual of Mental Disorders*. 5th ed. Arlington, VA: American Psychiatric Publishing; 2013.)

What is the rationale for the diagnosis?

The patient meets the proposed criteria of engaging in intentional self-inflicted harm to her body (cutting) of a sort that may induce pain with the expectation that the injury will lead to only minor physical harm. She is engaged in the self-injurious behavior with the intent to resolve interpersonal difficulty (with her mother). The self-injury is associated with depressive and angry thoughts before the behavior. The cutting is not a socially sanctioned behavior. It does not seem to cause clinically significant distress at this time. It is not associated with substance intoxication, psychosis, or neurodevelopmental disorder. Therefore, if NSSI were a diagnostic category in the next edition of the *DSM*, she would likely meet the criteria.

What test or tools should be considered to help identify the correct diagnosis?

Patient interview will be used to assess the extent of suicidality. The therapeutic alliance and detailed interviewing are the best means to evaluate symptoms in an inpatient setting. However, using a Hamilton Depression Scale is another option. The Self-Injurious Thoughts and Behaviors Interview (SITBI) could be used to assess self-injurious behaviors.

Gathering collateral information from the family and prior hospital records would be integral to assessing the patient. Because of the short stay in inpatient units, it may not be practical to obtain school records and records from previous outpatient providers, even though these would be useful sources of information in formulating the diagnosis and subsequent treatment.

What differential diagnosis (or diagnoses) should be considered?

None.

FORMULATING THE TREATMENT STRATEGY

What treatment would you prescribe and what is the rationale?

Psychopharmacology: Fluoxetine 10 mg daily. This medication is FDA approved to treat major depressive disorder for ages 8 to 18.

Consider Naltrexone 25 mg daily for self-injurious behaviors. Naltrexone is used off-label for self-injurious behaviors. The patient should be monitored for increase or decrease in self-injurious behavior.

Diagnostic Tests: All routine blood work and pregnancy test. If any symptoms of sexually transmitted infections (STIs) become apparent, then appropriate testing and referrals can be made.

Referrals: Because the patient is currently hospitalized on an inpatient unit, a family meeting with the social worker will address psychodynamic stressors. Patient will be referred for continued medication management and psychotherapy following discharge from the psychiatric hospital.

Type of Psychotherapy: Group therapy with peers on the inpatient unit.

Psychoeducation: There is an FDA warning on all selective serotonin reuptake inhibitor (SSRI) medications regarding risk of increased suicidality when prescribing antidepressant medications for people up to age 25.

Educate the patient and the family about the medication and psychotherapy to improve treatment adherence and to address any concerns they may have.

What standard guidelines would you use to treat or assess this patient?

AACAP Practice parameter for the assessment and treatment of children and adolescents with depressive disorders. *J Am Acad Child Adolesc Psychiatry.* 2007;46(11):1503-1526.

CLINICAL NOTE

- Cultural influences, including gendered expectations, may contribute to additional stressors in certain ethnic populations. This should be evaluated on a case-by-case basis. Cultural awareness is vital in treating patients and families who are members of minority populations.

REFERENCES/RECOMMENDED READINGS

American Psychiatric Association. *Diagnostic and Statistical Manual of Mental Disorders.* 5th ed. Arlington, VA: American Psychiatric Publishing; 2013.

Askew M, Byrne MW. Biopsychosocial approach to treating self-injurious behaviors: an adolescent case study. *J Child Adolesc Psychiatr Nurs.* 2009;22(3):115-119.

McGoldrick M, Giordano J, Garcia-Preto N. *Ethnicity and Family Therapy.* New York, NY: Guilford Press; 2005.

Nock MK, Holmberg EB, Photos VI, Michel BD. Self-injurious thoughts and behaviors interview: development, reliability, and validity in an adolescent sample. *Psychol Assess.* 2007;19(3):309-317.

CASE 9

Intrusive Thoughts

IDENTIFICATION: The patient is a 17-year-old white female residing at home with her biologic parents. She is a high school student. This is her first psychiatric hospitalization. She insisted that she needed to go to the hospital because she is mentally ill. She was referred to the inpatient unit from the emergency department because she reported suicidal and homicidal thoughts.

CHIEF COMPLAINT: "Because I think I need help."

HISTORY OF CHIEF COMPLAINT: Patient reports she needs help because she is overthinking everything and thinks she has mental illness. Intrusive, obsessive thoughts started when she was 14 years old. She reports watching a television show about sex offenders and began to think that she would engage in the behaviors she saw on the TV show. She reports thoughts that she might hurt or kill her parents and she was very frightened by these thoughts. She started having suicidal thoughts so that she wouldn't hurt other people and felt the need to punish herself for those thoughts. She tries to distract herself with other thoughts in order to avoid the homicidal and suicidal thoughts. She denies history of self-injurious behavior or eating disorders.

PAST PSYCHIATRIC HISTORY: No prior psychiatric treatment.

MEDICAL HISTORY: No acute or chronic medical conditions. Reports regular menstrual period. No history of sexual relationships. Urine toxicity negative and pregnancy test negative upon admission. No incidence of tic disorder.

HISTORY OF DRUG OR ALCOHOL ABUSE: Patient denied.

FAMILY HISTORY: Patient denied.

PERSONAL HISTORY

Perinatal: Not assessed.

Childhood: No known learning disabilities.

Adolescence: Reports good academic functioning. Reports some difficulty making friends. Identifies as bisexual. Prefers individual activities such as reading and watching TV rather than spending time with peers.

TRAUMA/ABUSE HISTORY: Denies bullying or other trauma.

MENTAL STATUS EXAMINATION

Appearance: White, female with short haircut wearing androgynous clothing.

Behavior and psychomotor activity: Calm, cooperative, forthcoming in reporting symptoms, tapping foot throughout assessment.

Consciousness:	Alert.
Orientation:	To person, place, time.
Memory:	Not assessed, but appeared intact.
Concentration and attention:	Somewhat distracted by her own thoughts, but generally attentive.
Visuospatial ability:	Not assessed.
Abstract thought:	Not assessed, but seemed within normal limits.
Intellectual functioning:	Average or above.
Speech and language:	Mildly pressured, regular volume.
Perceptions:	No evidence of perceptual disturbance.
Thought processes:	Mildly circumstantial.
Thought content:	Obsessive and intrusive thoughts about harming family members or self.

Reports feeling that people may be watching her or judging her.

Suicidality or homicidality: Reports suicidal and homicidal thoughts of an intrusive and obsessive nature. Denies any plan or intent.

Risk assessment: The patient does not indicate that she is currently at high risk of harm to self or others when evaluating risk factors. There is no history of violence toward others, lack of substance abuse, lack of history of threats toward others, lack of psychotic disorder, or lack of suspiciousness. She appears empathetic and seems to be future oriented and shows some insight into the fact that she is having abnormal thoughts. She is very distressed by having these thoughts (ie, the suicidal and homicidal thoughts are ego dystonic).

Mood: Anxious and depressed.

Affect: Constricted.

Impulse control: Moderate to good because patient is able to resist acting on any of the obsessive, intrusive thoughts she is experiencing.

Judgment: Limited.

Insight: Poor.

Reliability: Good.

FORMULATING THE DIAGNOSIS

Which diagnosis (or diagnoses) should be considered?

300.3 (F42.2) Obsessive-Compulsive Disorder

Diagnostic Criteria

A. Presence of obsessions, compulsions, or both:
- Obsessions are defined by (1) and (2):
  1. Recurrent and persistent thoughts, urges, or images that are experienced, at some time during the disturbance, as intrusive and

unwanted, and that in most individuals cause marked anxiety or distress.

2. The individual attempts to ignore or suppress such thoughts, urges, or images, or to neutralize them with some other thought or action (ie, by performing a compulsion).

- Compulsions are defined by (1) and (2):
  1. Repetitive behaviors (eg, hand washing, ordering, checking) or mental acts (eg, praying, counting, repeating words silently) that the individual feels driven to perform in response to an obsession or according to rules that must be applied rigidly.
  2. The behaviors or mental acts are aimed at preventing or reducing anxiety or distress, or preventing some dreaded event or situation; however, these behaviors or mental acts are not connected in a realistic way with what they are designed to neutralize or prevent, or are clearly excessive.

     Note: Young children may not be able to articulate the aims of these behaviors or mental acts.

B. The obsessions or compulsions are time consuming (eg, take more than 1 hour per day) or cause clinically significant distress or impairment in social, occupational, or other important areas of functioning.

C. The obsessive-compulsive symptoms are not attributable to the physiologic effects of a substance (eg, a drug of abuse, a medication) or another medical condition.

D. The disturbance is not better explained by the symptoms of another mental disorder (eg, excessive worries, as in generalized anxiety disorder; preoccupation with appearance, as in body dysmorphic disorder; difficulty discarding or parting with possessions, as in hoarding disorder; hair pulling, as in trichotillomania [hair-pulling disorder]; skin picking, as in excoriation [skin-picking] disorder; stereotypies, as in stereotypic movement disorder; ritualized eating behavior, as in eating disorders; preoccupation with substances or gambling, as in substance-related and addictive disorders; preoccupation with having an illness, as in illness anxiety disorder; sexual urges or fantasies, as in paraphilic disorders; impulses, as in disruptive, impulse-control, and conduct disorders; guilty ruminations, as in major depressive disorder; thought insertion or delusional preoccupations, as in schizophrenia spectrum and other psychotic disorders; or repetitive patterns of behavior, as in autism spectrum disorder).

Specify if:

- **With good or fair insight:** The individual recognizes that obsessive-compulsive disorder beliefs are definitely or probably not true or that they may or may not be true.
- **With poor insight:** The individual thinks obsessive-compulsive disorder beliefs are probably true.

- **With absent insight/delusional beliefs:** The individual is completely convinced that obsessive-compulsive disorder beliefs are true.

Specify if:

- **Tic-related:** The individual has a current or past history of a tic disorder.

(Reprinted with permission from the *Diagnostic and Statistical Manual of Mental Disorders*. 5th ed. Arlington, VA: American Psychiatric Publishing; 2013.)

What is the rationale for the diagnosis?

The patient reports obsessive intrusive thoughts that she finds very upsetting. She attempts to ignore them or replace them with other thoughts. She denies compulsions. The obsessions cause clinically significant distress and are not attributable to the physiologic effects of a substance. The obsessions are not better explained by the symptoms of another mental disorder.

What test or tools should be considered to help identify the correct diagnosis?

For ongoing assessment, the Children's Yale-Brown Obsessive-Compulsive Scale (CY-BOCS) could be used.

What differential diagnosis (or diagnoses) should be considered?

At the present time, no specific comorbid disorders are apparent, but often individuals with obsessive-compulsive disorder (OCD) tend to have other anxiety disorders so this should continue to be assessed. This kind of ongoing evaluation would most likely take place on an outpatient basis following discharge from the inpatient setting.

FORMULATING THE TREATMENT STRATEGY

What treatment would you prescribe and what is the rationale?

Psychopharmacology: Fluoxetine 10 mg. Selective serotonin reuptake inhibitors (SSRIs) are standard treatment for moderate to severe pediatric OCD. Similar to treatment in adults, higher dose ranges are usually necessary to effectively treat OCD symptoms. Fluoxetine may need to be titrated to close to 60 mg slowly over time while monitoring carefully for adverse effects, including a conversion to mania/hypomania or increased suicidality.

Diagnostic Tests: CY-BOCS.

Referrals: Cognitive Behavioral Therapy (CBT).

Type of Psychotherapy: CBT is the first line of treatment for mild to moderate symptoms. For moderate to severe levels of symptoms, medication is indicated in addition to CBT. CBT is helpful to improve self-esteem and to improve recognition of how thoughts affect behaviors and devise techniques to gain control over thoughts and behaviors.

Psychoeducation: Discussing the diagnosis and treatment with the patient and parents/guardians is essential when working with pediatric patients in order to obtain informed consent for medications and to improve treatment adherence.

There is a FDA black box warning on all SSRI medications for patients up to age 25 due to possibility of increased suicidality. Therefore, these medications require careful monitoring when prescribed for children and adolescents.

What standard guidelines would you use to treat or assess this patient?

Armstrong C. AACAP updates recommendations on diagnosis and treatment of obsessive-compulsive disorder in children. *Am Fam Physician.* 2012;85(11):1107.
Can be accessed at: http://www.aafp.org/afp/2012/0601/p1107.pdf

CLINICAL NOTE

- The practitioner should evaluate the symptomatology from a holistic perspective rather than focusing solely on the thoughts of harming self or others. The nature of the thoughts must be carefully evaluated to identify the pattern of obsessive and intrusive thoughts in order to arrive at the most accurate diagnosis and treatment plan.
- It is important to remember that with OCD the intensity of the symptoms may occur in an episodic nature and may fluctuate with stressors.
- There is likely to be a first-degree relative with OCD so obtaining information about family history of mental illness from the patient's parents/guardians is important.

REFERENCES/RECOMMENDED READINGS

American Psychiatric Association. *Diagnostic and Statistical Manual of Mental Disorders*. 5th ed. Arlington, VA: American Psychiatric Publishing; 2013.

Geller DA, Hoog SL, Heiligenstein JH, et al; Fluoxetine Pediatric OCD Study Team. Fluoxetine treatment for obsessive-compulsive disorder in children and adolescents: a placebo-controlled clinical trial. *J Am Acad Child Adolesc Psychiatry.* 2001;40(7):773-779.

CASE 10

Depressed Adolescent

IDENTIFICATION: The patient is a 17-year-old female of Philippine descent who resides at home with her mother, her maternal grandmother, her mother's brother, his wife, and their 5-year-old son. She is seen for the psychiatric evaluation on an inpatient crisis unit. Collateral information was obtained from the patient's mother.

CHIEF COMPLAINT: "I sort of had a mental breakdown yesterday."

HISTORY OF CHIEF COMPLAINT: Patient reports that she intentionally cut her forearm at school yesterday before music class. She realized that she would not be able to participate in class because the cuts were bleeding too much, so she went to the school nurse's office. The school nurse referred her for evaluation at the emergency department. In the emergency department it was decided to admit her to the inpatient unit due to imminent risk of harm to self because she made suicidal statements prior to arrival at the hospital.

The patient reports that she engaged in nonsuicidal self-injury (NSSI) due to feeling abandoned by her boyfriend. She states that he is not emotionally supportive. She reports that NSSI began 10 months ago and she uses a disposable razor to cut her upper arm or forearm. She reports problems with sleep onset and states that she cries herself to sleep on most nights. She reports disordered eating where she may at times binge eat and at other times restrict her food intake. She reports low self-esteem and low energy level. She endorsed a history of two prior suicide attempts by taking a palm-full of ibuprofen; the most recent attempt was 2 months ago. She did not tell anyone about either attempt and denies serious adverse effects. Her last suicidal ideation was yesterday prior to going to the hospital for evaluation. She reports that triggers for her depression include conflict with her mother and family members and pressure they put on her to get good grades and get into a good college, pressure she puts on herself to finish all her schoolwork, and low self-esteem. She used to participate in the school choir, but stopped attending rehearsals about 2 months ago because she was no longer interested.

Patient's mother expressed frustration and difficulty understanding why the patient treats her disrespectfully when she gives the patient everything the patient wants, such as clothing and money to go out with friends. The patient's mother acknowledged that she works a lot and is infrequently at home, but stated that when she tries to spend time with the patient and express interest in her life, the patient shuts her out or states that she does not have time to spend with her because she needs to finish her homework. Patient's mother additionally expresses confusion about why the patient behaves so differently than she did at that age, reporting that she was expected to be respectful and comply with her mother's requests.

PAST PSYCHIATRIC HISTORY: No prior psychotherapy or trials of psychiatric medication.

MEDICAL HISTORY: Several cuts noted on patient's right forearm, which appear to be healing. No known allergies. No acute or chronic medication conditions. Patient denies physical complaints at this time. Patient appears to be average height and weight. She denies any recent changes in weight. Regular menstruation. Patient reports she is expecting to start her menses soon.

HISTORY OF DRUG OR ALCOHOL ABUSE: Patient reports drinking alcohol at a wedding 1 year ago. States that she tried marijuana once 2 weeks ago. Denies use of any other illicit substances.

FAMILY HISTORY: Patient's parents were both born in the Philippines. The patient was born in the United States. Patient reports that her parents got divorced when she was 5 years old. Her father currently lives in Chicago and she has minimal contact with him. Both of her parents work at hair salons. Family history of mental illness denied.

PERSONAL HISTORY

Perinatal: No known perinatal complications.

Childhood/Adolescence: The patient attends the local public high school where she used to get good grades in her classes, mostly As and Bs; however, she states her grades have declined recently and she is in danger of failing several classes. She reports recent loss of close friends due to interpersonal conflict. She states she would like to be friends with them again but they are still angry at her. She identifies as pansexual and is currently dating a male peer. They have been dating for the past 2 months. She states that she would like to have sex with him, but he is not ready yet.

TRAUMA/ABUSE HISTORY: Patient denies trauma or abuse history.

MENTAL STATUS EXAMINATION

Appearance: Good grooming and hygiene. Cooperative with the assessment.

Behavior and psychomotor activity: Sits with legs pulled up on the chair in front of her. Makes moderate eye contact.

Consciousness:	Alert.
Orientation:	To person, place, time.
Memory:	Not formally assessed, but appears to be intact based on patient's ability to relate details from the past.
Concentration and attention:	Not formally assessed, but no indication of abnormalities.
Visuospatial ability:	Not formally assessed.
Abstract thought:	Intact.
Intellectual functioning:	Appears to be average or above average.
Speech and language:	Quiet volume, regular rate and rhythm.
Perceptions:	No evidence of perceptual disturbance. Patient denies auditory and visual hallucinations.
Thought processes:	Coherent and goal directed.
Thought content:	Distressed about peer relationships.
Suicidality or homicidality:	Denies current suicidal or homicidal ideation; however, reports suicidal thoughts yesterday on the way to the hospital.
Mood:	"Down."
Affect:	Constricted.

Impulse control: Limited as evidenced by impulsive self-injurious behavior.

Judgment/Insight/Reliability: Poor/Poor/Fair.

FORMULATING THE DIAGNOSIS

Which diagnosis (or diagnoses) should be considered?

296.23 (F32.2) Major depressive disorder, severe, single episode without psychotic features

Diagnostic Criteria

A. Five (or more) of the following symptoms have been present during the same 2-week period and represent a change from previous functioning; at least one of the symptoms is either (1) depressed mood or (2) loss of interest or pleasure.

   Note: Do not include symptoms that are clearly attributable to another medical condition.

   1. Depressed mood most of the day, nearly every day, as indicated by either subjective report (eg, feels sad, empty, hopeless) or observation made by others (eg, appears tearful). (Note: In children and adolescents, can be irritable mood.)
   2. Markedly diminished interest or pleasure in all, or almost all, activities most of the day, nearly every day (as indicated by either subjective account or observation).
   3. Significant weight loss when not dieting or weight gain (eg, a change of more than 5% of body weight in a month), or decrease or increase in appetite nearly every day. (Note: In children, consider failure to make expected weight gain.)
   4. Insomnia or hypersomnia nearly every day.
   5. Psychomotor agitation or retardation nearly every day (observable by others, not merely subjective feelings of restlessness or being slowed down).
   6. Fatigue or loss of energy nearly every day.
   7. Feelings of worthlessness or excessive or inappropriate guilt (which may be delusional) nearly every day (not merely self-reproach or guilt about being sick).
   8. Diminished ability to think or concentrate, or indecisiveness, nearly every day (either by subjective account or as observed by others).
   9. Recurrent thoughts of death (not just fear of dying), recurrent suicidal ideation without a specific plan, or a suicide attempt or a specific plan for committing suicide.

B. The symptoms cause clinically significant distress or impairment in social, occupational, or other important areas of functioning.
C. The episode is not attributable to the physiologic effects of a substance or another medical condition.

Note: Criteria A–C represent a major depressive episode (MDE).

Note: Responses to a significant loss (eg, bereavement, financial ruin, losses from a natural disaster, a serious medical illness or disability) may include feelings of intense sadness, rumination about the loss, insomnia, poor appetite, and weight loss noted in Criterion A, which may resemble a depressive episode. Although such symptoms may be understandable or considered appropriate to the loss, the presence of an MDE in addition to the normal response to a significant loss should also be carefully considered. This decision inevitably requires the exercise of clinical judgment based on the individual's history and the cultural norms for the expression of distress in the context of loss.

In distinguishing grief from an MDE, it is useful to consider that in grief the predominant affect is feelings of emptiness and loss, while in an MDE it is persistent depressed mood and the inability to anticipate happiness or pleasure. The dysphoria in grief is likely to decrease in intensity over days to weeks and occurs in waves, the so-called pangs of grief. These waves tend to be associated with thoughts or reminders of the deceased. The depressed mood of an MDE is more persistent and not tied to specific thoughts or preoccupations. The pain of grief may be accompanied by positive emotions and humor that are uncharacteristic of the pervasive unhappiness and misery characteristic of an MDE. The thought content associated with grief generally features a preoccupation with thoughts and memories of the deceased, rather than the self-critical or pessimistic ruminations seen in an MDE. In grief, self-esteem is generally preserved, whereas in an MDE feelings of worthlessness and self-loathing are common. If self-derogatory ideation is present in grief, it typically involves perceived failings vis-à-vis the deceased (eg, not visiting frequently enough, not telling the deceased how much he or she was loved). If a bereaved individual thinks about death and dying, such thoughts are generally focused on the deceased and possibly about "joining" the deceased, whereas in an MDE such thoughts are focused on ending one's own life because of feeling worthless, undeserving of life, or unable to cope with the pain of depression.

D. The occurrence of the MDE is not better explained by schizoaffective disorder, schizophrenia, schizophreniform disorder, delusional disorder, or other specified and unspecified schizophrenia spectrum and other psychotic disorders.
E. There has never been a manic episode or a hypomanic episode.
    Note: This exclusion does not apply if all of the manic-like or hypomanic-like episodes are substance induced or are attributable to the physiologic effects of another medical condition.

(Reprinted with permission from the *Diagnostic and Statistical Manual of Mental Disorders*. 5th ed. Arlington, VA: American Psychiatric Publishing; 2013.)

What is the rationale for the diagnosis?

The patient reports depressed mood for most days over the past 2 weeks. She has experienced loss of interest in usual activities and recent impairment in social functioning. She reports insomnia on most days and crying herself to sleep, as well as loss of energy and low self-esteem. In addition, she has two prior suicidal gestures and recurrent suicidal thoughts. These symptoms are causing impairment in functioning as evidenced by inability to attend class and loss of social relationships. These symptoms are not due to any medical condition. Therefore, she meets criteria for Major Depressive Disorder.

What test or tools should be considered to help identify the correct diagnosis?

Beck Depression Inventory.

What differential diagnosis (or diagnoses) should be considered?

307.50 (F50.9) Unspecified Feeding or Eating Disorder

Due to her reports of problems with eating, consider further evaluation for eating disorder. At this time because patient denies changes in weight or menstruation and does not report body image as a concern, this diagnosis will not be made.

301.83 (F60.3) Borderline Personality Disorder

Borderline personality disorder may be considered because the patient reports instability in interpersonal relationships (such as friends are angry at her), concerns with abandonment by her boyfriend, impulsivity as evidenced by binge eating, and recurrent suicidal gestures and self-injurious behavior. For individuals younger 18 years, symptoms of a personality disorder must have been present for at least 1 year for a diagnosis to be made (except for Antisocial Personality Disorder that cannot be diagnosed before age 18). Because at the time of this evaluation not enough information is known about the duration of these symptoms, this diagnosis will only be considered as a differential.

FORMULATING THE TREATMENT STRATEGY

What treatment would you prescribe and what is the rationale?

Safety Precautions: This patient was evaluated for imminent risk to self due to recent suicidality. She was able to contract for safety so routine observation for the inpatient unit (every 15 minutes) was ordered. However, if increased risk of harm to self were identified she would be put on more frequent observation such as one-to-one observation. On inpatient psychiatric units, all sharp objects and other objects that could represent a potential risk of harm, such as shoelaces and belts, are typically removed to ensure patient safety.

Psychopharmacology: Initiate fluoxetine 10 mg to target symptoms of depression. Fluoxetine is a selective serotonin reuptake inhibitor medication that is FDA approved to treat major depressive disorder for ages 8 to 18 years. The dose may be increased to 20 mg after 1 week, depending on the patient's tolerance of the medication and symptom presentation.

Diagnostic Tests: Per standing hospital admission protocol.

Referrals: Refer for Cognitive Behavioral Therapy and family therapy. Consider referral for Dialectical Behavioral Therapy depending on whether the Borderline Personality Disorder diagnosis is supported during further evaluation.

Type of Psychotherapy: Cognitive Behavioral Therapy. Family therapy to address family problems and improve communication in the family system.

Psychoeducation: Education regarding indication for medication and risks, benefits, and potential side effects of fluoxetine. Provide education on the FDA Black Box warning about increased risk of suicidality-associated antidepressant medications when prescribed to patients under age 25.

What standard guidelines would you use to treat or assess this patient?

AACAP Practice parameter for the assessment and treatment of children and adolescents with depressive disorders.

CLINICAL NOTE

- Parents may have difficulty understanding their adolescent's symptoms and challenges, particularly if they grew up in a different sociocultural environment.
- Nonsuicidal self-injury often occurs in the context of multiple stressors and may decrease when other stressors are addressed.

REFERENCES/RECOMMENDED READINGS

American Psychiatric Association. *Diagnostic and Statistical Manual of Mental Disorders*. 5th ed. Arlington, VA: American Psychiatric Publishing; 2013.

Birmaher B, Brent D, AACAP Work Group on Quality Issues. Practice parameter for the assessment and treatment of children and adolescents with depressive disorders. *J Am Acad Child Adolesc Psychiatry*. 2007;46(11):1503-1526

Emslie GJ, Heiligenstein JH, Wagner KD, et al. Fluoxetine for acute treatment of depression in children and adolescents: a placebo-controlled, randomized clinical trial. *J Am Acad Child Adolesc Psychiatry*. 2002;41(10):1205-1215.

Linehan MM, Comtois KA, Murray AM, et al. Two-year randomized controlled trial and follow-up of dialectical behavior therapy vs therapy by experts for suicidal behaviors and borderline personality disorder. *Arch Gen Psychiatry*. 2006;63(7):757-766.

March JS, Vitiello B. Clinical messages from the treatment for adolescents with depression study (TADS). *Am J Psychiatry*. 2009;166(10):1118-1123.

Sadock BJ, Sadock VA. *Kaplan and Sadock's Synopsis of Psychiatry: Behavioral Sciences/Clinical Psychiatry*. Philadelphia, PA: Lippincott Williams & Wilkins; 2011.

SECTION II

Adult Case Studies

CASE 11

Test Taking Anxiety

IDENTIFICATION: The patient is an 18-year-old, white, single, female college student.

CHIEF COMPLAINT: "I knew everything. I made stupid mistakes. I couldn't think when I took the test."

HISTORY OF CHIEF COMPLAINT: The patient experienced severe anxiety after failing a test 1 week ago. The student had never had trouble academically before. She felt she knew all the information, but became extremely anxious when the professor emphasized how important the test was. She couldn't focus on the test questions. Later when talking to her adviser her chest tightened and she felt her heart pounding and started sweating profusely.

PAST PSYCHIATRIC HISTORY: History of minor anxiety in high school. Denied any history of panic symptoms. No history of any psychiatric hospitalizations or treatment. No suicidal or assaultive history. No history of eating disorders or self-injurious behaviors.

MEDICAL HISTORY: No operations or acute or chronic medical conditions.

HISTORY OF DRUG OR ALCOHOL ABUSE: Denied.

FAMILY HISTORY: The patient is the oldest of four children. Was raised by both parents who were born in the United States. No significant family medical or psychiatric history.

PERSONAL HISTORY: The patient is a freshman in college and lives on campus. Currently unemployed. No military or legal history.

TRAUMA/ABUSE HISTORY: Denied.

MENTAL STATUS EXAMINATION

Appearance: Casual clothing. Well groomed.

Behavior and psychomotor activity: Cooperative. No motor abnormalities.

Consciousness: Alert.

Orientation: To place, person, and time.

Memory: Intact.

Concentration and attention: Good.

Visuospatial ability: Not assessed.

Abstract thought: Satisfactory.

Intellectual functioning: Average or above.

Speech and language: Normal rate and volume.

Perceptions: No abnormal perceptions elicited.

Thought processes: Organized. Linear.

Thought content: Expresses worry about upcoming tests.

Suicidality and homicidality: Denied.

Mood: Mildly anxious.

Affect: Congruent to mood.

Impulse control: Not observed.

Judgment/Insight/Reliability: Good.

FORMULATING THE DIAGNOSIS

What diagnosis should be considered?

300.23 (F40.10) Social Anxiety Disorder, Performance Only

Diagnostic Criteria

A. Marked fear or anxiety about one or more social situations in which the individual is exposed to possible scrutiny by others. Examples include

social interactions (eg, having a conversation, meeting unfamiliar people), being observed (eg, eating or drinking), and performing in front of others (eg, giving a speech).
Note: In children, the anxiety must occur in peer settings and not just during interactions with adults.

B. The individual fears that he or she will act in a way or show anxiety symptoms that will be negatively evaluated (ie, will be humiliating or embarrassing; will lead to rejection or offend others).
C. The social situations almost always provoke fear or anxiety.
Note: In children, the fear or anxiety may be expressed by crying, tantrums, freezing, clinging, shrinking, or failing to speak in social situations.
D. The social situations are avoided or endured with intense fear or anxiety.
E. The fear or anxiety is out of proportion to the actual threat posed by the social situation and to the sociocultural context.
F. The fear, anxiety, or avoidance is persistent, typically lasting for 6 months or more.
G. The fear, anxiety, or avoidance causes clinically significant distress or impairment in social, occupational, or other important areas of functioning.
H. The fear, anxiety, or avoidance is not attributable to the physiologic effects of a substance (eg, a drug of abuse, a medication) or another medical condition.
I. The fear, anxiety, or avoidance is not better explained by the symptoms of another mental disorder, such as panic disorder, body dysmorphic disorder, or autism spectrum disorder.
J. If another medical condition (eg, Parkinson's disease, obesity, disfigurement from burns or injury) is present, the fear, anxiety, or avoidance is clearly unrelated or is excessive.

Specify if:

- **Performance only:** The fear is only restricted to speaking or performing in public.

(Reprinted with permission from the *Diagnostic and Statistical Manual of Mental Disorders*. 5th ed. Arlington, VA: American Psychiatric Publishing; 2013.)

What is your rationale for the diagnosis?

This patient developed extreme anxiety that interfered significantly with her normal ability to take tests and thus is interfering with her academic functioning. Test taking anxiety can be identified as a form of Social Anxiety Disorder which is supported by the literature (see Bögels et al, 2010 for further details).

What tests or tools should be considered to help identify the correct diagnosis?

None.

What differential diagnosis should be considered?

None.

FORMULATING THE TREATMENT STRATEGY

What treatment would you prescribe and what is the rationale?

Psychopharmacology: Propranolol 10 mg PO TID PRN to be taken half an hour prior to test taking.

Propranolol, a beta blocker, has been found to be effective in reducing cognitive dysfunction related to test taking.

Diagnostic Tests: None indicated.

Referrals: None indicated.

Type of Psychotherapy: None indicated unless the anxiety persists.

Psychoeducation: Advise regarding the potential for hypotension with subsequent dizziness or loss of balance. Advise to try the propranolol at home prior to taking it before a test.

What standard guidelines would you use to assess or treat the patient?

None.

CLINICAL NOTE

- The patient should be specifically interviewed for any history of asthma or obstructive lung disease as beta blockers are contraindicated with these conditions. However, cardioselective beta blockers, such as atenolol and metoprolol, have a negligible risk for respiratory complications and may be considered acceptable if discussed with the patient's primary care provider.

REFERENCES/RECOMMENDED READINGS

American Psychiatric Association. *Diagnostic and Statistical Manual of Mental Disorders*. 5th ed. Arlington, VA: American Psychiatric Publishing; 2013.

Bögels SM, Alden L, Beidel DC, et al. Social anxiety disorder: questions and answers for the DSM-V. *Depress Anxiety*. 2010;27(2):168-189.

Faigel HC. The effect of beta blockade on stress-induced cognitive dysfunction in adolescents. *Clin Pediatr*. 1991;30(7):441-445.

Soeter M, Kindt M. An abrupt transformation of phobic behavior after a post-retrieval amnesic agent. *Biol Psychiatry*. 2015;78(12):880-886.

Zuckerman M, Spielberger CD. *Emotions and Anxiety (PLE: Emotion): New Concepts, Methods, and Applications*. Vol 12. New York, NY: Psychology Press; 2015.

CASE 12

Stimulants and Mania

IDENTIFICATION: The patient is a 19-year-old, single, white male referred by his college counselor and seen in the college counseling center.

CHIEF COMPLAINT: "I don't like how the medication is making me so tired, so I'm only taking it at night."

HISTORY OF CHIEF COMPLAINT: The patient was combining "Adderall, Focalin, and Vyvanse." The patient described himself as "reckless," as "playing around with drugs," and was in with a "bad crowd." He took nootropics (cognitive-enhancing drugs) that he obtained over the internet. He started taking "Klonopin or Xanax to sleep and calm down." The student said he was engaged in "high finance in the stock market" and didn't think he needed to be in college. He thought he had supernatural powers and had visions of his deceased aunt. The patient started hearing people talking in his head. He tried to stop the stimulants at one point, but "lost his emotions." He couldn't get out of bed for 3 days and was afraid that he couldn't stop the stimulants on his own. He wanted to go to a detox program and so went to a mental health center. The mental health center clinician called 911 because he "thought I was a danger to myself." He was then taken by ambulance to the local emergency room. He recalls how he was "chained down" while in the emergency room. He was admitted to the inpatient psychiatric unit. After 1 week, he was released on olanzapine 5 mg HS and valproic acid 500 mg BID. The patient states that he stopped taking the morning dose of valproic acid because it was making him tired. The college counselor set up an appointment for the student to be followed by a private psychiatrist. In the meantime, the college counselor referred the student to this psychiatric provider at the college counseling center because he was complaining about side effects from the medication.

PAST PSYCHIATRIC HISTORY: No psychiatric hospitalizations prior to the admission described above. He was discharged from the psychiatric unit

10 days ago. No history of suicidal or assaultive behavior. No developmental delays or learning difficulties.

MEDICAL HISTORY: Average height and weight. No allergies. No operations.

HISTORY OF DRUG OR ALCOHOL ABUSE: See History of Chief Complaint.

FAMILY HISTORY: Raised by both parents who were born in America. He has two siblings. Has a good relationship with family, although his father is very strict. Was raised Catholic. No known medical or psychiatric disorders in the family.

PERSONAL HISTORY

Perinatal: Full-term vaginal birth. No complications.

Childhood: Had many friends.

Adolescence: The patient participated in the Boy Scouts of America. He stated that he was very popular in high school and described his involvement in high school as "the best in everything." He stated, "Everybody liked me." He played on the lacrosse team.

Adulthood: The patient is currently enrolled as a Junior in college. He has always liked school and denied any problem making friends. He is not currently in a romantic relationship. The student is struggling to complete courses because he missed classes while hospitalized. During the summer, he worked as a cashier. He has no military history and no legal history.

TRAUMA/ABUSE HISTORY: Denied.

MENTAL STATUS EXAMINATION

Appearance: Casual attire. Good eye contact.

Behavior and psychomotor activity: Cooperative. Leg tapping nervously during the beginning of the interview, but it subsided as the interview progressed.

Consciousness: Alert.

Orientation: Oriented to all three spheres.

Memory:	Grossly intact. Not clear about dates or time immediately prior to hospitalization.
Concentration and attention:	Fair.
Visuospatial ability:	Not assessed.
Abstract thought:	WNL.
Intellectual functioning:	Average or above.
Speech and language:	Slightly rapid initially but normal rate as the interview progressed.
Perceptions:	No altered perceptions.
Thought processes:	Some tangentiality noted.
Thought content:	No obsessions or compulsions reported. Preoccupied with academic concerns.
Mood:	Anxious.
Affect:	Full range.
Impulse control:	Good.
Judgment:	Fair.
Insight:	Starting to question whether or not he had supernatural powers prior to his hospitalization, so his insight is improving.
Reliability:	Fair.

FORMULATING THE DIAGNOSIS

What diagnosis should be considered?

292.84 (F15.24) Substance/Medication-induced Bipolar and Related Disorder, Amphetamine

Diagnostic Criteria

A. A prominent and persistent disturbance in mood that predominates in the clinical picture and is characterized by elevated, expansive, or irritable mood, with or without depressed mood, or markedly diminished interest or pleasure in all, or almost all, activities.

B. There is evidence from the history, physical examination, or laboratory findings of both (1) and (2):
   1. The symptoms in Criterion A developed during or soon after substance intoxication or withdrawal or after exposure to a medication.
   2. The involved substance/medication is capable of producing the symptoms in Criterion A.
C. The disturbance is not better explained by a bipolar or related disorder that is not substance/medication induced. Such evidence of an independent bipolar or related disorder could include the following:
   - The symptoms precede the onset of the substance/medication use; the symptoms persist for a substantial period of time (eg, about 1 month) after the cessation of acute withdrawal or severe intoxication; or there is other evidence suggesting the existence of an independent nonsubstance/medication-induced bipolar and related disorder (eg, a history of recurrent nonsubstance/medication-related episodes).

The disturbance does not occur exclusively during the course of a delirium.
The disturbance causes clinically significant distress or impairment in social, occupational, or other important areas of functioning.

(Reprinted with permission from the *Diagnostic and Statistical Manual of Mental Disorders*. 5th ed. Arlington, VA: American Psychiatric Publishing; 2013.)

What is your rationale for the diagnosis?

The patient reports symptoms of impaired judgment, hyperactivity, auditory hallucinations, and grandiosity following extreme stimulant use. There seems to be a causal relationship between the use of the stimulants and the occurrence of the manic and psychotic symptoms. It is possible that the patient was also experiencing symptoms of delirium as evidenced by his report of visual hallucinations. Typically, the manic symptoms resolve within hours or days after ingestion of stimulants. Whether his manic symptoms would have continued without taking the antimanic medications (olanzapine and valproic acid) is not able to be determined.

What tools or tests should be considered to help identify the correct diagnosis?

Collateral history from the family would help clarify the diagnosis.

Obtain consent to obtain hospital records.

The Mood Disorder Questionnaire can be administered to identify a history of bipolar symptoms (see Appendix 1).

What differential diagnosis should be considered?

296.80 (F31.9) Unspecified Bipolar and Related Disorder

There is limited history or collateral information; however, the patient describes a history of risk-taking behavior and poor judgment which may have occurred prior to the excessive use of stimulants. This may indicate hypomanic/manic symptoms which occurred separate from his stimulant use. However, the information is insufficient to make a specific bipolar diagnosis, so the unspecified category will be considered as a differential.

FORMULATING THE TREATMENT STRATEGY

What treatment would you prescribe and what is the rationale?

Psychopharmacology: Until further history can be obtained with which to determine if there is a concurrent diagnosis of hypomanic/manic disorder, the antimanic medications should be continued.

Olanzapine 5 mg HS: Olanzapine is an atypical antipsychotic that is FDA approved for treatment of acute mania/mixed mania as monotherapy or as an adjunct to lithium or valproate. If continued, this antipsychotic may increase the risk for diabetes mellitus and dyslipidemia so these values would need to be monitored. These conditions can be part of a metabolic syndrome, which can be evaluated using the following chart: http://www.cqaimh.org/pdf/tool_metabolic.pdf

Valproic acid 500 mg BID: The patient would be encouraged to take the full dose of the valproic acid. Valproic acid is an anticonvulsant, voltage-sensitive sodium channel modulator that is FDA approved for acute mania and mixed episodes. Platelet counts and liver function tests should be monitored before and during treatment. If withdrawal is abrupt, seizures may occur.

There is limited evidence that a combination of multiple medications for treatment of bipolar maintenance is beneficial, although the practice is widespread.

Diagnostic Test: Because the patient has been started on valproic acid, liver function tests should be done at baseline, 1 month, and then every 6 to 12 months if there are no abnormalities. Complete blood count with platelet count is done at baseline, 1 month after starting treatment, and then every 6 to 12 months unless abnormal.

(A pregnancy test should be ordered for females. However, as a general rule, valproic acid should be avoided with females as there is an increased risk of polycystic ovary syndrome.)

Referral: Advise the patient to keep his scheduled psychiatric appointment for ongoing medication management. Communicate findings of the evaluation with the psychiatrist who will be following the patient.

Psychotherapy: Advise the patient to continue with his current counselor at college.

Psychoeducation: The potential for relapse should be evaluated with the patient. At this point the patient is motivated to abstain from any substance use. However, the potential for relapse should be an ongoing part of therapy and treatment.

The patient should be informed of the risks and benefits with olanzapine and valproic acid.

What standard guideline would you use to treat or assess this patient?

None.

CLINICAL NOTE

- When the patient reported that he was also taking nootropics he was referring to cognitive enhancers or "smart drugs" bought on the internet marketed as dietary supplements. They are produced by several companies and the ingredients are not consistent. Nonetheless, they may have some CNS stimulant effects and can be abused.

REFERENCES/RECOMMENDED READINGS

American Psychiatric Association. *Diagnostic and Statistical Manual of Mental Disorders.* 5th ed. Arlington, VA: American Psychiatric Publishing; 2013.

Caton CLM, Samet S, Hasin DS. When acute-stage psychosis and substance use co-occur: differentiating substance-induced and primary psychotic disorders. *J Psychiatr Pract.* 2000;6(5):256-266.

CASE 12 APPENDIX

Mood Disorder

SCORING THE MOOD DISORDER QUESTIONNAIRE (MDQ)

The MDQ (Table 12-1) was developed by a team of psychiatrists, researchers, and consumer advocates to address a critical need for timely and accurate diagnosis of bipolar disorder, which can be fatal if left untreated. The questionnaire takes about 5 minutes to complete, and can provide important insights into diagnosis and treatment. Clinical trials have indicated that the MDQ has a high rate of accuracy; it is able to identify seven out of ten people who have bipolar disorder and screen out nine out of ten people who do not.[1]

A recent National DMDA survey revealed that nearly 70% of people with bipolar disorder had received at least one misdiagnosis and many had waited more than 10 years from the onset of their symptoms before receiving a correct diagnosis. National DMDA hopes that the MDQ will shorten this delay and help more people to get the treatment they need, when they need it.

The MDQ screens for Bipolar Spectrum Disorder (which includes Bipolar I, Bipolar II, and Bipolar NOS).

If the patient answers:

1. "**Yes**" to seven or more of the 13 items in question number 1;
   AND
2. "**Yes**" to question number 2;
   AND
3. "**Moderate**" or "**Serious**" to question number 3;

[1]Hirschfeld RM, Williams JB, Spitzer RL, Calabrese JR, Flynn L, Keck PE Jr, et al. "Development and validation of a screening instrument for bipolar spectrum disorder: The Mood Disorder Questionnaire." *Am J Psychiatry*. 2000;157(11):1873-1875.

The Mood Disorder Questionnaire

Instructions: Please answer each question to the best of your ability.

	YES	NO
1. Has there ever been a period of time when you were not your usual self and ...		
...you felt so good or so hyper that other people thought you were not your normal self or you were so hyper that you got into trouble?	☐	☐
...you were so irritable that you shouted at people or started fights or arguments?	☐	☐
...you felt much more self-confident than usual?	☐	☐
...you got much less sleep than usual and found you didn't really miss it?	☐	☐
...you were much more talkative or spoke much faster than usual?	☐	☐
...thoughts raced through your head or you couldn't slow your mind down?	☐	☐
...you were so easily distracted by things around you that you had trouble concentrating or staying on track?	☐	☐
...you had much more energy than usual?	☐	☐
...you were much more active or did many more things than usual?	☐	☐
...you were much more social or outgoing than usual, for example, you telephoned friends in the middle of the night?	☐	☐
...you were much more interested in sex than usual?	☐	☐
...you did things that were unusual for you or that other people might have thought were excessive, foolish, or risky?	☐	☐
...spending money got you or your family into trouble?	☐	☐
2. If you checked YES to more than one of the above, have several of these ever happened during the same period of time?	☐	☐
3. How much of a problem did any of these cause you—like being unable to work; having family, money or legal troubles; getting into arguments or fights? *Please circle one response only.* No Problem Minor Problem Moderate Problem Serious Problem		
4. Have any of your blood relatives (i.e. children, siblings, parents, grand-parents, aunts, uncles) had manic-depressive illness or bipolar disorder?	☐	☐
5. Has a health professional ever told you that you have manic-depressive illness or bipolar disorder?	☐	☐

you have a positive screen. All three of the criteria above should be met. A positive screen should be followed by a comprehensive medical evaluation for Bipolar Spectrum Disorder.

ACKNOWLEDGEMENT: This instrument was developed by a committee composed of the following individuals: Chairman, Robert M.A. Hirschfeld, MD—University of Texas Medical Branch; Joseph R. Calabrese, MD—Case Western Reserve School of Medicine; Laurie Flynn—National Alliance for the Mentally Ill; Paul E. Keck, Jr., MD—University of Cincinnati College of Medicine; Lydia Lewis—National Depressive and Manic-Depressive Association; Robert M. Post, MD—National Institute of Mental Health; Gary S. Sachs, MD—Harvard University School of Medicine; Robert L. Spitzer, MD—Columbia University; Janet Williams, DSW—Columbia University and John M. Zajecka, MD—Rush Presbyterian-St. Luke's Medical Center.

CASE 13

Depressed and Anxious in College

IDENTIFICATION: The patient is a 19-year-old, single, white female college freshman living on campus referred by her college counselor for evaluation and treatment of depression. Additional information about the patient's history was obtained from the patient's mother via phone with the patient's consent.

CHIEF COMPLAINT: "I'm not sure how to handle things."

HISTORY OF CHIEF COMPLAINT: The patient reports feeling depressed and anxious. She said she started feeling this way in high school. She hears a voice in the back of her head, which is "getting nasty." The voice tells her to "give up on life." She says the voice is triggered by stress. The patient reports low self-worth. Beck Depression Inventory (BDI) was administered and her score was 25 which indicates "moderately depressed."

PAST PSYCHIATRIC HISTORY: The patient reported that she was diagnosed with Asperger syndrome as a child. She states, "I have a weird time expressing my emotions." Had remedial classes in elementary and middle school. She thought the voices started in elementary school, but she did not report them. Was on lisdexamfetamine in middle school. She reports social isolation, stating, "I didn't hang out with anyone." Reports a suicide attempt by trying to hang herself at age 13, but never told anyone. During high school, she saw a counselor after she told her parents she wanted to kill herself.
Her pediatrician started her on fluoxetine to treat depression, but she stopped it after 2 months because it increased the voices. She continued to feel depressed and anxious. No further suicide attempts, but continued to have mood-congruent voices that spoke to her in a derogatory manner and would tell her to kill herself. The voices became worse with stress. She identified a

history of past obsessions with fear that she might harm herself, violent and horrific images, excessive concerns about contamination with animal contact, somatic obsessions with her appearance, checking that nothing terrible did or will happen, checking that she did not make mistakes, obsessions with the need to know or remember, fear of losing things, and lucky/unlucky numbers. No psychiatric hospitalizations.

MEDICAL HISTORY: Reports fatigue, however, all recent labs for routine screening were negative. History of mononucleosis in high school. No operations or chronic medical conditions.

HISTORY OF DRUG OR ALCOHOL ABUSE: Denied.

FAMILY HISTORY: The patient was raised with two brothers with whom she does not get along. The mother has a history of depression. The mother reports that the younger brother has "pervasive developmental disorder" (autism spectrum disorder, according to *DSM-5*).

PERSONAL HISTORY

Perinatal: (Information obtained from the mother.) The patient was a full-term vaginal birth.

Childhood: Started walking at 13 months. Speech identified as "echolalia" when she was young. Before age 3 years would only say "mommy–daddy" but not separate the two words and did not recognize her own name. She would set up crayons in perfect rows. If a door was open, she had to shut it. The parents called county children's services to evaluate her at 32 months and she was screened for developmental disorders. She was diagnosed at 34 months with autism, moderate. Received Applied Behavioral Analysis full-day treatment. Attended a private specialized school from age 3 to 5, which the mother thought was excellent. Went to full-day kindergarten where she was assigned her own behavioral assistant. Unfortunately, the next year she did not have an assistant in the classroom. After the mother obtained legal representation, the school provided an Individualized Education Program and the patient received excellent behavioral and educational support. Patient had difficulty developing peer relationships. Patient states she "didn't fit in." Sat at the boys table at lunch because they played video games and she could relate to that. Everyone thought she was "weird." Was bullied. Older brother tried to protect her.

Adolescence: In middle school, she received partial supportive services in the classroom. Then in high school she was partially mainstreamed into regular education. She maintained a good academic record with a grade point average of 2.9 throughout high school.

Adulthood: Counselor in high school recommended attending a small college. Enrolled as a freshman and she is currently living in a dorm with a roommate. Has one friend at college. Connected with a boyfriend online and is sexually active. Is happy to be at college, but struggles academically. Embarrassed to go to tutors. Decided to see a counselor for depression and anxiety and then was referred by the counselor for this psychiatric evaluation.

TRAUMA/ABUSE HISTORY: History of being bullied.

MENTAL STATUS EXAMINATION

Appearance: Posture is slouched. Slumped in the chair. Wearing mismatched clothes that look ill fitting. Hair is scraggly and long.

Behavior and psychomotor activity	Cooperative. No abnormal movements.
Consciousness:	Alert.
Orientation:	To person, place, and time.
Memory:	Not formally assessed but is grossly intact.
Concentration and attention:	Not formally assessed but seems satisfactory. Does not appear easily distracted or preoccupied with internal or external stimuli. However, she reports that she is struggling academically. Feels it is hard to manage her time and all the demands.
Visuospatial ability:	Not assessed.
Abstract thought:	Adequate.
Intellectual functioning:	Average or above.
Speech and language:	Normal rate and volume and spontaneous.
Perceptions:	Auditory hallucinations described as “nasty” and telling her to harm herself. Not apparent during the interview.
Thought processes:	Linear and organized. Logical.

Thought content: The patient has significant obsessive thoughts. When administered the Yale–Brown Obsessive Compulsive Scale (Y-BOCS), she reported obsessions related to aggressive impulses toward herself, and contamination, as well as lucky/unlucky numbers and somatic obsessions. She reported compulsions regarding the need to confess, the need to tap or rub objects, and rituals involving blinking and staring.

Suicidality or homicidality: Although the patient hears voices telling her to harm herself and she is feeling depressed, she says she feels better because she is coming for help. Says the counseling makes her feel better. Denies any suicidal plan or intent.

Mood: "Depressed."

Affect: Appears depressed.

Impulse control: Good.

Judgment: Fair.

Insight: Fair.

Reliability: Good.

FORMULATING THE DIAGNOSIS

Which diagnosis (or diagnoses) should be considered?

300.4 (F34.1) Persistent Depressive Disorder (Dysthymia), with Mood-Congruent Psychotic Features

Diagnostic Criteria

This disorder represents a consolidation of *DSM-IV*-defined chronic major depressive disorder and dysthymic disorder.

A. Depressed mood for most of the day, for more days than not, as indicated by either subjective account or observation by others, for at least 2 years.
   - **Note:** In children and adolescents, mood can be irritable and duration must be at least 1 year.

B. Presence, while depressed, of two (or more) of the following:
   1. Poor appetite or overeating
   2. Insomnia or hypersomnia
   3. Low energy or fatigue
   4. Low self-esteem
   5. Poor concentration or difficulty making decisions
   6. Feelings of hopelessness.
C. During the 2-year period (1 year for children or adolescents) of the disturbance, the individual has never been without the symptoms in Criteria A and B for more than 2 months at a time.
D. Criteria for a major depressive disorder may be continuously present for 2 years.
E. There has never been a manic episode or a hypomanic episode, and criteria have never been met for cyclothymic disorder.
F. The disturbance is not better explained by a persistent schizoaffective disorder, schizophrenia, delusional disorder, or other specified or unspecified schizophrenia spectrum and other psychotic disorder.
G. The symptoms are not attributable to the physiologic effects of a substance (eg, a drug of abuse, a medication) or another medical condition (eg, hypothyroidism).
H. The symptoms cause clinically significant distress or impairment in social, occupational, or other important areas of functioning.

Note: Because the criteria for a major depressive episode include four symptoms that are absent from the symptom list for persistent depressive disorder (dysthymia), a very limited number of individuals will have depressive symptoms that have persisted longer than 2 years but will not meet criteria for persistent depressive disorder. If full criteria for a major depressive episode have been met at some point during the current episode of illness, they should be given a diagnosis of major depressive disorder. Otherwise, a diagnosis of other specified depressive disorder or unspecified depressive disorder is warranted.

Specify if:

- With anxious distress
- With mixed features
- With melancholic features
- With atypical features
- With mood-congruent psychotic features
- With mood-incongruent psychotic features
- With peripartum onset

(Reprinted with permission from the *Diagnostic and Statistical Manual of Mental Disorders*. 5th ed. Arlington, VA: American Psychiatric Publishing; 2013.)

What is the rationale for the diagnosis?

The patient reports a depressed mood for more than 2 years, with low self-esteem and low energy. She has not been without the symptoms for more than a 2-month period and the symptoms cannot be better explained by a psychotic disorder, and are not substance related or the result of a medical condition. The symptoms contribute to significant distress and impaired functioning as evidenced by her seeking counseling for her depressed mood. It is possible that her symptoms may have met the criteria for major depressive disorder, but information is not available to support that diagnosis at the time of the evaluation because she did not meet five of the nine symptom criteria for major depressive disorder. The auditory hallucinations, which the patient describes, contribute to her low self-esteem and feelings of worthlessness, so they are considered to be mood congruent. Therefore, the diagnosis of persistent depressive disorder with mood-congruent psychotic features was chosen.

Which diagnosis (or diagnoses) should be considered?

299.00 (F84.0) Autism Spectrum Disorder, without Accompanying Intellectual Impairment or Language Impairment

Diagnostic Criteria

A. Persistent deficits in social communication and social interaction across multiple contexts, as manifested by all of the following, currently or by history (examples are illustrative, not exhaustive; see text):
   1. Deficits in social-emotional reciprocity, ranging, for example, from abnormal social approach and failure of normal back-and-forth conversation to reduced sharing of interests, emotions, or affect; to failure to initiate or respond to social interactions.
   2. Deficits in nonverbal communicative behaviors used for social interaction, ranging, for example, from poorly integrated verbal and nonverbal communication to abnormalities in eye contact and body language or deficits in understanding and use of gestures; to a total lack of facial expressions and nonverbal communication.
   3. Deficits in developing, maintaining, and understanding relationships, ranging, for example, from difficulties adjusting behavior to suit various social contexts to difficulties in sharing imaginative play or in making friends; to absence of interest in peers.

Specify current severity:

- **Severity is based on social communication impairments and restricted, repetitive patterns of behavior.**

B. Restricted, repetitive patterns of behavior, interests, or activities, as manifested by at least two of the following, currently or by history (examples are illustrative, not exhaustive; see text):
   1. Stereotyped or repetitive motor movements, use of objects, or speech (eg, simple motor stereotypies, lining up toys or flipping objects, echolalia, idiosyncratic phrases).
   2. Insistence on sameness, inflexible adherence to routines, or ritualized patterns of verbal or nonverbal behavior (eg, extreme distress at small changes, difficulties with transitions, rigid thinking patterns, greeting rituals, need to take same route or eat same food every day).
   3. Highly restricted, fixated interests that are abnormal in intensity or focus (eg, strong attachment to or preoccupation with unusual objects, excessively circumscribed or perseverative interests).
   4. Hyper- or hyporeactivity to sensory input or unusual interest in sensory aspects of the environment (eg, apparent indifference to pain/temperature, adverse response to specific sounds or textures, excessive smelling or touching of objects, visual fascination with lights or movement).

Specify current severity:

- **Severity is based on social communication impairments and restricted, repetitive patterns of behavior.**

C. Symptoms must be present in the early developmental period (but may not become fully manifest until social demands exceed limited capacities, or may be masked by learned strategies in later life).
D. Symptoms cause clinically significant impairment in social, occupational, or other important areas of current functioning.
E. These disturbances are not better explained by intellectual disability (intellectual developmental disorder) or global developmental delay. Intellectual disability and autism spectrum disorder frequently co-occur; to make comorbid diagnoses of autism spectrum disorder and intellectual disability, social communication should be below that expected for general developmental level.

Note: Individuals with a well-established DSM-IV diagnosis of autistic disorder, Asperger disorder, or pervasive developmental disorder not otherwise specified should be given the diagnosis of autism spectrum disorder. Individuals who have marked deficits in social communication but whose symptoms do not otherwise meet criteria for autism spectrum disorder should be evaluated for social (pragmatic) communication disorder.

Specify if:

- With or without accompanying intellectual impairment
- With or without accompanying language impairment
- Associated with a known medical or genetic condition or environmental factor (**Coding note:** Use additional code to identify the associated medical or genetic condition.)

- Associated with another neurodevelopmental, mental, or behavioral disorder (**Coding note:** Use additional code[s] to identify the associated neurodevelopmental, mental, or behavioral disorder[s].)
- With catatonia (refer to the criteria for catatonia associated with another mental disorder) (**Coding note:** Use additional code 293.89 [F06.1] for catatonia associated with autism spectrum disorder to indicate the presence of the comorbid catatonia.)

(Reprinted with permission from the *Diagnostic and Statistical Manual of Mental Disorders.* 5th ed. Arlington, VA: American Psychiatric Publishing; 2013.)

What is the rationale for the diagnosis?

The patient has persistent deficits in her social interactions at home and at school as evidenced by her lack of friends. She has restricted, repetitive behaviors exhibited by a history of echolalia and lining up objects. She has restricted interests limited to video games and drawing animated figures (has not been able to complete other art courses involving human drawing, etc.). These symptoms were present in her early development according to her mother. These symptoms have caused significant impairment in her social and academic functioning. These disturbances are not better attributed to an intellectual disability or a global developmental delay. Therefore, she meets the criteria for autism spectrum disorder.

What test or tools should be considered to help identify the correct diagnosis?

The BDI can help evaluate the severity of the depression.

The Y-BOCS can help evaluate the presence of obsessive compulsive disorder symptoms.

Consultation with the patient's former therapist is indicated to obtain additional information to inform the diagnosis. The patient gave written consent for this interprofessional collaboration.

What differential diagnosis (or diagnoses) should be considered?

300.3 (F42.2) Obsessive Compulsive Disorder

Although the patient has numerous obsessions and a history of compulsive behavior, they are considered part of the autism spectrum disorder symptomatology. Therefore, the diagnosis of obsessive compulsive disorder is not applicable.

FORMULATING THE TREATMENT STRATEGY

What treatment would you prescribe and what is the rationale?

Psychopharmacology: Lurasidone 20 mg daily was ordered to treat the psychotic symptoms. Most guidelines recommend a combination of an antipsychotic and an antidepressant or an antidepressant as monotherapy for depressive disorder with psychotic features. Because dysthymia with psychotic features appears to be in a similar diagnostic category, the same treatment approach seems appropriate. However, because the auditory hallucinations increased when this patient had a trial of fluoxetine, an antipsychotic as monotherapy is the preferred initial medication.

Diagnostic Tests: None.

Referrals: Referred to the college center for disabilities for academic accommodations and additional support. However, the patient does not want to connect with these services. She wants to maintain her independence and is concerned about stigma.

Type of Psychotherapy: Individual psychotherapy to help her manage stress and improve her organizational skills.

Psychoeducation: The mother will be referred to "Autism Speaks," a national community and support group for individuals and their families. More information can be found at https://www.autismspeaks.org/

What standard guidelines would you use to treat or assess this patient?

The Guidelines for treatment of Patients with Major Depressive Disorder can be accessed at http://psychiatryonline.org/pb/assets/raw/sitewide/practice_guidelines/guidelines/mdd-guide.pdf

CLINICAL NOTE

- This case presented challenges in identifying the correct diagnoses. Additionally, there is a variety of opinions as to whether depression with psychotic features is a subset of major depressive disorder or is a separate diagnosis entity. It is not uncommon that a patient's presentation and history may make diagnosing difficult. Changes in the patient's presentation or the addition of relevant history may indicate a different diagnosis and subsequently a new direction in treatment.
- There is an increasing number of individuals with autism who are applying to college and universities. There may be a better likelihood of them completing their college degree if they attend a school with programs that provide additional supportive services for this population.

REFERENCES/RECOMMENDED READINGS

Adreon D, Durocher JS. Evaluating the college transition needs of individuals with high-functioning autism spectrum disorders. *Intervent School Clinic*. 2007;42(5):271-279.

American Psychiatric Association. *Diagnostic and Statistical Manual of Mental Disorders*. 5th ed. Arlington, VA: American Psychiatric Publishing; 2013.

Hewitt LE. Assessment considerations for college students with autism spectrum disorder. *Topics Language Disord*. 2015;35(4):313-328.

Rothschild AJ. Challenges in the treatment of major depressive disorder with psychotic features. *Schizophrenia Bull*. 2013;39(4):787-796. doi:10.1093/schbul/sbt046.

CASE 14

Depressed and Voices Say to Kill Myself

IDENTIFICATION: The patient is a 20-year-old single, third-generation, American-born Caucasian female of Jewish heritage who is one of three children. She has never been married, has no children, and lives independently in a one-bedroom apartment for the past 10 months until 2 weeks ago when her mother moved in. She is being evaluated on the inpatient psychiatric unit to which she has recently been admitted on a voluntary status.

CHIEF COMPLAINT: "I am hearing voices to kill myself and my mom and boyfriend."

HISTORY OF CHIEF COMPLAINT: This is the sixth inpatient admission for this 20-year-old female. She presented to the crisis center last night on a voluntary basis after a recommendation by her private psychiatrist. She reports being plagued with command auditory hallucination to cut her wrist with a razor or a knife and to kill her mother and boyfriend with a knife or a gun. She reports experiencing these command auditory hallucinations of a man's voice at least 10 to 20 times daily for the past 2 weeks along with paranoid delusions of others laughing and talking about her. She denies any past or present suicide or homicide attempts. She denies access to weapons. She alleges that she has not been able to work for the past 2 weeks because of her symptoms. However, as per collateral from her mother, the patient has not been able to work consistently for the past 3 months due to multiple hospitalizations. The patient reports irritability, racing thoughts, feelings of sadness, lack of interest in usual activities, poor appetite, fatigue, lack of motivation, interrupted sleep of 4 hours per night, increased anxiety, and fears about the future for the past 2 weeks. She reports sporadic compliance with topiramate and risperidone for the past 2 weeks. She attributes the auditory hallucinations to medication changes from lithium and valproic acid to topiramate and risperidone due to her declining renal status. Recent stressors include her mother moving in with her 2 weeks ago after mother broke up with her own boyfriend. Mother has been voicing her disapproval of the patient's boyfriend since moving in, which the patient identifies as being stressful. The patient is requesting to be placed back on lithium and valproic acid. Her psychotropic medications prior to admission include topiramate 100 mg PO HS, risperidone 1 mg PO BID, trazodone 100 mg PO HS, and hydroxyzine 50 mg PO Q4h PRN.

PAST PSYCHIATRIC HISTORY

The patient was initially diagnosed with bipolar disorder 5 years ago at age 15 during her sophomore year when she was first hospitalized at a psychiatric hospital due to aggressive behavior toward her mother and sister. She was treated with lithium 600 mg PO BID and valproic acid 1000 mg PO HS. Following her hospitalization, she was treated by a private therapist and psychiatrist.

Her second psychiatric hospitalization was at the age of 16 for depression related to her father's death and regret that she did not confront him about past sexual abuse. Prior to the hospitalization, she confronted her mother about the abuse, and the mother denied ever knowing about the abuse and expressed remorse.

A third inpatient psychiatric hospitalization occurred when she was 18 for depression. During this hospitalization, there were no medication changes and she was discharged to outpatient treatment after a few days.

The fourth hospitalization occurred a year ago (when she was 19) for manic symptoms and her first episode of command auditory hallucinations to hurt random people. During that admission, her medication was changed because of declining renal status from valproic acid 1000 mg PO HS and lithium 600 mg PO BID to topiramate 100 mg PO HS and paliperidone 6 mg PO BID.

The paliperidone helped eliminate her homicidal thoughts and voices for about 2 months; however, symptoms returned and precipitated her fifth psychiatric admission. She reports that the paliperidone was discontinued. She was then started on haloperidol 5 mg PO BID which was stopped due to EPS after 2 days and then started on risperidone 1 mg PO BID. Trazodone 100 mg PO HS, and hydroxyzine 50 mg PO Q4h PRN were also ordered during the hospitalization.. The patient reports that she was discharged after a week to her outpatient therapist and private psychiatrist. Two weeks ago her symptoms returned.

MEDICAL HISTORY

Review of previous hospital admission records indicates electrocardiogram (ECG) findings with slight QTc prolongation of 460 ms.

No known allergies, medical hospitalizations, or surgeries.
The patient has a history of:
- Hypertension currently treated with carvedilol 3.125 mg PO BID and losartan 50 mg PO BID.
- Type II diabetes currently treated with glipizide 5 mg PO AM.
- Hyperlipidemia
- Obesity
- Gout treated with allopurinol 300 mg PO AM.

She was diagnosed with sleep apnea 6 months ago and uses a continuous positive airway pressure machine at HS.

HISTORY OF DRUG OR ALCOHOL ABUSE: She denies past or present use of substances including tobacco and alcohol.

FAMILY HISTORY: The patient is one of three children. Her non-Hassidic Orthodox Jewish maternal grandparents severed ties with her mom when she married her dad who was not very religious even though of a non-Hassidic Orthodox Jewish background. She states her family only went to the temple occasionally during holidays while growing up. Her father died when the patient was 18 years old. Her mother is currently living with her. No known psychiatric illnesses in the family.

PERSONAL HISTORY

Perinatal: No known perinatal complications.

Childhood: No history of head banging, rocking, attachment issues, intellectual or motor skill deficits, separation anxiety, gender identity development, friendship difficulties, learning disabilities, nightmares, phobias, bedwetting, fire setting, or cruelty to animals.

Adolescence: Attended public school as opposed to a Jewish school, which she later regretted and was jealous about her sister attending a Jewish school. She was a sophomore in high school when she was initially admitted to a psychiatric hospital for aggressiveness toward her mother and sister. The patient was able to graduate high school with a B average. She reports having had a few friends in high school.

Adulthood

She got a job in the Jewish community center as a youth worker shortly after high school.

The patient subscribes to the Jewish religion. She currently observes Rosh Hashanah and Yom Kippur.

The patient has never been married, has no children, and has lived independently in a one-bedroom apartment for the past 10 months until 2 weeks ago when her mother who recently broke up with her boyfriend moved in. The patient has a boyfriend who is American born of Italian heritage. She has been seeing him for 9 months and he spent weekends at her apartment until her mother moved in. The patient met her boyfriend at work. The patient denies any criminal or delinquent history and has never served in the military.

TRAUMA/ABUSE HISTORY: As a child, the patient experienced sexual abuse by her father. She never spoke about the sexual abuse to anyone until she saw a therapist for the first time when she was 15 and was admitted to a psychiatric unit. She did not want to provide any details about the sexual abuse, such as the frequency or length of time, to this provider at the time of this evaluation.

MENTAL STATUS EXAMINATION

Appearance: Disheveled with poor ADLs.

Behavior and psychomotor activity: Apathetic and reluctant to answer questions. Normal motor activity with poor eye contact.

Consciousness:	Fully alert.
Orientation:	Oriented to person, place, and date.
Memory:	Intact immediate, recent, and remote recall.
Concentration and attention:	Unimpaired; serial 7s intact.
Visuospatial ability:	Not assessed.
Abstract thought:	Adequate proverb interpretation.
Intellectual functioning:	Average.
Speech and language:	Slow rate with normal volume.
Perceptions:	Command auditory hallucinations of a male voice telling her to hurt herself and others.
Thought processes:	Logical and coherent, reports racing thoughts.

Thought content: Paranoid delusions of others talking and laughing at her.

Suicidality or homicidality: Reports thoughts to cut wrist for the past 2 weeks due to the voices that resolved after arrival at the hospital. Reports thoughts to kill mother and boyfriend for the past 2 weeks due to the voices.

Mood: Dysphoric and anxious.

Affect: Flat.

Impulse control: Good during the interview. No history of impulsiveness.

Judgment: Poor. Needed others to coax her to seek help.

Insight: Fair, understands present mental state.

Reliability: Generally seems to be a reliable historian.

FORMULATING THE DIAGNOSIS

Which diagnosis (or diagnoses) should be considered?

296.44 (F31.44) Bipolar Disorder, Current Episode Depressed, with Mood-Congruent Psychotic Features

Diagnostic Criteria

For a diagnosis of bipolar I disorder, it is necessary to meet the following criteria for a manic episode. The manic episode may have been preceded by and may be followed by hypomanic episode or major depressive episodes (MDEs).

Manic Episode

A. A distinct period of abnormally and persistently elevated, expansive, or irritable mood and abnormally and persistently increased activity or energy, lasting at least 1 week and present most of the day, nearly every day (or any duration if hospitalization is necessary).
B. During the period of mood disturbance and increased energy or activity, three (or more) of the following symptoms (four if the mood is only irritable) are present to a significant degree and represent a noticeable change from usual behavior:

1. Inflated self-esteem or grandiosity
2. Decreased need for sleep (eg, feels rested after only 3 hours of sleep)
3. More talkative than usual or pressure to keep talking
4. Flight of ideas or subjective experience that thoughts are racing
5. Distractibility (ie, attention too easily drawn to unimportant or irrelevant external stimuli), as reported or observed
6. Increase in goal-directed activity (socially, at work or school, or sexually) or psychomotor agitation (ie, purposeless non–goal-directed activity)
7. Excessive involvement in activities that have a high potential for painful consequences (eg, engaging in unrestrained buying sprees, sexual indiscretions, or foolish business investments)

C. The mood disturbance is sufficiently severe to cause marked impairment in social or occupational functioning or to necessitate hospitalization to prevent harm to self or others, or there are psychotic features.
D. The episode is not attributable to the physiologic effects of a substance (eg, a drug of abuse, a medication, other treatment) or another medical condition.
   - **Note:** A full manic episode that emerges during antidepressant treatment (eg, medication, electroconvulsive therapy) but persists at a fully syndromal level beyond the physiologic effect of that treatment is sufficient evidence for a manic episode and, therefore, a bipolar I diagnosis.

Note: Criteria A–D constitute a manic episode. At least one lifetime manic episode is required for the diagnosis of bipolar I disorder.

Hypomanic Episode

A. A distinct period of abnormally and persistently elevated, expansive, or irritable mood and abnormally and persistently increased activity or energy, lasting at least 4 consecutive days and present most of the day, nearly every day.
B. During the period of mood disturbance and increased energy and activity, three (or more) of the following symptoms (four if the mood is only irritable) have persisted, represent a noticeable change from usual behavior, and have been present to a significant degree:
   1. Inflated self-esteem or grandiosity
   2. Decreased need for sleep (eg, feels rested after only 3 hours of sleep)
   3. More talkative than usual or pressure to keep talking
   4. Flight of ideas or subjective experience that thoughts are racing
   5. Distractibility (ie, attention too easily drawn to unimportant or irrelevant external stimuli), as reported or observed
   6. Increase in goal-directed activity (socially, at work or school, or sexually) or psychomotor agitation

7. Excessive involvement in activities that have a high potential for painful consequences (eg, engaging in unrestrained buying sprees, sexual indiscretions, or foolish business investments)

C. The episode is associated with an unequivocal change in functioning that is uncharacteristic of the individual when not symptomatic.
D. The disturbance in mood and the change in functioning are observable by others.
E. The episode is not severe enough to cause marked impairment in social or occupational functioning or to necessitate hospitalization. If there are psychotic features, the episode is, by definition, manic.
F. The episode is not attributable to the physiologic effects of a substance (eg, a drug of abuse, a medication, other treatment) or another medical condition.
   - **Note:** A full hypomanic episode that emerges during antidepressant treatment (eg, medication, electroconvulsive therapy) but persists at a fully syndromal level beyond the physiologic effect of that treatment is sufficient evidence for a hypomanic episode diagnosis. However, caution is indicated so that one or two symptoms (particularly increased irritability, edginess, or agitation following antidepressant use) are not taken as sufficient for diagnosis of a hypomanic episode, nor necessarily indicative of a bipolar diathesis.

Note: Criteria A–F constitute a hypomanic episode. Hypomanic episodes are common in bipolar I disorder but are not required for the diagnosis of bipolar I disorder.

Major Depressive Episode

A. Five (or more) of the following symptoms have been present during the same 2-week period and represent a change from previous functioning; at least one of the symptoms is either (1) depressed mood or (2) loss of interest or pleasure.
   - **Note:** Do not include symptoms that are clearly attributable to another medical condition.
     1. Depressed mood most of the day, nearly every day, as indicated by either subjective report (eg, feels sad, empty, or hopeless) or observation made by others (eg, appears tearful). (Note: In children and adolescents, can be irritable mood.)
     2. Markedly diminished interest or pleasure in all, or almost all, activities most of the day, nearly every day (as indicated by either subjective account or observation).
     3. Significant weight loss when not dieting or weight gain (eg, a change of more than 5% of body weight in a month), or decrease or increase in appetite nearly every day. (Note: In children, consider failure to make expected weight gain.)
     4. Insomnia or hypersomnia nearly every day.

5. Psychomotor agitation or retardation nearly every day (observable by others; not merely subjective feelings of restlessness or being slowed down).
6. Fatigue or loss of energy nearly every day.
7. Feelings of worthlessness or excessive or inappropriate guilt (which may be delusional) nearly every day (not merely self-reproach or guilt about being sick).
8. Diminished ability to think or concentrate, or indecisiveness, nearly every day (either by subjective account or as observed by others).
9. Recurrent thoughts of death (not just fear of dying), recurrent suicidal ideation without a specific plan, or a suicide attempt or a specific plan for committing suicide.

B. The symptoms cause clinically significant distress or impairment in social, occupational, or other important areas of functioning.
C. The episode is not attributable to the physiologic effects of a substance or another medical condition.

Note: Criteria A–C constitute an MDE. MDEs are common in bipolar I disorder but are not required for the diagnosis of bipolar I disorder.

Note: Responses to a significant loss (eg, bereavement, financial ruin, losses from a natural disaster, a serious medical illness or disability) may include the feelings of intense sadness, rumination about the loss, insomnia, poor appetite, and weight loss noted in Criterion A, which may resemble a depressive episode. Although such symptoms may be understandable or considered appropriate to the loss, the presence of an MDE in addition to the normal response to a significant loss should also be carefully considered. This decision inevitably requires the exercise of clinical judgment based on the individual's history and the cultural norms for the expression of distress in the context of loss.

In distinguishing grief from an MDE, it is useful to consider that in grief the predominant affect is feelings of emptiness and loss, while in an MDE it is persistent depressed mood and the inability to anticipate happiness or pleasure. The dysphoria in grief is likely to decrease in intensity over days to weeks and occurs in waves, the so-called pangs of grief. These waves tend to be associated with thoughts or reminders of the deceased. The depressed mood of an MDE is more persistent and not tied to specific thoughts or preoccupations. The pain of grief may be accompanied by positive emotions and humor that are uncharacteristic of the pervasive unhappiness and misery characteristic of an MDE . The thought content associated with grief generally features a preoccupation with thoughts and memories of the deceased, rather than the self-critical or pessimistic ruminations seen in an MDE. In grief, self-esteem is generally preserved, whereas in an MDE, feelings of worthlessness and self-loathing are common. If self-derogatory ideation is present in grief, it typically involves perceived failings vis-à-vis the deceased (eg, not visiting frequently enough, not telling the deceased how much he or she was loved). If a bereaved individual thinks about death and dying, such thoughts are generally focused on the deceased and possibly about "joining" the deceased, whereas in an MDE such thoughts are focused on ending one's own life because of feeling worthless, undeserving of life, or unable to cope with the pain of depression.

Bipolar I Disorder

A. Criteria have been met for at least one manic episode (Criteria A–D under "Manic Episode" above).
B. The occurrence of the manic episode and MDE(s) is not better explained by schizoaffective disorder, schizophrenia, schizophreniform disorder, delusional disorder, or other specified or unspecified schizophrenia spectrum and other psychotic disorder.

Specify:

- With anxious distress
- With mixed features
- With rapid cycling
- With melancholic features
- With atypical features
- With mood-congruent psychotic features
- With mood-incongruent psychotic features
- With catatonia (**Coding note:** Use additional code 293.89 (F06.1))
- With peripartum onset
- With seasonal pattern

(Reprinted with permission from the *Diagnostic and Statistical Manual of Mental Disorders*. 5th ed. Arlington, VA: American Psychiatric Publishing; 2013.)

What is the rationale for the diagnosis?

The patient has a history of manic episodes. She meets more than the five required criteria for a depressed episode. For the past 2 weeks, she has had a depressed mood and suicidal ideations, feelings of sadness, fatigue, loss of appetite, insomnia, avolition, and anhedonia. Her symptom presentation also meets the criteria for psychotic features due to presence of auditory hallucinations telling her to kill herself and others.

Which diagnosis (or diagnoses) should be considered?

309.81 (F43.10) Posttraumatic Stress Disorder

Diagnostic Criteria

Posttraumatic Stress Disorder

- **Note:** The following criteria apply to adults, adolescents, and children older than 6 years. For children 6 years and younger, see corresponding criteria below.

A. Exposure to actual or threatened death, serious injury, or sexual violence in one (or more) of the following ways:
   1. Directly experiencing the traumatic event(s).
   2. Witnessing, in person, the event(s) as it occurred to others.
   3. Learning that the traumatic event(s) occurred to a close family member or close friend. In cases of actual or threatened death of a family member or friend, the event(s) must have been violent or accidental.
   4. Experiencing repeated or extreme exposure to aversive details of the traumatic event(s) (eg, first responders collecting human remains; police officers repeatedly exposed to details of child abuse).
      - **Note:** Criterion A4 does not apply to exposure through electronic media, television, movies, or pictures, unless this exposure is work related.

B. Presence of one (or more) of the following intrusion symptoms associated with the traumatic event(s), beginning after the traumatic event(s) occurred:
   1. Recurrent, involuntary, and intrusive distressing memories of the traumatic event(s).
      - **Note:** In children older than 6 years, repetitive play may occur in which themes or aspects of the traumatic event(s) are expressed.
   2. Recurrent distressing dreams in which the content and/or affect of the dream are related to the traumatic event(s).
      - **Note:** In children, there may be frightening dreams without recognizable content.
   3. Dissociative reactions (eg, flashbacks) in which the individual feels or acts as if the traumatic event(s) were recurring. (Such reactions may occur on a continuum, with the most extreme expression being a complete loss of awareness of present surroundings.)
      - **Note:** In children, trauma-specific reenactment may occur in play.
   4. Intense or prolonged psychological distress at exposure to internal or external cues that symbolize or resemble an aspect of the traumatic event(s).
   5. Marked physiologic reactions to internal or external cues that symbolize or resemble an aspect of the traumatic event(s).

C. Persistent avoidance of stimuli associated with the traumatic event(s), beginning after the traumatic event(s) occurred, as evidenced by one or both of the following:
   1. Avoidance of or efforts to avoid distressing memories, thoughts, or feelings about or closely associated with the traumatic event(s).
   2. Avoidance of or efforts to avoid external reminders (people, places, conversations, activities, objects, situations) that arouse distressing memories, thoughts, or feelings about or closely associated with the traumatic event(s).

D. Negative alterations in cognitions and mood associated with the traumatic event(s), beginning or worsening after the traumatic event(s) occurred, as evidenced by two (or more) of the following:
   1. Inability to remember an important aspect of the traumatic event(s) (typically due to dissociative amnesia and not to other factors such as head injury, alcohol, or drugs).
   2. Persistent and exaggerated negative beliefs or expectations about oneself, others, or the world (eg, "I am bad," "No one can be trusted," "The world is completely dangerous," "My whole nervous system is permanently ruined").
   3. Persistent, distorted cognitions about the cause or consequences of the traumatic event(s) that lead the individual to blame himself/herself or others.
   4. Persistent negative emotional state (eg, fear, horror, anger, guilt, or shame).
   5. Markedly diminished interest or participation in significant activities.
   6. Feelings of detachment or estrangement from others.
   7. Persistent inability to experience positive emotions (eg, inability to experience happiness, satisfaction, or loving feelings).
E. Marked alterations in arousal and reactivity associated with the traumatic event(s), beginning or worsening after the traumatic event(s) occurred, as evidenced by two (or more) of the following:
   1. Irritable behavior and angry outbursts (with little or no provocation) typically expressed as verbal or physical aggression toward people or objects
   2. Reckless or self-destructive behavior
   3. Hypervigilance
   4. Exaggerated startle response
   5. Problems with concentration
   6. Sleep disturbance (eg, difficulty falling or staying asleep or restless sleep)
F. Duration of the disturbance (Criteria B, C, D, and E) is more than 1 month.
G. The disturbance causes clinically significant distress or impairment in social, occupational, or other important areas of functioning.
H. The disturbance is not attributable to the physiologic effects of a substance (eg, medication, alcohol) or another medical condition.

Specify whether:

- With dissociative symptoms: The individual's symptoms meet the criteria for posttraumatic stress disorder (PTSD), and in addition, in response to the stressor, the individual experiences persistent or recurrent symptoms of either of the following:
   1. Depersonalization: Persistent or recurrent experiences of feeling detached from, and as if one were an outside observer of, one's mental processes or body (eg, feeling as though one were in a dream; feeling a sense of unreality of self or body or of time moving slowly).

2. Derealization: Persistent or recurrent experiences of unreality of surroundings (eg, the world around the individual is experienced as unreal, dreamlike, distant, or distorted).
   - **Note:** To use this subtype, the dissociative symptoms must not be attributable to the physiologic effects of a substance (eg, blackouts, behavior during alcohol intoxication) or another medical condition (eg, complex partial seizures).

Specify if:

- With delayed expression: The full diagnostic criteria are not met until at least 6 months after the event (although the onset and expression of some symptoms may be immediate).

(Reprinted with permission from the *Diagnostic and Statistical Manual of Mental Disorders*. 5th ed. Arlington, VA: American Psychiatric Publishing; 2013.)

What is the rationale for the diagnosis?

The patient's symptoms meet criteria for this diagnosis. She experienced a traumatic childhood event of sexual abuse by her father; she attempts to avoid conversations about the event; she has difficulty falling and staying asleep; she has had periods of impaired social and occupational functioning; and the event occurred more than a month ago. The patient spoke about having flashbacks of the sexual abuse after the death of her father. Therefore, the diagnosis of PTSD is being assigned.

What test or tools should be considered to help identify the correct diagnosis?

Hamilton Depression Scale (HAM-D), which can help identify the level of depression. (http://www.assessmentpsychology.com/HAM-D.pdf)

Hamilton Anxiety Scale (HAM-A), which can help identify the level of anxiety. (http://dcf.psychiatry.ufl.edu/files/2011/05/HAMILTON-ANXIETY.pdf)

PTSD CheckList—Civilian Version (PCL-C), which can be diagnostic of PTSD. (http://www.mirecc.va.gov/docs/visn6/3_PTSD_CheckList_and_Scoring.pdf)

Brief Psychiatric Rating Scale (BRPS), which can indicate the presence of mood, behavioral, or psychotic symptoms. (http://www.public-health.uiowa.edu/icmha/outreach/documents/BPRS_expanded.PDF)

What differential diagnosis (or diagnoses) should be considered?

None indicated at this time.

FORMULATING THE TREATMENT STRATEGY

What treatment would you prescribe and what is the rationale?

Safety Precautions: Q15 minute observation checks. If there is indication of increased risk of harm to self or others then initiate one-to-one observation.

Psychopharmacology/Pharmacology: Discontinue risperidone due to renal impairment because it requires renal dosing.

Discontinue topiramate because there is limited evidence for this medication's efficacy in treating bipolar disorder or PTSD.

Valproic acid 500 mg PO HS and titrate up gradually until mood stabilizes at a therapeutic level as per serum valproic levels and patient symptoms. No renal dosing is required for valproic acid.

Trazodone 100 mg PO HS for sleep. As a weak antidepressant, this drug is used for its side effect of somnolence due to its blockade of histamine and alpha adrenergic-1 receptors.

Fluphenazine 5 mg PO BID to treat auditory hallucination and anxiety.

This high-potency first-generation antipsychotic was chosen because of the reduced potential for weight gain that is associated with metabolic syndrome. Even though atypical antipsychotics are first-line treatment for psychotic symptoms due to less dopamine blockade effects, a first-generation antipsychotic was chosen due to the risk of increasing the symptoms of metabolic syndrome with this patient (she has a high BMI and has a recent history of an elevated glucose in her previous admissions). Ziprasidone, which has a better metabolic side effect profile, was not considered due to this patient's history of a slight QTc prolongation.

Hydroxyzine 50 mg PO PRN Q4h for anxiety. There is no dose adjustment necessary in renal impairment. A clinical trial by Ferreri and Hantouche (1998) showed that hydroxyzine was efficacious in treating anxiety comparable to lorazepam. Moreover, a greater cognitive improvement was seen with hydroxyzine than lorazepam. In addition, lorazepam has the potential to develop tolerance and dependence.

Continue current medications for medical conditions:

Carvedilol 3.125 mg PO BID and losartan 50 mg PO BID—Monitor blood pressure twice daily.
Glipizide 5 mg PO daily—Monitor fingersticks twice daily.
Allopurinol 300 mg PO daily.

Diagnostic Tests: Besides conducting routine laboratory tests, pregnancy test, and urine drug screen, obtain renal function tests (blood urea nitrogen, creatinine, glomerular filtration rate) upon admission, and to be followed up by renal specialist. Liver function should be evaluated closely as well because valproic acid may have potential for hepatotoxicity. Glucose should also be evaluated closely as metabolic syndrome is a potential complication of treatment with antipsychotic medication.

AIMS daily to assess for extrapyramidal effects.

Periodic liver function tests.

Valproic acid level in 5 days after steady state to monitor for toxicity and drug efficacy. Monitor periodically.

CBC with platelet counts to monitor for agranulocytosis and thrombocytopenia.

ECG to monitor for arrhythmias.

Monitor for metabolic syndrome by tracking abdominal obesity, triglycerides, HDL cholesterol, fasting glucose, and blood pressure.

The patient's menstrual history should be obtained as she may be at risk for polycystic ovary syndrome with the use of valproic acid.

Consultations: Hospitalist consult for declining renal function.

Dietary consult for elevated BMI and declining renal function.

Referrals: Refer for gynecology consult with recommendation for birth control because there is risk for impaired fetal development with the use of valproic acid.

Referral to a psychotherapist experienced with Bowen family therapy and cognitive behavioral therapy (CBT).

Type of Psychotherapy: A combination of Bowen family therapy and cognitive behavioral therapy will be recommended to treat this patient. The patient may benefit from Bowen family therapy by achieving goals of self-differentiation and detriangulation. Several studies have supported CBT as a form of evidence-based treatment modality for posttraumatic syndrome in relation to sexual abuse.

Psychoeducation: Advise regarding the risk of fetal complications with the use of valproic acid during pregnancy.

Recommend patient to see her gynecologist to be started on some form of birth control.

CLINICAL NOTE

- There is no known family history of bipolar disorder or schizophrenia, which suggests that the sexual abuse trauma may have been a contributing factor to the development of the patient's psychiatric symptoms. Research findings support the hypothesis that childhood sexual abuse can have an impact on mental health ranging from mood disorders to personality disorders.

REFERENCES/RECOMMENDED READINGS

American Psychiatric Association. *Diagnostic and Statistical Manual of Mental Disorders.* 5th ed. Arlington, VA: American Psychiatric Publishing; 2013.

Becker-Weidman A. Treatment for children with trauma-attachment disorders: dyadic developmental psychotherapy. *Child Adolesc Social Work J.* 2006;23(2):147-171.

Berkson W. Jewish family values today. *J Jewish Communal Service.* 1996;54(3).

Chard KM. An evaluation of cognitive processing therapy for the treatment of post traumatic stress disorder related to childhood sexual abuse. *J Consult Clin Psychol.* 2005;73(5):965-971.

Davis LL, Bartolucci A, Petty F. Divalproex in the treatment of bipolar depression: placebo-controlled study. *J Affective Disord.* 2005;85(3):259-266.

Dawson TE. A lifespan comparison of early attachment experiences to current attachment and psychological well being in an elderly population. *Dissertation Abstr Int: Sect B, Sci Eng* 2001;61(7–B):3838.

Epstein NB, Bishop D, Ryan C, Miller L, Keitner G. The McMaster Model View of Healthy Family Functioning. In Froma Walsh (Eds.), *Normal Family Processes* (pp. 138-160). New York/London: The Guilford Press; 1993.

Feldman RS. *Development across the Lifespan.* 5th ed. Upper saddle River, NJ: Prentice Hall; 2008.

Ferreri M, Hantouche EG. Recent trial of hydroxyzine in generalized anxiety disorder. *Acta Psychiatr Scandinavica.* 1998;98(393):102-108.

Foa EB, Rothbaum BO. *Treating the Trauma of Rape: Cognitive behavioral Therapy for PTSD.* New York: Gilford Press; 1998.

Liem JH, Boudewyn AC. Contextualizing the effects of childhood sexual abuse on adult self- and social functioning: an attachment theory perspective. *Child Abuse Neglect.* 1999;23(11):1141-1157.

McDonagh A, Friedman M, McHugo G, et al. Randomized trial of cognitive behavioral therapy for chronic post traumatic stress disorder in adult female survivors of childhood sexual abuse. *J Consult Clinical Psychol.* 2005;73(3):515-524.

Noller P, Fitzpatrick MA. Marital communication in the eighties. *J Marriage Fam.* 1990;52:832-843.

Norton RW. Foundation of a communication style construct. *Hum Commun Res.* 1978;4(2):99-112.

Resick PA, Nishith P, Griffin GM. How well does cognitive behavioral therapy treat symptoms of complex PTSD? An examination of sexual abuse survivors within a clinical trial. *CNS Spectr.* 2003;8(5):340-355.

Sadock B, Sadock V. *Kaplan & Sadock's Synopsis of Psychiatry.* 11th ed. Philadelphia, PA: Lippincott, William and Wilkins; 2015.

Stahl SS. *Essential Psychopharmacology. The Prescriber's Guide.* 4th ed. New York: Cambridge University Press; 2012.

Surcinelli P, Rossi N, Montebarrocci O, Baldaro B. Adult attachment style and psychological disease: examining the mediating role of personality traits. *J Psychol: Interdisciplinary Appl.* 2010;144(6):523-535.

Wieselberg H. Family therapy and ultra-orthodox Jewish families: a structural approach. *J Fam Therapy.* 1992;14:305-329.

CASE 15

Not Doing Well in College

IDENTIFICATION: This 20-year-old, single male is a full-time college student living with his parents in a suburban middle class community where he grew up. He is of Italian descent and was raised in the Catholic faith although chooses to be agnostic. He is self-referred at this time. He is being evaluated at a private psychiatric practice.

CHIEF COMPLAINT: "I am struggling with anxiety and focusing. I also want to be more independent."

HISTORY OF CHIEF COMPLAINT: The patient reports recognizing he has difficulties in several areas of his functioning. He states he has considered himself to be "very bright" but does not always feel "sharp." He states, "I am not doing as well as I can do." Patient states his mind wanders: "I get lost in my thoughts and lose track of time." Patient states that while completing simple tasks such as in the shower, cooking, anything that takes longer than 15 minutes, he gets offtrack. He recognizes that sometimes the thoughts are a waste of time and that it took years for him to realize this. He states he experiences lost time with no recollection. He reports he tries to train his mind to focus deeply such as when driving, but sometimes becomes overfocused on details or distracted and misses things, especially when he is tired.

Patient reports he has difficulty starting large tasks and has trouble with envisioning the final project, particularly when it comes to schoolwork. He believes he overanalyzes things especially when writing. He then procrastinates and feels very anxious. "The act of trying to start makes me feel anxious." In class, he listens to the professor, then gets sidetracked from what is being said and is lost. He will study for an exam "when I have no choice, at the last minute, I force myself and run out of time and I don't finish the material." Patient also reports being forgetful and losing information such as due dates.

He additionally reports feeling anxious in social situations and when he needs to participate in class. He describes holding back socially in conversation because of lack of confidence and not being sure if what he wants to say is relevant. Patient reports avoiding social situations in which he needs to participate in small group discussions, meeting new people, attending parties, or being the center of attention. He reports moderate to severe anxiety in social situations such as when being observed, entering a room, expressing an opinion, returning items in a store, or talking to people in authority.

PAST PSYCHIATRIC HISTORY: Presented at age 7 with a diagnosis of attention-deficit–hyperactivity disorder (ADHD) made by psychiatrist after demonstrating difficulties with attention, listening, adjusting to change, disruptive behaviors, and poor social skills (impulsive and attention-seeking behaviors) with onset prior to kindergarten. He was treated with amphetamine/dextroamphetamine (Adderall), which led to persistent vocal tics that were further interfering with his functioning academically and socially. Most trials of psychostimulants led to increased tics and obsessive thinking. Atomoxetine (Strattera) seemed to be the best tolerated although not producing the most robust control of symptoms of ADHD. Prior to college, the patient made the decision to stop taking medication to see how he could function.

MEDICAL HISTORY: The patient has no known allergies, no head trauma, seizures, infectious diseases, or any other major medical disorders. He has had one injury while engaging in sports that culminated in a cast to right leg.

HISTORY OF DRUG OR ALCOHOL ABUSE: Patient denies use of drugs or alcohol.

FAMILY HISTORY: Patient reports that his father had difficulties as a child and adolescent with academics related to lack of focus and keeping up with his studies; however, he was never evaluated, diagnosed, or treated. Several cousins of patient on father's side have some academic issues although details are unknown. Maternal family history of anxiety disorders.

PERSONAL HISTORY

Perinatal: The patient was born full term. No birth complications or developmental delays reported.

Childhood: Academic performance was satisfactory but did require parental supervision to get work done. Had friends in school and neighborhood, and was active in some recreational sports.

Adolescence: Continued with close group of friends and select recreational sports.

Adulthood: Patient has a long distance relationship with a girl his age. He reports not seeing friends or engaging in college social life. Spends his free time on computer or playing video games.

TRAUMA/ABUSE HISTORY: Trauma and abuse are denied by the patient.

MENTAL STATUS EXAMINATION

Appearance: The patient is well groomed and clothed appropriately for climate. His posture demonstrates a level of comfort and openness to discussion. He is polite and pleasant in attitude toward examiner.

Behavior and psychomotor activity: The patient demonstrates appropriate eye contact, no hyperactivity, or abnormal motor or verbal activity.

Consciousness:	Patient is alert.
Orientation:	Patient is oriented to person, place, and time.
Memory:	Through examination patient exhibits no deficits in recent, remote, or immediate retention memory.
Concentration and attention:	The patient has no deficits in concentration and attention during the examination. However, while completing self-assessment questionnaires on anxiety and ADHD checklist, the patient worked slowly to complete as he thought through each item and asked for points of clarification while he considered each answer. Patient stated he felt unsure how to generalize his responses and that he was overanalyzing the items.
Visuospatial ability:	The patient demonstrated no deficits in visuospatial ability.
Abstract thought:	Patient was able to provide good responses to abstractions.

Intellectual functioning:	Patient speaks in an articulate manner with excellent vocabulary and above average fund of knowledge.
Speech and language:	Patient has normal rate and rhythm of speech. He is thoughtful in his responses.
Perceptions:	The patient denies perceptual abnormalities.
Thought processes:	The patient does not demonstrate abnormal thought processes.
Thought content:	The patient reports experiencing anxious thoughts in social situations where he states he hesitates to speak up because of feelings of low self-esteem and lack of confidence. He repeatedly rethinks what he should say and how he should behave when planning to attend a social situation, such as a party. Patient does not identify any particular obsessive thoughts that might indicate a clear diagnosis of obsessive-compulsive disorder (OCD).
Suicidality or homicidality:	The patient denies suicidal or homicidal thoughts or tendencies.
Mood:	Mood is neutral with no history of significant mood alterations. However, of note is patient's report that he sometimes feels down about his awareness that he is not functioning to his highest potential.
Affect:	The patient demonstrates affect that is congruent with mood and content of discussion.
Impulse control:	No impulse control problems noted during the interview; however, patient reports poor impulse control related to playing video games when he needs to do chores or schoolwork.

Judgment: There appear to be no impairments in judgment regarding societal boundaries/expectations. Judgment is impaired related to time management.

Insight: Patient reports he has gained insight into his difficulties in functioning independently and socially in the past year while he was away at college and since returning home. Insight is above average.

Reliability: Patient appears to be a reliable historian.

FORMULATING THE DIAGNOSIS

Which diagnosis (or diagnoses) should be considered?

314.00 (F90.0) Attention-Deficit/Hyperactivity Disorder, Predominantly Inattentive Presentation

Diagnostic Criteria

A. A persistent pattern of inattention and/or hyperactivity–impulsivity that interferes with functioning or development, as characterized by (1) and/or (2):
   1. Inattention: Six (or more) of the following symptoms have persisted for at least 6 months to a degree that is inconsistent with developmental level and that negatively impacts directly on social and academic/occupational activities:
      - **Note:** The symptoms are not solely a manifestation of oppositional behavior, defiance, hostility, or failure to understand tasks or instructions. For older adolescents and adults (age 17 and older), at least five symptoms are required.
        a. Often fails to give close attention to detail or makes careless mistakes in schoolwork, at work, or during other activities (eg, overlooks or misses details, work is inaccurate).
        b. Often has difficulty sustaining attention in tasks or play activities (eg, has difficulty remaining focused during lectures, conversations, or lengthy reading).
        c. Often does not seem to listen when spoken to directly (eg, mind seems elsewhere, even in the absence of any obvious distraction).
        d. Often does not follow through on instructions and fails to finish schoolwork, chores, or duties in the workplace (eg, starts tasks but quickly loses focus and is easily sidetracked).

   e. Often has difficulty organizing tasks and activities (eg, difficulty managing sequential tasks; difficulty keeping materials and belongings in order; messy, disorganized work; has poor time management; fails to meet deadlines).
   f. Often avoids, dislikes, or is reluctant to engage in tasks that require sustained mental effort (eg, schoolwork or homework; for older adolescents and adults, preparing reports, completing forms, reviewing lengthy papers).
   g. Often loses things necessary for tasks or activities (eg, school materials, pencils, books, tools, wallets, keys, paperwork, eyeglasses, mobile phones).
   h. Is often easily distracted by extraneous stimuli (for older adolescents and adults, may include unrelated thoughts).
   i. Is often forgetful in daily activities (eg, doing chores, running errands; for older adolescents and adults, returning calls, paying bills, keeping appointments).
2. Hyperactivity and impulsivity: Six (or more) of the following symptoms have persisted for at least 6 months to a degree that is inconsistent with developmental level and that negatively impacts directly on social and academic/occupational activities:
   - **Note:** The symptoms are not solely a manifestation of oppositional behavior, defiance, hostility, or a failure to understand tasks or instructions. For older adolescents and adults (age 17 and older), at least five symptoms are required.
     a. Often fidgets with or taps hands or feet or squirms in seat.
     b. Often leaves seat in situations when remaining seated is expected (eg, leaves his or her place in the classroom, in the office or other workplace, or in other situations that require remaining in place).
     c. Often runs about or climbs in situations where it is inappropriate. (Note: In adolescents or adults, may be limited to feeling restless.)
     d. Often unable to play or engage in leisure activities quietly.
     e. Is often "on the go," acting as if "driven by a motor" (eg, is unable to be or uncomfortable being still for extended time, as in restaurants, meetings; may be experienced by others as being restless or difficult to keep up with).
     f. Often talks excessively.
     g. Often blurts out an answer before a question has been completed (eg, completes people's sentences; cannot wait for turn in conversation).
     h. Often has difficulty waiting his or her turn (eg, while waiting in line).
     i. Often interrupts or intrudes on others (eg, butts into conversations, games, or activities; may start using other people's things

without asking or receiving permission; for adolescents and adults, may intrude into or take over what others are doing).

B. Several inattentive or hyperactive-impulsive symptoms were present prior to age 12 years.
C. Several inattentive or hyperactive-impulsive symptoms are present in two or more settings (eg, at home, school, or work; with friends or relatives; in other activities).
D. There is clear evidence that the symptoms interfere with, or reduce the quality of, social, academic, or occupational functioning.
E. The symptoms do not occur exclusively during the course of schizophrenia or another psychotic disorder and are not better explained by another mental disorder (eg, mood disorder, anxiety disorder, dissociative disorder, personality disorder, substance intoxication or withdrawal).

Specify whether:

- 314.01 (F90.2) Combined presentation: Both Criterion A1 (inattention) and Criterion A2 (hyperactivity–impulsivity) are met for the past 6 months.
- 314.00 (F90.0) Predominantly inattentive presentation: Criterion A1 (inattention) is met but Criterion A2 (hyperactivity–impulsivity) is not met for the past 6 months.
- 314.01 (F90.1) Predominantly hyperactive/impulsive presentation: Criterion A2 (hyperactivity–impulsivity) is met and Criterion A1 (inattention) is not met for the past 6 months.

Specify if:

- In partial remission: When full criteria were previously met, fewer than the full criteria have been met for the past 6 months, and the symptoms still result in impairment in social, academic, or occupational functioning.

Specify current severity:

- Mild: Few, if any, symptoms in excess of those required to make the diagnosis are present, and symptoms result in no more than minor impairments in social or occupational functioning.
- Moderate: Symptoms or functional impairment between "mild" and "severe" is present.
- Severe: Many symptoms in excess of those required to make the diagnosis, or several symptoms that are particularly severe, are present, or the symptoms result in marked impairment in social or occupational functioning.

(Reprinted with permission from the *Diagnostic and Statistical Manual of Mental Disorders*. 5th ed. Arlington, VA: American Psychiatric Publishing; 2013.)

What is the rationale for the diagnosis?

This patient presented in childhood with ADHD including difficulties with attention, listening, adjusting to change, disruptive behaviors, and poor social skills (impulsive and attention-seeking behaviors) noted prior to kindergarten. As a college student, he chose not to initially continue with treatment and began to notice difficulties including problems staying focused, completing work or tasks, being easily distracted, and difficulty paying attention. His presentation was primarily inattentive, not hyperactive at this time.

These difficulties exacerbate anxiety by patient's report of avoiding or procrastinating behaviors as he is aware of how he is struggling to manage his symptoms. In turn, feelings of diminished confidence contributed to his social anxiety.

Which diagnosis (or diagnoses) should be considered?

300.23 (F40.10) Social Anxiety Disorder

Diagnostic Criteria

A. Marked fear or anxiety about one or more social situations in which the individual is exposed to possible scrutiny by others. Examples include social interactions (eg, having a conversation, meeting unfamiliar people), being observed (eg, eating or drinking), and performing in front of others (eg, giving a speech).

Note: In children, the anxiety must occur in peer settings and not just during interactions with adults.

B. The individual fears that he or she will act in a way or show anxiety symptoms that will be negatively evaluated (ie, will be humiliating or embarrassing; will lead to rejection or offend others).
C. The social situations almost always provoke fear or anxiety.
    - **Note:** In children, the fear or anxiety may be expressed by crying, tantrums, freezing, clinging, shrinking, or failing to speak in social situations.
D. The social situations are avoided or endured with intense fear or anxiety.
E. The fear or anxiety is out of proportion to the actual threat posed by the social situation and to the sociocultural context.
F. The fear, anxiety, or avoidance is persistent, typically lasting for 6 months or more.
G. The fear, anxiety, or avoidance causes clinically significant distress or impairment in social, occupational, or other important areas of functioning.
H. The fear, anxiety, or avoidance is not attributable to the physiologic effects of a substance (eg, a drug of abuse, a medication) or another medical condition.

I. The fear, anxiety, or avoidance is not better explained by the symptoms of another mental disorder, such as panic disorder, body dysmorphic disorder, or autism spectrum disorder.

J. If another medical condition (eg, Parkinson disease, obesity, disfigurement from burns or injury) is present, the fear, anxiety, or avoidance is clearly unrelated or is excessive.

Specify if:

- Performance only: The fear is restricted to speaking or performing in public.

(Reprinted with permission from the *Diagnostic and Statistical Manual of Mental Disorders*. 5th ed. Arlington, VA: American Psychiatric Publishing; 2013.)

What is the rationale for the diagnosis?

The patient meets the criteria for social anxiety disorder because he reports feeling anxious in social situations and when he needs to participate in class. He describes holding back socially in conversation because of lack of confidence and not being sure if what he wants to say is relevant. Patient reports avoiding social situations in which he needs to participate in small group discussions, meeting new people, attending parties, or being the center of attention. He reports moderate to severe anxiety in social situations such as when being observed, entering a room, expressing an opinion, returning items in a store, or talking to people in authority.

What test or tools should be considered to help identify the correct diagnosis?

The following tools were used for this patient although the reader is encouraged to evaluate tools that they consider relevant and valid for use within their practice setting and based on patient presentation:

Adult ADHD Self-Report Scale (ASRS-v1.1) Symptom Checklist (https://add.org/wp-content/uploads/2015/03/adhd-questionnaire-ASRS111.pdf)

The Liebowitz Social Anxiety Scale (LSAS) (https://psychology-tools.com/liebowitz-social-anxiety-scale/).

What differential diagnosis (or diagnoses) should be considered?

307.20 (F95.9) Unspecified Tic Disorder

314.01 (F90.2) ADHD combined type

300.3 (F42.2) OCD

The patient's symptoms do not currently meet the criteria for these diagnoses so they are being considered as differentials.

FORMULATING THE TREATMENT STRATEGY

What treatment would you prescribe and what is the rationale?

Psychopharmacology: Fluoxetine 10 mg PO daily with reassessment and dose titration as indicated.

The social anxiety will be treated first in this case with fluoxetine followed by reassessment of symptoms as studies show medications in the selective serotonin reuptake inhibitor category can be effective in the treatment of social anxiety disorder. Because anxiety can contribute to impaired concentration, will treat the anxiety disorder first.

Once patient is on fluoxetine for 4 to 8 weeks, will reassess to determine severity of ADHD symptoms. If ADHD symptoms are still present, will plan a trial of methylphenidate extended release (Concerta) 18 mg and titrate up to effectively treat symptoms. Then reassess to monitor any onset of motor or vocal tics or obsessive thinking based on prior history of side effects on psychostimulants.

Diagnostic Tests: Because all routine lab results have been negative, no additional testing is ordered. The patient denied any history of cardiac abnormalities with himself or a history of sudden death in his family, so no cardiac testing (electrocardiogram) was indicated.

Referrals: No referrals made as the psychiatric-mental health practitioner is conducting psychotherapy and medication management.

Type of Psychotherapy: Supportive psychotherapy and Cognitive Behavioral Therapy as both are indicated in the treatment of social anxiety disorder and attention-deficit disorder (ADD). A combination of medication and therapy is considered to be more effective than one without the other.

Psychoeducation: Educate patient about ADD/ADHD as a disorder of executive function and self-regulation, which affects time management and management of emotional reactions. Further information can be found at https://add.org/adhd-facts/

Recommend he join Attention Deficit Disorders Association (ADDA) (add.org), the support organization for adults with ADHD. One of ADDA's foci is college students, and they have frequent webinars.

What standard guidelines would you use to treat or assess this patient?

An example of a practice guideline for the treatment of patients with ADHD can be retrieved at http://www.aafp.org/afp/2012/0501/p890.html. Although this article suggests starting with treatment for the ADHD, individuals should be evaluated for the severity of symptoms with the most distressing symptoms targeted first with medication.

CLINICAL NOTE

- ADHD is a disorder of self-regulation which can lead to anxiety. One is likely to exacerbate the other if both disorders are present. Assessment should include careful exploration of patient history, behavior patterns, and functioning across all domains. Determining which disorder to target with medication first is based on a discussion between patient and provider while education is provided.

REFERENCES/RECOMMENDED READINGS

American Psychiatric Association. *Diagnostic and Statistical Manual of Mental Disorders.* 5th ed. Arlington, VA: American Psychiatric Publishing; 2013.

Brown TE. *Attention Deficit Disorder: the Unfocused Mind in Children and Adults*. New Haven, CT: Yale University Press; 2005.

Brown TE. *A New Understanding of ADHD in Children and Adults: Executive Function Impairments*. New York: Routledge; 2013.

Epstein JN, Loren REA. Changes in the definition of ADHD in DSM-5: subtle but important. *Neuropsychiatry*. 2013;3(5):455-458. http://doi.org/10.2217/npy.13.59

Posner J, Kass E, Hulvershorn L. Using stimulants to treat ADHD-related emotional lability. *Curr Psychiatry Rep*. 2014;16(10):478. http://doi.org/10.1007/s11920-014-0478-4

Shaw P, Stringaris A, Nigg J, Leibenluft E. Emotional dysregulation and attention-deficit/hyperactivity disorder. *Am J Psychiatry*. 2014;171(3):276-293. http://doi.org/10.1176/appi.ajp.2013.13070966

CASE 16

Depressed and Anxious

IDENTIFICATION: The patient is a 20-year-old, single, white, female college student referred by the college counselor for an outpatient psychiatric evaluation.

CHIEF COMPLAINT: "Depressed and anxious."

HISTORY OF CHIEF COMPLAINT: Felt depressed a few months ago but then started feeling better until 2 weeks ago. Now getting more depressed so she went to see a counselor. Has a low mood, low motivation, and suicidal thoughts.

PAST PSYCHIATRIC HISTORY: The student noticed depression 2 years ago. She could not identify any particular situations that contributed to it. She started cutting her forearms, but has not been cutting for the past year. She has always been preoccupied with her weight. The patient reports no psychiatric hospitalizations, suicidal attempts, or assaultive behavior. No history of treatment or medications other than seeing a counselor recently.

MEDICAL HISTORY: Two years ago, the patient developed menstrual irregularities and went to her gynecologist. Was diagnosed with hyperprolactinemia. Had severe headaches. Went to a neurologist and was diagnosed with microadenoma. Was started on cabergoline. Recently, her endocrinologist doubled her cabergoline dose because of her elevated prolactin.

HISTORY OF DRUG OR ALCOHOL ABUSE: Denies.

FAMILY HISTORY: Raised by an intact family with a younger sister with anxiety. No other psychiatric or medical conditions known regarding her family.

PERSONAL HISTORY

Perinatal: Full-term birth. No known complications.

Childhood: Able to socialize. No anxiety reported.

Adolescence: Very active in school activities. Honor roll student.

Adulthood: Freshman student in college. Has average grades. Works part time in a convenience store. Lives on campus.

TRAUMA/ABUSE HISTORY: Denies

MENTAL STATUS EXAMINATION

Appearance: Well groomed. Good eye contact.

Behavior and psychomotor activity: Cooperative. No abnormal movements.

Consciousness:	Alert.
Orientation:	Times three.
Memory:	Intact.
Concentration and attention:	Although she can concentrate generally, her motivation is low and she has no interest in reading or focusing on her academic work.
Visuospatial ability:	Not assessed.
Intellectual functioning:	Average or above.
Speech and language:	Clear and concise.
Perceptions:	No hallucinations, delusions.
Thought processes:	Linear, logical, no obsessions or compulsions.
Thought content:	See below.

Suicidality and homicidality: Intermittent thoughts about how she might kill herself, running into a tree, overdose, cutting her wrists. However, she tells herself she's not going to do anything.

Mood: Depressed and anxious.

Affect: Congruent to mood.

Impulse control: Good.

Judgment/insight/reliability: Good.

FORMULATING THE DIAGNOSIS

Which diagnosis should be considered?

293.83 (F06.32) Depressive Disorder due to Another Medical Condition (with Major Depressive-Like Episode)

Diagnostic Criteria

A. A prominent and persistent period of depressed mood or markedly diminished interest or pleasure in all, or almost all, activities that predominate in the clinical picture.
B. There is evidence from the history, physical examination, or laboratory findings that the disturbance is the direct pathophysiologic consequence of another medical condition.
C. The disturbance is not better explained by another mental disorder (eg, adjustment disorder, with depressed mood, in which the stressor is a serious medical condition).
D. The disturbance does not occur exclusively during the course of a delirium.
E. The disturbance causes clinically significant distress or impairment in social, occupational, or other important areas of functioning.

Coding note: The *ICD-9-CM* code for depressive disorder due to another medical condition is **293.83**, which is assigned regardless of the specifier. The *ICD-10-CM* code depends on the specifier (see below).

Specify if:

- **(F06.31) With depressive features:** Full criteria are not met for a major depressive episode.
- **(F06.32) With major depressive-like episode:** Full criteria are met (except Criterion C) for a major depressive episode.

- **(F06.34) With mixed features**: Symptoms of mania or hypomania are also present but do not predominate in the clinical picture.
- **Coding note:** Include the name of the other medical condition in the name of the mental disorder (eg, 293.83 [F06.31] depressive disorder due to hypothyroidism, with depressive features). The other medical condition should also be coded and listed separately immediately before the depressive disorder due to the medical condition (eg, 244.9 [E03.9] hypothyroidism; 293.83 [F06.31] depressive disorder due to hypothyroidism, with depressive features).

(Reprinted with permission from the *Diagnostic and Statistical Manual of Mental Disorders*. 5th ed. Arlington, VA: American Psychiatric Publishing; 2013.)

What is your rationale for the diagnosis?

The patient's symptoms meet the criteria for (A) with a persistent period of depressed mood and (B) evidence from her history that the depression correlates with the diagnosis of hyperprolactinemia, (C) the depression is not better explained by another mental disorder, (D) did not occur during the course of delirium, and (E) the depression causes significant impairment in her social functioning.

What tests or tools should be considered to help identify the correct diagnosis?

Drawing a timeline with the start of the depressive symptoms and the identification of the start of the hyperprolactinemia might show if there is a temporal association.

The Hamilton Depression Scale or the Beck Depression Inventory should be used to obtain a baseline severity of depression and administered later to evaluate treatment.

What differential diagnosis should be considered?

296.20 (F32.9) Major Depressive Disorder, Unspecified

The patient's symptoms meet all the criteria for a major depressive disorder. However, there is a strong possibility that her symptoms may be related to her hyperprolactinemia. Her symptoms began around the same time she was experiencing menstrual irregularities and was subsequently diagnosed with hyperprolactinemia. Her symptoms have waxed and waned and do not seem to be related to any situational stress or loss. Nonetheless, a diagnosis of major depressive disorder cannot be entirely ruled out.

FORMULATING THE TREATMENT STRATEGY

What treatment would you prescribe and what is the rationale?

Consultation with her endocrinologist is imperative to coordinate treatment.

The patient should be encouraged to follow up regularly with her endocrinologist.

Psychopharmacology: Bupropion extended release 150 mg QAM. Due to the severity of her symptoms and risk for suicide, antidepressant medication should be considered. Bupropion does not increase prolactin like tricyclic antidepressants and selective serotonin reuptake inhibitors do. However, bupropion may increase anxiety so the patient should be monitored for anxiety and an antianxiety medication such as clonazepam may be indicated.

Diagnostic Tests: Pertinent laboratory tests will be completed by the endocrinologist and communicated to the psychiatric practitioner.

Referrals: None indicated.

Psychotherapy: Individual psychotherapy is indicated to help the patient avoid any unnecessary stress as she is already in a stressed state. Relaxation techniques would be helpful.

Collaboration with the counselor to monitor for increased depression or suicidality is indicated.

Psychoeducation: Information regarding hyperprolactinemia and cabergoline should be reviewed along with risks and benefits of bupropion.

Advise that antidepressant use in patients under 25 may increase risk of suicidal thoughts and behavior.

What standard guidelines would you use to treat or assess this patient?

None indicated.

CLINICAL NOTE

- The patient should be assessed for any history of seizures or ongoing eating disorders as bupropion may lower the seizure threshold.
- This patient should be monitored closely for any increase in suicidal thoughts.
- Depression along with other mood changes has been identified as a result hyperprolactinemia in case studies.

REFERENCES/RECOMMENDED READINGS

American Psychiatric Association. *Diagnostic and Statistical Manual of Mental Disorders*. 5th ed. Arlington, VA: American Psychiatric Publishing; 2013.

Fava GA, Fava M, Kellner R, Serafini E, Mastrogiacomo I. Depression, hostility and anxiety in hyperprolactinemic amenorrhea. *Psychother Psychosom*. 1981;36(2):122-128.

Gomes J, Sousa A, Lima G. Hyperprolactinemia: effect on mood? *Eur Psychiatry*. 2015;30:714.

Liao WT, Bai YM. Major depressive disorder induced by prolactinoma—a case report. *Gen Hosp Psychiatry*. 2014;36(1):e121-125.e122.

CASE 17

Hates Everyone, Angry Everyday

IDENTIFICATION: The patient is a 21-year-old single, white, female enrolled in a community college. She is seen for the assessment in an outpatient mental health clinic.

CHIEF COMPLAINT: "Upset. Don't like myself."

HISTORY OF CHIEF COMPLAINT: The patient was treated a year ago by a psychiatrist for complaints of "anxiety, depression, obsessive–compulsive disorder, and attention deficit disorder." Her friend encouraged her to get help. She started skipping work. Had a decreased appetite. Was crying frequently. Felt angry all the time "for no reason." Had episodes of hyperactivity where she did not sleep much and felt "on the go." During these periods she was shopping impulsively and overspending. She had a history of panic attacks whereby she was short of breath, she felt nauseous, her heart was racing, and she felt dizzy. She also reported her thoughts as "jumping," and having difficulty staying focused. Had a history of passive suicidal thoughts thinking "What if I were dead?" Never had any specific plan or intention to hurt herself. She had been treated with aripiprazole and then ziprasidone but could not remember how she responded. Next she had been prescribed lurasidone 20 mg, which improved her mood partially.

Currently taking lurasidone 20 mg daily for depressed, anxious mood after being diagnosed with bipolar depression. Mood continues to be mildly agitated and depressed, but generally improved. Previous increase of lurasidone to 40 mg caused a complaint of "couldn't stand being in my own skin." The complaint probably represented a side effect (akathisia) because the uncomfortable sensation ceased when the lurasidone was decreased to 20 mg daily. She was angry at her previous psychiatric provider and therefore is seeing this nurse practitioner.

PAST PSYCHIATRIC HISTORY: No hospitalizations or suicidal or assaultive behavior.

MEDICAL HISTORY: Multiple food allergies. Reported being diagnosed with polycystic ovary syndrome. Current medications: birth control pill (does not know the name).

HISTORY OF DRUG OR ALCOHOL ABUSE: Denies.

FAMILY HISTORY: Was adopted as a baby. Does not have any knowledge of biologic parents. Has a positive relationship with her adoptive parents who are very supportive. No siblings.

PERSONAL HISTORY

Perinatal: Information not known because she was adopted as a baby.

Childhood: Attached to her adoptive parents. Normal childhood developmental achievements.

Adolescence: Graduated high school. Identifies as heterosexual.

Adulthood: In training to become an emergency medical technician. No current boyfriend. Works part-time in a pet store. Attends community college part-time.

TRAUMA/ABUSE HISTORY: Reports history of being raped when in high school.

MENTAL STATUS EXAMINATION

Appearance: Casual attire. No motor abnormalities.

Behavior and psychomotor activity: Cooperative. Good eye contact.

Consciousness:	Alert.
Orientation:	Times three.
Memory:	Grossly intact.
Concentration and attention:	Fair.
Visuospatial ability:	Not assessed.

Abstract thought:	Apparent.
Intellectual functioning:	Average.
Speech and language:	Clear, normal rate and volume.
Perception:	No hallucinations or delusions.
Thought processes:	Organized.
Thought content:	Appropriate to subject.
Suicidality and homicidality:	Denies.
Mood:	Depressed, irritable, angry.
Affect:	Congruent to mood.
Impulse control:	Good.
Judgment/Insight/Reliability:	May be misinterpreting comments from others, thereby affecting her judgment. Insight is fair. Reliability is questionable and therefore the information may not be accurate.

FORMULATING THE DIAGNOSIS

Which diagnosis should be considered?

296.80 (F31.9) Unspecified Bipolar and Related Disorder; with Mixed Features

Diagnostic Criteria

This category applies to presentations in which symptoms characteristic of a bipolar and related disorder that cause clinically significant distress or impairment in social, occupational, or other important areas of functioning predominate but do not meet the full criteria for any of the disorders in the bipolar and related disorders diagnostic class. The unspecified bipolar and related disorder category is used in situations in which the clinician chooses not to specify the reason that the criteria are not met for a specific bipolar and related disorder, and includes presentations in which there is insufficient information to make a more specific diagnosis (eg, in emergency room settings).

(Reprinted with permission from the *Diagnostic and Statistical Manual of Mental Disorders*. eth ed. Arlington, VA: American Psychiatric Publishing; 2013.)

What is your rationale for the diagnosis?

The patient presents with symptoms characteristic of a bipolar and related disorder. Her agitated and angry, depressed mood causes clinically significant distress, but does not meet the full criteria for a diagnosis of any specific bipolar and related disorder and there is not enough information to make a more specific diagnosis. Patient has a history of episodic mood changes. She has mixed features of depression and agitation therefore she does not meet the criteria for cyclothymia or other bipolar disorders.

What tests or tools should be considered to help identify the correct diagnosis?

Mood Disorder Questionnaire (MDQ), a brief self-report screening tool for bipolar disorder.

What differential diagnosis should be considered?

None indicated.

FORMULATING THE TREATMENT PLAN

What treatment would you prescribe and what is the rationale?

Psychopharmacology: Continue lurasidone 20 mg daily with food.

The patient experienced akathisia at 40 mg daily so the dose can't be increased without the potential for this side effect reoccurring. Lurasidone is indicated as an adjunct with lithium for the treatment of bipolar depression.

Start lithium carbonate ER 150 mg HS to help stabilize mood.

Recommended starting lamotrigine instead of lithium but the patient was too fearful to take it due to the potential for Stevens–Johnson syndrome.

Diagnostic Tests: Thyroid-stimulating hormone, free triiodothyronine and thyroxine, creatinine, blood urea nitrogen, electrolytes as baseline and every 4 to 6 months thereafter when treatment with lithium is indicated. A pregnancy test is indicated because she is of childbearing age.

Lithium level should be checked within 4 to 7 days after initiating treatment and with every increase thereafter routinely every 4 to 6 months thereafter. Therapeutic lithium level 0.5 to 1.5 mEq/L.

Advise the patient to obtain the blood sample to check lithium level 12 hours after the last dose.

Comprehensive metabolic panel, A1C, and complete blood count with differential and platelets should be obtained at least yearly for anyone taking an antipsychotic medication due to the risk for metabolic syndrome or other complications.

Abnormal Involuntary Movement Scale (AIMS) should be recorded at baseline and routinely at least every 6 months. Although second-generation antipsychotic drugs have been reported to have a lower incidence of movement disorders, they still do occur even with low doses.

Barnes Akathisia Rating Scale can be used to evaluate any future symptoms of akathisia (see Appendix).

Referrals: None indicated.

Type of Psychotherapy: Trauma-focused therapy after the patient's mood has been stabilized may indicated as she describes a history of rape as a teenager.

Psychoeducation: Advise the patient of the risks and benefits of lithium and about symptoms of lithium toxicity. Advise of the need to prevent dehydration. Advise of need to obtain lithium blood levels with every dose increase in the beginning of treatment and routinely thereafter at a minimum of every 4 to 6 months. Thyroid and renal function will also be monitored due to the potential for altered thyroid and renal function with the use of lithium.

What standard guidelines would you use to treat or assess this patient?

Practice Guidelines from the American Psychiatric Association for the Treatment of Patients with Bipolar Disorder can be retrieved from http://psychiatryonline.org/pb/assets/raw/sitewide/practice_guidelines/guidelines/bipolar.pdf

CLINICAL NOTE

- The clinician should use clinical judgment in assessing for lithium toxicity. Even within the therapeutic range of 0.5 to 1.5 mEq/L, elderly individuals may develop toxicity. Some patients may achieve therapeutic results on doses lower than the therapeutic range. In these cases, treat the patient and not the laboratory results, especially if symptoms are not extreme.
- There is much controversy about which formulation of lithium is least likely to cause damage to the kidney. Generally, patients are more likely to be medication adherent if dosing is once daily. Extended release formulations may cause less gastric distress than immediate release formulations.

REFERENCES/RECOMMENDED READINGS

American Psychiatric Association. *Diagnostic and Statistical Manual of Mental Disorders.* 5th ed. Arlington, VA: American Psychiatric Publishing; 2013.

Cipriani A, Hawton K, Stockton S, Geddes JR. Lithium in the prevention of suicide in mood disorders: Updated systematic review and meta-analysis. *The BMJ* 2013;346:1–13.

CASE 17 APPENDIX

Barnes Akathisia Rating Scale (BARS)[1]

NAME: ______________________________ DATE: ____________

Barnes Akathisia Rating Scale (BARS)

Instructions: Patient should be observed while they are seated, and then standing while engaged in neutral conversation (for a minimum of two minutes in each position). Symptoms observed in other situations, for example while engaged in activity on the ward, may also be rated. Subsequently, the subjective phenomena should be elicited by direct questioning.

Objective

0 Normal, occasional fidgety movements of the limbs

1 Presence of characteristic restless movements: shuffling or tramping movements of the legs/feet, or swinging of one leg while sitting, *and/or* rocking from foot to foot or "walking on the spot" when standing, but movements present for less than half the time observed

2 Observed phenomena, as described in (1) above, which are present for at least half the observation period

3 Patient is constantly engaged in characteristic restless movements, *and/or* has the inability to remain seated or standing without walking or pacing, during the time observed

---

[1]Reprinted with permission from Barnes TR. A rating scale for drug-induced akathisia. *Br J Psychiatry.* 1989;154:672-676.

Subjective

Awareness of restlessness

0 Absence of inner restlessness

1 Non-specific sense of inner restlessness

2 The patient is aware of an inability to keep the legs still, or a desire to move the legs, *and/or* complains of inner restlessness aggravated specifically by being required to stand still

3 Awareness of intense compulsion to move most of the time *and/or* reports strong desire to walk or pace most of the time

Distress related to restlessness

0 No distress

1 Mild

2 Moderate

3 Severe

Global Clinical Assessment of Akathisia

0 *Absent.* No evidence of awareness of restlessness. Observation of characteristic movements of akathisia in the absence of a subjective report of inner restlessness or compulsive desire to move the legs should be classified as pseudoakathisia

1 *Questionable.* Non-specific inner tension and fidgety movements

2 *Mild akathisia.* Awareness of restlessness in the legs *and/or* inner restlessness worse when required to stand still. Fidgety movements present, but characteristic restless movements of akathisia not necessarily observed. Condition causes little or no distress.

3 *Moderate akathisia.* Awareness of restlessness as described for mild akathisia above, combined with characteristic restless movements such as rocking from foot to foot when standing. Patient finds the condition distressing.

4 *Marked akathisia.* Subjective experience of restlessness includes a compulsive desire to walk or pace. However, the patient is able to remain seated for at least five minutes. The condition is obviously distressing.

5 *Severe akathisia.* The patient reports a strong compulsion to pace up and down most of the time. Unable to sit or lie down for more than a few minutes. Constant restlessness which is associated with intense distress and insomnia.

SCORING THE BARNES AKATHISIA RATING SCALE (BARS)

The Barnes Akathisia Rating Scale is scored as follows:

Objective Akathisia, Subjective Awareness of Restlessness, and Subjective Distress Related to Restlessness are rated on a 4-point scale from 0 to 3 and are summed yielding a total score ranging from 0 to 9.

The Global Clinical Assessment of Akathisia uses a 6-point scale ranging from 0 to 5.

CASE 18

Anxiety and Insomnia

IDENTIFICATION: The patient is a 22-year-old, single, white male seen in a private outpatient mental health office. Patient was referred by his mother.

CHIEF COMPLAINT: "I feel really anxious and angry and I have trouble breathing."

HISTORY OF CHIEF COMPLAINT: Besides feeling anxious, the patient also reports feeling depressed and angry. Has not been sleeping and does not have an appetite. He reports episodes of shaking, shortness of breath, nausea, and sweating which occur suddenly. The symptoms started a month ago after a breakup with his girlfriend. She said she did not want to see him anymore and then she started dating his best friend. He started thinking about her all the time and couldn't focus on his studies. He is worried he will fail his exams. He has been avoiding his friends because he does not want to be around people. He sought help at the urging of his family.

PAST PSYCHIATRIC HISTORY: None.

MEDICAL HISTORY: No acute or chronic medical conditions. Average height and weight. Poor appetite.

HISTORY OF DRUG OR ALCOHOL ABUSE: Denied.

FAMILY HISTORY: The patient was raised by his mother and father with his older brother. His father and older brother have a history of panic attacks. Father was very encouraging about the benefits of medication for his panic attacks.

PERSONAL HISTORY

Perinatal: Full-term vaginal birth. No complications.

Childhood: Normal developmental achievements.

Adolescence: Did well academically in high school. Played hockey.

Adulthood: Currently enrolled as a junior in college. Unemployed. No military or legal history.

MENTAL STATUS EXAMINATION

Appearance: Casual dress.

Behavior and psychomotor activity: Good eye contact. Initially tapping his foot rapidly.

Consciousness:	Alert.
Orientation:	Oriented to person, place, and time.
Memory:	Intact.
Concentration and attention:	Attentive during interview. Describes poor concentration with school work. Worried about failing an exam.
Visuospatial ability:	Not assessed.
Intellectual functioning:	Average or above.
Speech and language:	Normal rate and volume.
Perception:	No abnormalities evident.
Thought process:	Has been obsessing about his ex-girlfriend.
Thought content:	His thoughts center on his ex-girlfriend and these thoughts were confused and angry. He fears that he will fail his exams because he cannot concentrate enough to study.

Suicidality and homicidality: Denied.

Mood: Anxious, depressed.

Affect: Congruent to mood.

Impulse control: Good.

Judgment/Insight/Reliability: Good.

FORMULATING THE DIAGNOSIS

What diagnosis should be considered?

309.28 (F43.23) Adjustment Disorder with Mixed Anxiety and Depressed Mood and with Panic Attacks.

Diagnostic Criteria

A. The development of emotional or behavioral symptoms in response to an identifiable stressor(s) occurring within 3 months of the onset of the stressor(s).
B. These symptoms or behaviors are clinically significant, as evidenced by one or both of the following:
   1. Marked distress that is out of proportion to the severity or intensity of the stressor, taking into account the external context and the cultural factors that might influence symptom severity and presentation.
   2. Significant impairment in social, occupational, or other important areas of functioning.
C. The stress-related disturbance does not meet the criteria for another mental disorder and is not merely an exacerbation of a preexisting mental disorder.
D. The symptoms do not represent normal bereavement.
E. Once the stressor or its consequences have terminated, the symptoms do not persist for more than an additional 6 months.

Specify whether:

- **309.0 (F43.21) With depressed mood:** Low mood, tearfulness, or feelings of hopelessness are predominant.
- **309.24 (F43.22) With anxiety:** Nervousness, worry, jitteriness, or separation anxiety is predominant.
- **309.28 (F43.23) With mixed anxiety and depressed mood:** A combination of depression and anxiety is predominant.
- **309.3 (F43.24) With disturbance of conduct:** Disturbance of conduct is predominant.

- **309.4 (F43.25) With mixed disturbance of emotions and conduct:** Both emotional symptoms (eg, depression, anxiety) and a disturbance of conduct are predominant.
- **309.9 (F43.20) Unspecified:** For maladaptive reactions that are not classifiable as one of the specific subtypes of adjustment disorder.

Specify if:

- **Acute:** If the disturbance lasts less than 6 months.
- **Persistent (chronic):** If the disturbance lasts for 6 months or longer.

(Reprinted with permission from the *Diagnostic and Statistical Manual of Mental Disorders*. 5th ed. Arlington, VA: American Psychiatric Publication; 2013.)

What is the rationale for the diagnosis?

The patient's symptoms of anxiety and depression appear to be in response to a specific stressor (the breakup with his girlfriend) that occurred within the past 3 months. The symptoms are clinically significant as evidenced by an impairment in his studies and avoiding friends. The symptoms do not meet the criteria for any other mental disorder and are not an exacerbation of a preexisting mental disorder. Panic attacks can occur with any mental disorder and can be added as a specifier. The panic attacks are not due to another medical condition or substance/medication-induced anxiety disorder and do not meet the full criteria for panic disorder. With this patient the panic attacks are related to the breakup with his girlfriend and the subsequent adjustment disorder with depression and anxiety.

What test or tools should be considered to help identify the correct diagnosis?

The Beck Depression Inventory (BDI) could be used to identify the severity of his depressive symptoms.

What differential diagnosis should be considered?

296.20 (F32.9) Major Depressive Disorder, Unspecified

This diagnosis requires at least five specific symptoms and this patient only presents with four: a depressed mood, a markedly diminished interest or pleasure in activities, a significant decrease in appetite, and a diminished ability to think or concentrate. Although the patient's symptoms do not meet the full criteria initially, there is the possibility that his symptoms may increase and if so the diagnosis should be changed to major depressive disorder.

FORMULATING THE TREATMENT STRATEGY

What treatment would you prescribe and what is the rationale?

Psychopharmacology: Sertraline 25 mg daily.

Sertraline is FDA indicated for the treatment of major depressive disorder, obsessive–compulsive disorder, panic disorder, social anxiety disorder, and premenstrual dysphoric disorder. This patient has symptoms of depression, some obsessive thinking about his ex-girlfriend, anxiety, and panic so he is likely to respond to sertraline.

Diagnostic Tests: A baseline weight is essential because the patient's appetite has decreased significantly.

Referrals: If the clinician is not able to provide ongoing therapy, a referral should be made for psychodynamic psychotherapy.

Type of Psychotherapy: Supportive psychotherapy should be provided initially. Psychodynamic psychotherapy is recommended because the conscious and the unconscious meaning of the stress and the patient's vulnerability need to be understood. Vulnerability can be increased by several factors including loss of a parent during infancy or being reared in a dysfunctional environment. Due to greater childhood trauma, some children may have less mature defense mechanisms and may be more vulnerable to trauma as adults. Therefore, it is important to further explore the patient's history to identify factors that may contribute to increased vulnerability.

Psychoeducation: The patient should be advised about the delayed response to antidepressants, which may be 4 to 6 weeks. Additionally, he should be informed that gastrointestinal side effects are common and usually transient. The potential for sexual side effects should be reviewed with the patient.

The patient should be informed of the FDA Black Box Warning, which states that antidepressants can increase the risk of suicidal thoughts for anyone 24 years old and younger. This patient should be followed closely to evaluate for any potential risk.

What standard guidelines would you use to assess or threat this patient?

None indicated.

CLINICAL NOTE

- The dose of sertraline may need to be adjusted depending on the patient's symptom presentation. Clonazepam 0.5 to 1 mg Q 12 hours, which will have an immediate effect, can be additionally prescribed if panic symptoms persist. However, the potential for dependence must be taken into consideration.
- Because adjustment disorders are associated with an increased risk of suicide, the patient's mental status should be monitored closely until his mood improves. Emergency services should be available to the patient if suicidal thoughts develop. In addition, if the patient is agreeable, the family should be informed of the risks regarding his condition and the treatment plan.

REFERENCES/RECOMMENDED READINGS

American Psychiatric Association. *Diagnostic and Statistical Manual of Mental Disorders.* 5th ed. Arlington, VA: American Psychiatric Publishing; 2013.

Sadock BJ, Sadock VA. *Kaplan and Sadock's Synopsis of Psychiatry: Behavioral Sciences/Clinical Psychiatry*. New York, NY: Lippincott Williams & Wilkins; 2011.

Wheeler K. *Psychotherapy for the Advanced Practice Psychiatric Nurse: A How-to Guide for Evidence-Based Practice*. New York, NY: Springer Publishing Company.

CASE 19

Stressed and Biting Fingers More

IDENTIFICATION: The patient is a 24-year-old, single, white female.

CHIEF COMPLAINT: "I don't want people noticing my scarred fingers."

HISTORY OF CHIEF COMPLAINT: She has been biting her fingers since she was young. Is in the orchestra and doesn't want people noticing her fingers. Is overwhelmed with the amount of work in graduate school, which she started 2 months ago. She states, "I'm worried about getting the work done. So I've been biting my fingers more." Has developed scars on fingers and has become self-conscious about how it looks but cannot stop.

PAST PSYCHIATRIC HISTORY: No previous psychiatric treatment or medications. No history of suicide attempts or assaultive behavior.

MEDICAL HISTORY: Takes birth control pills. No operations. No medical conditions. Feels tired for the past month. Having difficulty getting to sleep and staying asleep.

HISTORY OF DRUG OR ALCOHOL ABUSE: Denied.

FAMILY HISTORY: Raised by both American-born parents with a younger sister. Father has history of anemia.

PERSONAL HISTORY

Perinatal: Full-term vaginal birth.

Childhood: Started biting her fingers. Started playing in school orchestra.

Adolescence: Had many friends. Participated in a number of school organizations.

Adulthood: Graduate student in music education for the past 2 months. Unemployed. Had worked in retail sales. Identifies as a Methodist. Has the same boyfriend for the past 2 years. No military service or legal history.

TRAUMA/ABUSE HISTORY: Denied.

MENTAL STATUS EXAMINATION

Appearance: Well groomed. Fingers are visibly scarred above the proximal interphalangeal joint.

Behavior and psychomotor activity: Good eye contact. No motor abnormalities. Cooperative.

Consciousness:	Alert but appears tired.
Orientation:	Oriented to all three spheres.
Memory:	Grossly intact.
Concentration and attention:	Reports difficult concentrating. Pacing at night and unable to focus on her school requirements. Was generally attentive and focused during the interview.
Visuospatial ability:	Not assessed.
Abstract thought:	Not assessed formally but seems satisfactory.
Intellectual functioning:	Average or above.
Speech and language:	Normal rate and volume.
Perceptions:	No altered perceptions.
Thought processes:	Organized and logical.
Thought content:	Preoccupied with academic demands.
Suicidality and homicidality:	Denied.

Mood:	Anxious.
Affect:	Full range. Mood congruent.
Impulse control:	Good other than not being able to control biting her fingers.
Judgment/Insight/Reliability:	Good.

FORMULATING THE DIAGNOSIS

What diagnosis should be considered?

309.24 (F43.22) Adjustment Disorder with Anxiety

Diagnostic Criteria

A. The development of emotional or behavioral symptoms in response to an identifiable stressor(s) occurring within 3 months of the onset of the stressor(s).
B. These symptoms or behaviors are clinically significant, as evidenced by one or both of the following:
   1. Marked distress that is out of proportion to the severity or intensity of the stressor, taking into account the external context and the cultural factors that might influence symptom severity and presentation.
   2. Significant impairment in social, occupational, or other important areas of functioning.
C. The stress-related disturbance does not meet the criteria for another mental disorder and is not merely an exacerbation of a preexisting mental disorder.
D. The symptoms do not represent normal bereavement.
E. Once the stressor or its consequences have terminated, the symptoms do not persist for more than an additional 6 months.

Specify whether:

- **309.0 (F43.21) With depressed mood:** Low mood, tearfulness, or feelings of hopelessness are predominant.
- **309.24 (F43.22) With anxiety:** Nervousness, worry, jitteriness, or separation anxiety is predominant.
- **309.28 (F43.23) With mixed anxiety and depressed mood:** A combination of depression and anxiety is predominant.
- **309.3 (F43.24) With disturbance of conduct:** Disturbance of conduct is predominant.

- **309.4 (F43.25) With mixed disturbance of emotions and conduct:** Both emotional symptoms (eg, depression, anxiety) and a disturbance of conduct are predominant.
- **309.9 (F43.20) Unspecified:** For maladaptive reactions that are not classifiable as one of the specific subtypes of adjustment disorder.

Specify if:

- **Acute:** If the disturbance lasts less than 6 months.
- **Persistent (chronic):** If the disturbance lasts for 6 months or longer.

(Reprinted with permission from the *Diagnostic and Statistical Manual of Mental Disorders*. 5th ed. Arlington, VA: American Psychiatric Publication; 2013.)

What is the rationale for the diagnosis?

The anxiety with subsequent increase in finger biting is a response to an identifiable stressor (demands of graduate school) occurring within 3 months of the onset of the stressor. She is experiencing marked distress (not able to sleep, pacing) and significant impairment in an important area of functioning (not able to focus on school work). These stress-related disturbances do not meet criteria for another mental disorder and are not an exacerbation of a preexisting mental disorder. Her symptoms include anxiety and worry, which meet the specification for Adjustment Disorder with Anxiety.

What tests or tools should be considered to help identify the correct diagnosis?

None indicated.

What diagnosis should be considered?

300.3 (F42.8) Other Specified Obsessive–Compulsive and Related Disorder: Body-Focused Repetitive Behavior Disorder

This category applies to presentations in which symptoms characteristic of an obsessive–compulsive and related disorder that cause clinically significant distress or impairment in social, occupational, or other important areas of functioning predominate but do not meet the full criteria for any of the disorders in the obsessive–compulsive and related disorders diagnostic class. The other specified obsessive–compulsive and related disorder category is used in situations in which the clinician chooses to communicate the specific reason that the presentation does not meet the criteria for any specific obsessive–compulsive and related disorder. This is done by recording “other specified obsessive–compulsive and related disorder” followed by the specific reason (eg, “body-focused repetitive behavior disorder”).

Examples of presentations that can be specified using the "other specified" designation include the following:

1. **Body dysmorphic-like disorder with actual flaws:** This is similar to body dysmorphic disorder except that the defects or flaws in physical appearance are clearly observable by others (ie, they are more noticeable than "slight"). In such cases, the preoccupation with these flaws is clearly excessive and causes significant impairment or distress.
2. **Body dysmorphic-like disorder without repetitive behaviors:** Presentations that meet body dysmorphic disorder except that the individual has not performed repetitive behaviors or mental acts in response to the appearance concerns.
3. **Body-focused repetitive behavior disorder:** This is characterized by recurrent body-focused repetitive behaviors (eg, nail biting, lip biting, cheek chewing) and repeated attempts to decrease or stop the behaviors. These symptoms cause clinically significant distress or impairment in social, occupational, or other important areas of functioning and are not better explained by trichotillomania (hair-pulling disorder), excoriation (skin-picking) disorder, stereotypic movement disorder, or nonsuicidal self-injury.

(Reprinted with permission from the *Diagnostic and Statistical Manual of Mental Disorders*. 5th ed. Arlington, VA: American Psychiatric Publication; 2013.)

What is the rationale for the diagnosis?

The patient's finger biting behavior does not meet the full criteria for obsessive–compulsive disorder (OCD). She does not have obsessions and does not meet both criteria for compulsive behaviors. Although she has repetitive behavior (finger biting), it is not in response to an obsession or rules. These criteria must be met for OCD to be diagnosed. Her symptoms do meet the criteria for other specified obsessive–compulsive and related disorder: body-focused repetitive behavior disorder. Her symptoms are characteristic of an OCD and cause clinically significant distress in social areas but do not meet the full criteria for any of the disorders in the obsessive–compulsive and related disorder category.

What differential diagnosis should be considered?

300.3 (F42.2) Obsessive–Compulsive Disorder

The criteria for OCD require obsessions (which the patient does not report) or compulsions defined by repetitive behavior to perform in response to an obsession or according to rules. The patient does not describe her finger biting in this manner. She describes it as a habit, which is causing stress and she wants to stop it. Therefore, the diagnosis of OCD would not be appropriate.

FORMULATING THE TREATMENT PLAN

What treatment would you prescribe and what is the rationale?

Psychopharmacology: Sertraline 25 mg daily and titrate as tolerated.

Consider cyproheptadine 4 mg, one to two tabs taken a half hour prior to sexual activity.

Consider *N-acetylcysteine* (NAC) 600 mg BID.

Although the patient is experiencing an adjustment disorder, which may be transient, a selective serotonin reuptake inhibitor (SSRI) such as sertraline may be helpful in reducing her anxiety. Sertraline has been FDA approved to treat social anxiety and panic disorder. It can reduce the obsessive–compulsive symptoms that the patient is exhibiting. Sertraline is known to cause more gastrointestinal (GI) side effects than other SSRIs. Therefore, starting at lower dose allows for the tolerance for GI symptoms to develop. Sexual side effects are also common with SSRIs. In order to maintain compliance, this issue should be discussed with the patient and options to maintain typical sexual functioning offered.

Cyproheptadine can block the sexual side effects caused by SSRIs and is usually well tolerated. The patient should be informed that the sexual side effects are generally transient.

NAC, a glutamatergic agent, was found to demonstrate statistically significant reductions in trichotillomania behavior. Pharmacologic modulation of the glutamate system may prove to be useful in the control of a range of compulsive behaviors. Although there are no studies that identify the utility of NAC in treating biting compulsions, there is potential for a positive outcome due to the similarity of the disorders.

Diagnostic Tests: Routine laboratory tests to rule out any medical comorbidities that could contribute to symptoms of anxiety or fatigue.

Yale-Brown Obsessive Compulsive Scale (Y-BOCS) to identify any other obsessive–compulsive symptoms. The patient did not report any obsessive–compulsive symptom other than finger biting.

Referrals: Referral for specialized behavioral therapy, such as habit reversal.

Type of Psychotherapy: Individual psychotherapy to improve coping skills would be indicated. Habit reversal therapy, in combination with SSRIs, has been found to be effective.

Psychoeducation: Education about the benefits of exercise, relaxation techniques (such as deep breathing), and mindfulness is indicated to help reduce anxiety.

The patient should be informed of the FDA Black Box Warning, which states that antidepressants can increase the risk of suicidal thoughts for anyone 24 years old and younger. This patient should be followed up closely to evaluate for any potential risk.

What standard guidelines would you use to assess or treat this patient?

Although the patient does not meet the full criteria for OCD, the National Guideline Clearinghouse Practice guideline for the treatment of patients with obsessive–compulsive disorder may be helpful and can be accessed at https://www.guideline.gov/content.aspx?id = 11078.

CLINICAL NOTES

- The dose of medication for treatment of OCD needs to be higher and takes longer than the treatment of depression. Although clomipramine has been studied the most for the treatment of OCD and was the first to receive FDA approval, it is not generally tolerated as well as sertraline at higher doses. Other FDA-approved drugs for OCD include fluoxetine, fluvoxamine, and paroxetine.
- Typically, college students may not have substantial health insurance and may be limited in which medications they can afford. Older generic medications are generally more affordable. Sertraline is an older SSRI and is quite affordable. However, there are newer medications such as vilazodone that may have fewer sexual side effects and could be considered.

REFERENCES/RECOMMENDED READINGS

American Psychiatric Association. *Diagnostic and Statistical Manual of Mental Disorders.* 5th ed. Arlington, VA: American Psychiatric Publishing; 2013.

Ashton AK, Hamer R, Rosen RC. Serotonin reuptake inhibitor-induced sexual dysfunction and its treatment: a large-scale retrospective study of 596 psychiatric outpatients. *J Sex Marital Therapy.* 1997;23(3):165-175.

Craig AR. Self-administered behavior modification to reduce nail biting: incorporating simple technology to ensure treatment integrity. *Behavior Anal Pract.* 2010;3(2):38-41.

Grant JE, Odlaug BL, Kim, SW. N-Acetylcysteine, a glutamate modulator, in the treatment of trichotillomania: a double-blind, placebo-controlled study. *Arch Gen Psychiatry.* 2009;66(7):756-763.

Gupta S, Gargi PD. Habit reversal training for trichotillomania. *Int J Trichol.* 2012;4(1):39.

CASE 20

Stressed and Cutting

IDENTIFICATION: The patient is a 26-year-old, single, white female who lives with her boyfriend. She moved recently and needs a new psychiatric provider to prescribe her medications. She is scheduled to see a new dialectical behavioral therapist (DBT) in a few days.

CHIEF COMPLAINT: "Need a new psychiatrist."

HISTORY OF CHIEF COMPLAINT: The patient says she has been diagnosed with borderline personality disorder (BPD) and bipolar disorder. Has depression and anxiety, panic and anorexia. While out with her boyfriend in a restaurant, she became upset at a comment he made that she now thinks was not inflammatory but at the time she thought it was meant to be hostile toward her. She went to the restroom and used a fork to scratch herself until she broke her skin. Then when she went home, she went to the bathroom again and started cutting her arm with a knife. Shortly after, she told her boyfriend. The wounds have since closed and healed. Now, she thinks that there was really no reason for her to react the way she did, but at the time she interpreted his comments as a statement against her.

PAST PSYCHIATRIC HISTORY: The patient has had four psychiatric hospitalizations. The first hospitalization was when she was 13 years old after taking an overdose. The most recent hospitalization was 3 years ago. Denies any manic or psychotic symptoms. History of anorexia and cutting. Medication history includes sertraline, fluoxetine, trazodone (helped with sleeping), quetiapine, lorazepam, gabapentin, and citalopram. She is currently prescribed lamotrigine 200 mg daily and clonazepam 0.5 mg Q 12 hours.

MEDICAL HISTORY: No acute or chronic medical conditions.

Reports nightmares and night sweats. Problems with going to sleep and staying asleep. Takes over-the-counter diphenhydramine as needed for sleep. Appetite is reported to be fair. Weight is within low to normal limits.

Reports regular menses. Uses oral contraceptives for birth control; she does not know the name.

HISTORY OF DRUG OR ALCOHOL ABUSE: Only drank occasionally and has not drank at all for several years. Uses a nicotine vaporizer. Denies drinking caffeinated beverages.

FAMILY HISTORY: Raised by both her parents until they divorced when she was a teen and then lived with her mother and stepfather. Angry at her mother but adores her stepfather. Will talk to him on the phone but will not talk to her mother. Her father had a problem drinking when she was young. Has a good relationship with him now.

PERSONAL HISTORY

Perinatal: No known complications.

Childhood: No history of developmental delays or learning disorder. Never had any problem making friends. Has had nightmares off and on since a child. Always had difficulty falling asleep. Took an overdose when parents separated when she was 13 years old.

Adolescence: Graduated high school.

Adulthood: Went to college off and on and finally graduated in the past year. Has a job as a sales representative that she enjoys. Currently lives with her boyfriend and thinks they have a good relationship.

TRAUMA/ABUSE HISTORY: Patient made vague comments about emotional abuse by her parents, but was unable to describe any specific traumatic incident.

MENTAL STATUS EXAMINATION

Appearance: Petite, thin, dressed in attractive outfit. Appeared slightly anxious during the interview but did smile and laugh appropriately.

Behavior and psychomotor activity: No unusual movements.

Consciousness: Alert.

Orientation: Oriented times 3.

Memory: Good.

Concentration and attention: Not formally assessed but appeared within normal limits (WNL).

Visuospatial ability: Not assessed.

Abstract thought: WNL.

Intellectual functioning: Average or above.

Speech and language: Normal volume and rate and spontaneous.

Perceptions: No abnormalities elicited.

Thought processes: Circumstantial but logical and coherent. Says her "mind runs 24/7."

Thought content: WNL.

Suicidality or homicidality: No suicidal or homicidal ideas or urges but does report being very reactive to stress that triggers self-injurious behavior like cutting her arms.

Mood: Feel "steady" now.

Affect: Appears mildly anxious but otherwise neutral.

Impulse control: Good during the interview, but reports rapid impulse to cut when stressed.

Judgment: Good.

Insight: Good. Able to identify the nature of her disorder and seek appropriate treatment.

Reliability: Good.

FORMULATING THE DIAGNOSIS

Which diagnosis (or diagnoses) should be considered?

301.83 (F60.3) Borderline Personality Disorder

Diagnostic Criteria

A pervasive pattern of instability of interpersonal relationships, self-image, affects, and marked impulsivity, beginning by early adulthood and present in a variety of contexts, as indicated by five (or more) of the following:

1. Frantic efforts to avoid real or imagined abandonment. (Note: Do not include suicidal or self-mutilating behavior covered in Criterion 5.)

2. A pattern of unstable and intense interpersonal relationships characterized by alternating between extremes of idealization and devaluation.
3. Identity disturbance: markedly and persistently unstable self-image or sense of self.
4. Impulsivity in at least two areas that are potentially self-damaging (eg, spending, sex, substance abuse, reckless driving, binge eating). (Note: Do not include suicidal or self-mutilating behavior covered in Criterion 5.)
5. Recurrent suicidal behavior, gestures, threats, or self-mutilating behavior.
6. Affective instability due to a marked reactivity of mood (eg, intense episodic dysphoria, irritability, or anxiety usually lasting a few hours and only rarely more than a few days).
7. Chronic feelings of emptiness.
8. Inappropriate, intense anger or difficulty controlling anger (eg, frequent displays of temper, constant anger, recurrent physical fights).
9. Transient, stress-related paranoid ideation or severe dissociative symptoms.

(Reprinted with permission from the *Diagnostic and Statistical Manual of Mental Disorders*. 5th ed. Arlington, VA: American Psychiatric Publication; 2013.)

What is the rationale for the diagnosis?

The patient has a history of instability and impulsivity exhibited by her history of taking an overdose and cutting beginning as a teen and continuing to the present. She reports extreme mood reactivity resulting frequently in self-injurious behaviors (SIBs). She describes a long history of anger toward her mother and describes a positive relationship with the mother's husband, the patient's stepfather. She describes transient stress-related misinterpretations of events that border on paranoia. Therefore, this patient meets at least five of the criteria for the diagnosis of BPD.

What test or tools should be considered to help identify the correct diagnosis?

None indicated.

What differential diagnosis (or diagnoses) should be considered? Which diagnosis (or diagnoses) should be considered?

301.13 (F34.0) Cyclothymic Disorder or 296.89 (F31.81) Bipolar II Disorder

The patient reports that she has been diagnosed with Bipolar II disorder. However, she denies any hypomanic episodes. Although she does describe a history of anxiety, depression, and mood instability, it is not clear if she has a bipolar spectrum disorder. Additional medical records to evaluate her psychiatric history will need to be obtained in order to clarify the diagnosis.

FORMULATING THE TREATMENT STRATEGY

What treatment would you prescribe and what is the rationale?

Psychopharmacology: Continue lamotrigine 200 mg daily. The patient reports that other than intermittent episodes, her mood has been stable. She will be reminded of the importance of taking the medication regularly and not missing any doses. If she misses more than 3 days she should call as the titration may have to be resumed starting at 25 mg daily again to avoid the possibility of a Stevens–Johnson rash.

Additionally, she should inform her gynecologist that she is taking lamotrigine. Some literature recommends adjusting oral contraceptives while taking lamotrigine; however, other reports indicate that it is one of the few anticonvulsants that does not alter the concentration of the contraceptive.

Continue clonazepam 0.5 mg Q12 hours because the patient has been taking this medication prior to this evaluation and reports a stable mood. However, a gradual tapering with eventual discontinuation should be strongly considered as benzodiazepines are not recommended for individuals with BPD as they may have a disinhibiting effect.

Alpha-adrenergic blocker medications such as clonidine may be a better choice for treating anxiety in a patient with BPD.

Add naltrexone 50 mg QD. This opioid antagonist is used off-label for SIB. There is limited research to support its use other than case studies. However, because there are not any FDA-approved medications to reduce SIB, a trial of naltrexone is warranted.

Diagnostic Tests: Liver function tests needed for a baseline when prescribing naltrexone. Lamotrigine levels can be considered but are not required.

Referrals: Dialectical behavioral therapy (DBT).

Type of Psychotherapy: DBT.

Psychoeducation: Explain the rationale for the medication recommendations as stated earlier.

What standard guidelines would you use to treat or assess this patient?

Clinical practice guideline for the management of borderline personality disorder. In: *National Guideline Clearinghouse (NGC)*: Agency for Healthcare Research and Quality. Available at: https://www.guideline.gov/summaries/summary/48553.

CLINICAL NOTE

- While treating an individual with BPD maintain clear boundaries as the patient may be prone to misinterpret communication which may precipitate anxiety or transient paranoia.

REFERENCES/RECOMMENDED READINGS

American Psychiatric Association. *Diagnostic and Statistical Manual of Mental Disorders.* 5th ed. Arlington, VA: American Psychiatric Publishing; 2013.

Carl JS, Weaver SP, Tweed EM. Effect of antiepileptic drugs on oral contraceptives. *Clin Inquiries.* 2008;57(8).

Chapman AL. Dialectical behavior therapy: current indications and unique elements. *Psychiatry (Edgmont).* 2006;3(9):62-68.

https://www.ncbi.nlm.nih.gov/pmc/articles/PMC2963469/

Smith BD. Self-mutilation and pharmacotherapy. *Psychiatry (Edgmont).* 2005;2(10):28.

CASE 21

Migraines and Impaired

IDENTIFICATION: The patient is a 26-year-old, single female who works as a nurse in a hospital. She lives with her boyfriend who is unemployed. She was referred for an evaluation after she was reported to her licensing board on allegations that she was impaired at work.

CHIEF COMPLAINT: "I might lose my job. I got in trouble at work and was suspended from my job. I had a migraine and took my meds as prescribed. I had a confrontation with a patient's angry mother who reported me to my nurse manager and to one of the doctors … he [the doctor] said I was drunk."

HISTORY OF CHIEF COMPLAINT: The patient had been to a friend's birthday party the night before the incident and felt a migraine starting. She had forgotten to bring her headache medication and her friend gave her a pill that she said was "just like Fioricet (butalbital acetaminophen caffeine)." She took it. She admits it was poor judgment to do so and that the headache was probably triggered by alcohol and the tension of knowing she had to work the next morning. She went home, took her prescribed zolpidem, went to work the next morning, and within an hour had a migraine for which she then took her prescribed butalbital acetaminophen caffeine. She said she did not feel impaired at all. She was sent to the hospital human resource department by her nurse manager after she was reported and agreed to a toxicology screen that came up positive for opiates, barbiturates, and benzodiazepines.

PAST PSYCHIATRIC HISTORY: The patient has a long history of anxiety and difficulty sleeping. She reports that the anxiety causes her heart to pound and also leads to shortness of breath. She worries a lot normally, but she now is also worried about her financial situation because both she and her boyfriend are out of work. She describes herself as shy. She is inclined to be meticulous and perfectionistic to the point where it is difficult for her to start something unless she is certain it will be done perfectly. There is no history of psychiatric hospitalizations, suicidal attempts, or assaultive behavior.

MEDICAL HISTORY: The patient has a long history of chronic migraine headaches. The headaches are not accompanied by an aura, nausea, photosensitivity, or heightened sensory perceptions. Over the years, she has been prescribed a variety of medications including prophylactic beta blockers, triptans, antiseizure medications, barbiturates, and opiates to treat her chronic daily headaches. She is also prescribed benzodiazepine and a hypnotic by her medical providers for comorbid anxiety and disordered sleep and a stimulant for daytime drowsiness. She detailed her long-standing history of having migraine headaches "as far back as I can remember." Currently, these headaches occur on average 16 days a month and last for hours. She reports seasonal allergies noting that migraines are worse during allergy season, which used to be only during the spring, but now she is also affected in the fall, reporting rhinorrhea and nasal stuffiness. At times she wakes up with a headache and sometimes the headache awakens her. She states that her sleep is often disturbed by headaches and when she is not feeling well, she is not interested in eating.

Vital signs: BP 118/70, P = 90/min, R = 18/min
Height 5′4″, Weight 103 lb.
Current medications are as follows:

Topiramate extended release 100 mg daily
Armodafinil 250 mg daily
Alprazolam 1 mg QID PRN*
Alprazolam 1 mg TID PRN*
Zolpidem CR 12.5 mg HS
Zolmitriptan 5 mg PRN
Acetaminophen/oxycodone 10/350 mg BID PRN
Butalbital acetaminophen caffeine w codeine 50 mg/300 mg/40 mg/30 mg cap PRN, not to exceed six caps per 24 hour period.

*According to the State Prescription Drug Monitoring Program, the patient is prescribed alprazolam from both her primary care practitioner and her neurologist. The patient reported that the amount of alprazolam to relieve her anxiety symptoms was not enough so her primary care doctor wrote a prescription for alprazolam 1 mg QID PRN.

The patient thinks that the medication she takes for migraines and for anxiety may now be altering her moods. She is prescribed armodafinil for daytime drowsiness to counteract the side effects of topiramate. She takes alprazolam for anxiety. Over the week prior to our interview, she reported having taken "a Fioricet (butalbital acetaminophen caffeine) before bed and another one the next day and a Percocet (acetaminophen/oxycodone) once a day for 2 days."

She states she would like to wean off all the psychoactive medications because she does not "want it to look so bad with all these medications."

HISTORY OF DRUG OR ALCOHOL ABUSE: The patient's first alcoholic drink was at age 14 and she first got high on marijuana and alcohol when she was 15. When she was in high school and college, she used marijuana on a "fairly regular basis," and alcohol "maybe once a week." She claims that the most she ever drank was four drinks 3 days in a week. She claims that there was no pattern to it and her use never impacted her relationship with her boyfriend, other family members, neighbors, friends, or coworkers. She also denies any impact of alcohol or illegal drugs on her work performance, school performance, or finances and denies any current or past legal, work, or family problems related to substances.

She smokes cigarettes and would like to quit.

FAMILY HISTORY: The patient is of German-Irish decent. She describes her mother as "perfectionistic and uptight." She was a strict disciplinarian who died 3 years ago from a myocardial infarction. Her father was a "womanizer and would stay out drinking and carousing," and was very volatile when he was drunk or hung over. She describes her life at home as tense and a bit scary at times. Two uncles abused alcohol. Diabetes and cardiovascular disease afflicted aunts, uncles, and grandparents on both sides of the family. She is close with her younger sister who is also a nurse. No family history of psychiatric treatment or psychiatric hospitalizations.

PERSONAL HISTORY

Perinatal: The patient was born at term and bottle-fed.

Childhood: The patient describes herself as a somewhat timid and anxious child who worked hard and did well in elementary school.

Adolescence: The patient reports that she was an introvert and put a lot of effort into making friends. Her grades slipped in favor of her popularity but she maintained a B minus average. She was sexually active at 16.

Adulthood: The patient went to community college and achieved an associates degree in nursing. She was employed fulltime for 5 years in two hospitals. Patient is a nonpracticing Catholic, and had no history of legal issues.

TRAUMA/ABUSE HISTORY: Denied.

MENTAL STATUS EXAMINATION

Appearance: The patient arrived 40 minutes late dressed in casual, neat clothing that was appropriate to the weather and to the situation. She appeared to be her stated age. Her gait was normal.

Behavior: Mild psychomotor agitation: restlessness, fidgety. Interpersonally, she exhibited subdued mistrust, needing considerable support to build rapport.

Consciousness: Appeared tired and mentally sluggish. She explained that she was hot and headachy and that she had taken zolmitriptan 5 mg nasal spray on the way to the appointment and only had 5.5 hours of sleep the night before.

Orientation: Oriented to time, place, person, and situation. She was confused about the time for the appointment and the route to get there.

Memory: Patient's immediate memory was found to be impaired. After two prior rehearsals, she was only able to recall two out of five words in a five-word recall after 5 minutes. In number reversal, she could reverse three numbers but not five.

Patient's recent memory was impaired as she had trouble remembering if she ate breakfast that same morning, the highway she took to get to the appointment, and did not remember the time of the evaluation appointment.

Her remote memory was tested and found to be intact in that she was able to recall the last four presidents in order and she was able to recall the plots of her favorite childhood TV shows. She could name the days and months of the year albeit very slowly in reverse order with one mistake.

Concentration and attention: Story recall indicated mild impairment. The patient was unable to recall three details. Had difficulty doing serial 3s and was unable to do serial 7s.

Saint Louis University Mental Status (SLUMS) indicated moderate impairment.

Visuospatial ability: Was able to draw clock face, fine tremor noted.

Concentration and attention: Was able to spell "world" backward, but only able to do a 3-digit span.

Abstract thought: She had a concrete response to proverbs. "The grass is greener on the other side of the fence" question was answered "because ... uh maybe its watered more? I don't know."

Intellectual functioning: Appears to be of average intelligence, fund of knowledge was consistent with her education.

Speech and language: Speech was disorganized. Sometimes animated, but often slow, quiet, and impoverished.

Perceptions: There was no evidence of hallucinations, depersonalization, derealization, or formication.

Thought processes: The patient seemed to be able to comprehend all questions; however, her answers were often inconsistent, obtuse, and incomplete with most sentences truncated midstream to "... ya know what I mean?" with this examiner having to respond with, "No, I don't, can you tell me more about it?" Her communication was circumstantial. At times she answered questions that were not asked. For example, when asked about her anxiety, she gave a full account of her alprazolam without addressing the anxiety. And other times, it was nearly impossible to get her to give a clear answer to the question that was asked. For example, when asked how many headaches she gets a month, she gave an obtuse response about the medications she takes and how she takes them.

	Her responses to this examiner's questions were simplistic, concrete, and lacking in detail. Her thought process indicated some difficulty in conveying a line of reasoning. In recalling the plot of a recent movie, she said, "It was the usual boy meets girl and then. . .you know the rest."
Thought content:	Consisted of worries, with possible persecutory delusions that the physician who reported her was always yelling at her, and believed that he and other coworkers want to damage her reputation.
Suicidality or homicidality:	Denied.
Mood:	"Anxious."
Affect:	Exhibited range of emotions consistent with the content of the conversation. Seemed indifferent to her failure on test items such as serial 7s and 3s.
Impulse control:	No impulsiveness exhibited during the interview.
Judgment:	Poor, based on her explanation of what happened and the expected outcome. She claimed that she was "fine" and did not feel that she had been impaired at all. When asked, "Did you wonder what Dr. L. saw in you that made him think you were impaired at work?" she replied, "No, he sounds like he is yelling at me." Accepting an unknown drug at a party indicates some impairment of judgment.
Insight:	Poor insight. Expressed more concern about how it looks to list that she is on so many medications than concern about the impact these medications may be having on her cognitive functioning.
Reliability:	Questionable, given that the evaluation is required by her employer and she is not self-referred.

FORMULATING THE DIAGNOSIS

Which diagnosis (or diagnoses) should be considered?

292.81 (F19.921) Delirium, Unknown Substance, Without Use Disorder, Medication Induced (Unknown if Sedative, Hypnotic, or Anxiolytic and/or Opioid Medication)

Diagnostic Criteria

A. A disturbance in attention (ie, reduced ability to direct, focus, sustain, and shift attention) and awareness (reduced orientation to the environment).
B. The disturbance develops over a short period of time (usually hours to a few days), represents a change from baseline attention and awareness, and tends to fluctuate in severity during the course of a day.
C. An additional disturbance in cognition (eg, memory deficit, disorientation, language, visuospatial ability, or perception).
D. The disturbances in Criteria A and C are not better explained by another preexisting, established, or evolving neurocognitive disorder and do not occur in the context of a severely reduced level of arousal, such as coma.
E. There is evidence from the history, physical examination, or laboratory findings that the disturbance is a direct physiologic consequence of another medical condition, substance intoxication or withdrawal (ie, due to a drug of abuse or to a medication), or exposure to a toxin, or is due to multiple etiologies.

Specify whether:

- **Substance intoxication delirium:** This diagnosis should be made instead of substance intoxication when the symptoms in Criteria A and C predominate in the clinical picture and when they are sufficiently severe to warrant clinical attention.
  - **Coding note:** The *ICD-9-CM* and *ICD-10-CM* codes for the [specific substance] intoxication delirium are indicated in the table below. Note that the *ICD-10-CM* code depends on whether or not there is a comorbid substance use disorder present for the same class of substance. If a mild substance use disorder is comorbid with the substance intoxication delirium, the 4th position character is "1," and the clinician should record "mild [substance] use disorder" before the substance intoxication delirium (eg, "mild cocaine use disorder with cocaine intoxication delirium"). If a moderate or severe substance use disorder is comorbid with the substance intoxication delirium, the 4th position character is "2," and the clinician should record "moderate [substance] use disorder" or "severe [substance] use disorder," depending on the severity of the comorbid substance use disorder. If there is no comorbid substance use disorder (eg, after a one-time heavy use of the

substance), then the 4th position character is "9," and the clinician should record only the substance intoxication delirium.

(Reprinted with permission from the *Diagnostic and Statistical Manual of Mental Disorders*. 5th ed. Arlington, VA: American Psychiatric Publication; 2013.)

What is the rationale for the diagnosis?

The patient exhibits a disturbance in attention, memory deficits, disorientation, language, and perceptual disturbance that are not better accounted for by dementia. There is evidence from the history, physical examination, and laboratory findings that the disturbance is a direct physiologic consequence of an intoxication of a medication. It is not clear how long the disturbance has been developing; however, until recently the patient has been functioning without complications on her job, which typically requires a high degree of concentration and attention.

Which diagnosis (or diagnoses) should be considered?

G44.40 Medication Overuse Headache

(The *DSM-5* does not have a code for medication overuse headache. However, this disorder is identified in the *ICD-10*.)

Criteria

Headache present on >15 days/month.
Regular overuse for >3 months of one or more drugs that can be taken for acute and/or symptomatic treatment of headache.
Headache has developed or markedly worsened during medication overuse.
Headache resolves or reverts to its previous pattern within 2 months after discontinuation of overused medication.

(Reprinted with permission from the World Health Organization. *The ICD-10 Classification of Mental and Behavioural Disorders: Clinical Descriptions and Diagnostic Guidelines*. Geneva: World Health Organization; 1992.)

What is the rationale for the diagnosis?

The patient meets the criteria for this diagnosis because she has had headache present for over 15 days out of the month, describes an overuse of medication for symptomatic treatment of the headaches, and her headaches have become worse during this period.

What differential diagnosis (or diagnoses) should be considered?

304.10 (F13.20) Sedative, Hypnotic, or Anxiolytic Use Disorder, Moderate

The patient has not exhibited a problematic "pattern" (because she has no history of previous complications related to her sedative, hypnotic, or anxiolytic use leading to clinically significant impairment). She has only one known occurrence of problematic behavior occurring while at work. Therefore, this diagnosis would not be applicable without further supporting information.

However, her need for an increase in dose of anxiolytics (alprazolam) indicates tolerance, which is a prominent contributing factor in the development of sedative, hypnotic, anxiolytic use disorder. Therefore, she may be likely to meet criteria for this diagnosis depending on future pattern of use.

300.00 (F41.9) Unspecified Anxiety Disorder

The patient reports experiencing anxiety symptoms. However, there is not enough information to identify a specific anxiety disorder. Therefore, the diagnosis of Unspecified Anxiety Disorder is not currently appropriate.

What test or tools should be considered to help identify the correct diagnosis?

Saint Louis University Mental Status: This neurocognitive screening test is more sensitive than the MiniMental Status Exam and is therefore more apt to accurately identify possible delirium.

Substance Abuse Subtle Screening Inventory: A screening tool to identify individuals with substance use problems who are unwilling or unable to acknowledge substance misuse or symptoms associated with it.

The Drug Abuse Screening Test is a 10-item brief screening tool that can be administered by a clinician or self-administered.

Clinical Institute Withdrawal Assessment for Alcohol/Drugs is an eight-item scale for clinical quantification of the severity of withdrawal syndrome.

FORMULATING THE TREATMENT STRATEGY

What treatment would you prescribe and what is the rationale?

Refer to Inpatient Detoxification: Withdrawal protocol for benzodiazepines and opiates will be instituted by the inpatient provider. Medically assisted detoxification is only the first stage of treatment. Substance-related disorders are complex and have multiple causes and require individualized treatment.

This patient's history suggests a preexisting mental disorder, probably anxiety disorder.

Effective treatment should address all psychiatric comorbidities.

Psychopharmacology: Detox protocol while hospitalized usually involves a 5- to 7-day taper off benzodiazepines with either chlordiazepoxide or lorazepam. Opiate detox may include a gradual taper with an opiate or buprenorphine and medications to relieve the withdrawal symptoms such as clonidine.

Selective serotonin reuptake inhibitors should be considered for any ongoing anxiety symptoms because they are safer, not prone to misuse, and can be accompanied by cognitive-behavioral therapy (CBT) for long-term treatment of comorbid psychiatric diagnoses. Anxiety and insomnia either preexisted (co-occurring) or were caused by her prescribed medications (substance induced). Benzodiazepine for treatment of anxiety should be avoided with this patient due to the potential for dependence.

Diagnostic Tests: Routine lab tests as per hospital protocol.

Creatinine level is vital to obtain along with an estimated glomerular filtration rate (eGFR), as this may indicate impaired renal function. Impaired renal function would reduce the excretion of medications, which may predispose the patient to drug-induced delirium.

Referrals: The patient was advised to be evaluated and treated for possible co-occurring anxiety and/or other mental health issues following her medically assisted inpatient detoxification.

Type of Psychotherapy: SMART Recovery is based on Rational Emotive Therapy.

12-Step programs.

CBT to manage with cravings, to promote self-monitoring to recognize, avoid, and cope with the situations in which she is most likely to use drugs, improve coping and life skills, and deal with underlying anxiety disorder.

Family therapy addresses a range of influences on drug abuse patterns, designed to improve overall family functioning.

Motivational interviewing makes the most of people's readiness to change their behavior and enter treatment.

Motivational incentives (contingency management) uses positive reinforcement to encourage abstinence from drugs.

Psychoeducation: Educate about medication overuse headache.

What standard guidelines would you use to treat or assess this patient?

Collaborate with her other medical treatment providers to encourage the following practice parameters:

Evidence-Based Guidelines for Migraine Headache

The Centers for Disease Control and Prevention (CDC) Guideline for Prescribing Opioids for Chronic Pain

CLINICAL NOTE

- Diagnosis of medication overuse headache is important as it will help identify the appropriate treatment. A high percentage of patients with a history of headaches are likely to develop medication overuse headache. Some patients will only need to be educated about the consequences of overusing headache medication. However, individuals who are prone to addictive disorders may have more difficulty changing their pattern of use. The Severity of Dependence Scale (http://www.emcdda.europa.eu/attachements.cfm/att_7364_EN_english_sds.pdf) can provide an indication of those patients who may struggle more to manage their headache medication use.

REFERENCES/RECOMMENDED READINGS

American Psychiatric Association. *Diagnostic and Statistical Manual of Mental Disorders.* 5th ed. Arlington, VA: American Psychiatric Publishing; 2013.

Dowell D, Haegerich TM, Chou R. CDC guideline for prescribing opioids for chronic pain—United States, 2016. *JAMA.* 2016;315(15):1624-1645.

Goldstein RZ, Bechara A, Garavan H, Childress AR, Paulus MP, Volkow ND. The neurocircuitry of impaired insight in drug addiction. *Trends Cogn Sci.* 2009;13(9):372-380.

Loder E, Biondi D. Oral phenobarbital loading: a safe and effective method of withdrawing patients with headache from butalbital compounds. *Headache: J Head Face Pain.* 2003;43(8):904-909.

Pomeroy E. *Clinical Assessment Workbook: Balancing Strengths and Differential Diagnosis.* Boston, MA: Cengage Learning; 2014.

Prater CD, Zylstra RG, Miller KE. Successful pain management for the recovering addicted patient. *J Clin Psychiatry.* 2002;4(4):125.

Silberstein SD, Consortium US Headache. Practice parameter: evidence-based guidelines for migraine headache (an evidence-based review). Report of the Quality Standards Subcommittee of the American Academy of Neurology. *Neurology.* 2000;55(6):754-762.

World Health Organization. *The ICD-10 Classification of Mental and Behavioural Disorders: Clinical Descriptions and Diagnostic Guidelines.* Geneva: World Health Organization; 1992.

CASE 22

Night Terrors

IDENTIFICATION: The patient is a 27-year-old, single, Hispanic, male seen in an outpatient mental health office and is self-referred.

CHIEF COMPLAINT: "I think I have night terrors. I wake up 2–3 hours after going to sleep in utter panic. I've hurt myself on more than one occasion during an episode."

HISTORY OF CHIEF COMPLAINT: The patient had a history of eating in his sleep since he was a child. Described himself as always being anxious. The "night terrors" started approximately 5 to 6 years ago. He was working the night shift and his sleep was erratic. He would wake up but not feel completely awake and thought there were cockroaches all over the room. While he was away at graduate school he would wake up thinking someone was breaking into his apartment. He stated it felt real. Once he cut his arm when he hit a window. After returning home from college, these episodes subsided for a few months and then returned. He looked up his symptoms on the internet and thought they fit the diagnosis for night terrors.

PAST PSYCHIATRIC HISTORY: While in college, the patient went to the emergency room for complaints of chest pain. Was evaluated and then informed that what he was experiencing was anxiety. Two months ago his primary care provider prescribed alprazolam 0.5 mg at bedtime and it reduced the frequency and severity of the night terrors.

MEDICAL HISTORY: History of asthma treated with albuterol sulfate inhaler PRN. Obese. Denies any recent change in appetite.

For sleep history, see History of Chief Complaint.

HISTORY OF DRUG OR ALCOHOL ABUSE: Drinks 8 to 10 cups of coffee per day.

FAMILY HISTORY: Was adopted at birth. Became acquainted with biologic siblings but his biologic mother avoided any relationship with him. No specific medical or psychiatric history is known about his biologic mother or father, but he thinks his mother did have a psychiatric condition.

PERSONAL HISTORY

Prenatal: It is not known if his biologic mother used any alcohol or drugs during the prenatal period. Other details regarding his early history are not known either.

Childhood: No overt attachment issues but never had a close friend. He had a history of getting out of bed and eating in his sleep when he was a child. He also reported an insect phobia that started during his childhood.

Adolescence: He identifies as heterosexual. Never had a close friend, only acquaintances. Describes himself as having a low self-esteem. Compensated by focusing on his academics and excelled in that area.

Adulthood: Currently attending graduate school. Reports that his Catholic faith has helped him deal with issues related to his self-esteem.

TRAUMA/ABUSE HISTORY: No history of trauma or abuse.

MENTAL STATUS EXAMINATION

Appearance: Well groomed.

Behavior and psychomotor activity: Cooperative. No abnormal movements.

Consciousness:	Alert.
Orientation:	Times three.
Memory:	Grossly intact. Not formally assessed.
Concentration and attention:	Concentration and attention seem satisfactory during the interview.
Visuospatial ability:	Not formally assessed.

Abstract thought:	Not assessed but seems adequate.
Intellectual functioning:	Average or above.
Speech and language:	Fluent. Normal rate and volume.
Perceptions:	No abnormal perceptions elicited.
Thought processes:	No formal thought disorder identified.
Thought content:	Concerned about hurting himself when sleeping. No other psychosocial stressors identified.
Suicidality or homicidality:	None.
Mood:	Anxious.
Affect:	Full range. Mood congruent.
Impulse control:	No impulsivity noted during the interview or reported by the patient.
Judgment/insight/reliability:	Good/good/good.

FORMULATING THE DIAGNOSIS

What diagnosis should be considered?

307.46 (F51.4) Non-Rapid Eye Movement Sleep Arousal Disorders: Sleep Terror Type

Diagnostic Criteria

A. Recurrent episodes of incomplete awakening from sleep, usually occurring during the first third of the major sleep episode, accompanied by either one of the following:
   1. **Sleepwalking:** Repeated episodes of rising from bed during sleep and walking about. While sleepwalking, the individual has a blank, staring face; is relatively unresponsive to the efforts of others to communicate with him or her; and can be awakened only with great difficulty.
   2. **Sleep terrors:** Recurrent episodes of abrupt terror arousals from sleep, usually beginning with a panicky scream. There is intense fear and signs of autonomic arousal, such as mydriasis, tachycardia, rapid breathing, and sweating, during each episode. There is relative unresponsiveness to efforts of others to comfort the individual during the episodes.

B. No or little (eg, only a single visual scene) dream imagery is recalled.
C. Amnesia for the episodes is present.
D. The episodes cause clinically significant distress or impairment in social, occupational, or other important areas of functioning.
E. The disturbance is not attributable to the physiologic effects of a substance (eg, a drug of abuse, a medication).
F. Coexisting mental and medical disorders do not explain the episodes of sleepwalking or sleep terrors.

Coding note: For *ICD-9-CM*, code 307.46 for all subtypes. For *ICD-10-CM*, code is based on subtype.

Specify whether:

- **307.46 (F51.3) Sleepwalking type**

Specify if:

- **With sleep-related eating**
- **With sleep-related sexual behavior (sexsomnia)**
- **307.46 (F51.4) Sleep terror type**

(Reprinted with permission from the *Diagnostic and Statistical Manual of Mental Disorders*. 5th ed. Arlington, VA: American Psychiatric Publication; 2013.)

What is your rationale for the diagnosis?

The patient reports recurrent episodes of incomplete awakening from sleep ("would wake up and not be completely awake") which are occurring during the first 2 to 3 hours after falling asleep. He experiences intense fear. He describes some memory of the event ("thought there were cockroaches," "thought someone was breaking into the apartment"). Although he is able to describe the event, his recollection may not be complete. It is not known, unless collateral information can be obtained, if he has amnesia of the event. The episodes have caused significant distress because he has sought treatment for the disorder. Additionally, he sustained physical injury when he hit a window and cut his arm on one occasion. Although he describes periods of increased anxiety in his past, there is no clear causal relationship. A diagnosis of panic disorder is not indicated. Therefore, he meets the diagnostic criteria for non-rapid eye movement sleep arousal disorder: with sleep terror type.

What test or tools should be considered to help identify the correct diagnosis?

Collateral history from family members can provide more information to help identify the correct diagnosis.

Polysomnography can help provide more detailed information about the sleep pattern.

What differential diagnosis should be considered?

307.46 (F51.3) Non-Rapid Eye Movement Sleep Arousal Disorders: Sleepwalking type: with Sleep-Related Eating.

The patient's self-report of eating in his sleep since a child may indicate non-rapid eye movement sleep arousal disorder: sleepwalking type, with sleep-related eating. However, there is not enough specific information to make the diagnosis.

327.42 (G47.52) Rapid Eye Movement Sleep Behavior Disorder

This disorder may be difficult to distinguish from non-rapid eye movement (non-REM) sleep arousal disorder. Although the patient experiences repeated episodes of arousal during sleep, the episodes seem to occur in the first third of the sleep cycle, which is more indicative of non-REM sleep. Also the patient does not wake up from the episodes. These factors would preclude REM Sleep Behavior Disorder from being diagnosed.

It is unclear if the patient is having hallucinations upon waking. These hallucinations are known as hypnopompic hallucinations.

FORMULATING THE TREATMENT STRATEGY

What treatment would you prescribe and the rationale?

Psychopharmacology: Clonazepam 0.5 mg HS. Benzodiazepines have been shown to reduce symptoms of parasomnias.

Diagnostic Tests: Routine laboratory tests.

Referrals: A referral for a sleep study is indicated. Although a sleep study is not required for the diagnosis, other sleep disorders such as obstructive sleep apnea, periodic limb movement disorder, or restless leg syndrome may increase the frequency of parasomnias and should be identified and treated.

Type of Psychotherapy: Individual psychotherapy is recommended to address the patient's low self-esteem and anxiety. Emotional stress can increase the frequency of sleep parasomnias.

Psychoeducation: Sleep hygiene techniques should be reviewed and the patient should be instructed to avoid sleep deprivation. Reduction of caffeine intake is recommended to improve sleep.

What standard guidelines would you use to assess or treat the patient?

Practice Parameters for the Indications for Polysomnography and Related Procedures: An Update for 2005 can be accessed at http://www.aasmnet.org/Resources/PracticeParameters/PP_Polysomnography.pdf

CLINICAL NOTE

- New onset of adult parasomnias may indicate neurologic conditions and require a neurologic consultation.

REFERENCES/RECOMMENDED READINGS

American Psychiatric Association. *Diagnostic and Statistical Manual of Mental Disorders*. 5th ed. Arlington, VA: American Psychiatric Publishing; 2013.

Markov D, Jaffe F, Doghramji K. Update on parasomnias: a review for psychiatric practice. *Psychiatry (Edgmont)*. 2006;3(7):69.

Schenck CH, Mahowald MW. Long-term, nightly benzodiazepine treatment of injurious parasomnias and other disorders of disrupted nocturnal sleep in 170 adults. *Am J Med*. 1996;100(3):333-337.

CASE 23

Still Has Auditory Hallucinations with Olanzapine

IDENTIFICATION: The patient is a 27-year-old Filipina single woman accompanied by an aunt and uncle with whom she lives.

CHIEF COMPLAINT: "I have schizophrenia and I need my medications ordered."

HISTORY OF CHIEF COMPLAINT: The psychiatrist who has been treating the patient does not take her insurance any longer so she needs a new provider. She has been taking olanzapine 15 mg daily.

PAST PSYCHIATRIC HISTORY: The patient started hearing voices as a freshman in college. Initially, the voices were just chattering but then started saying they were going to hurt her. She said, "I thought people were stalking me." She was treated by a psychiatrist with olanzapine that helped. She thought she was fine and stopped the olanzapine. She relapsed and was hospitalized and was prescribed risperidone before being discharged, but she could not sleep. She was prescribed a variety of antipsychotic medication (ziprasidone, aripiprazole, quetiapine). They did not control the paranoid thinking and the voices were loud and threatening. Eventually, she was prescribed olanzapine again, which she described as the most effective. She has been taking the olanzapine consistently.

MEDICAL HISTORY: No acute or chronic medical conditions reported.

Appetite: Good.

Sleep: 7 to 8 hours at night.

Menstrual pattern: Has regular menses. Not sexually active.

Height: 5′0″.

Weight: 114 lb.

HISTORY OF DRUG OR ALCOHOL ABUSE: Denied.

FAMILY HISTORY: Lived with her mother until 5 years old when her mother died in a motor vehicle accident. Then she lived with her aunt and uncle. The patient considers her cousins to be her siblings. Her aunt and uncle are very supportive. The patient worries about her aunt because she has diabetes.

PERSONAL HISTORY: No known alcohol or drug use by her mother during the pregnancy. Normal vaginal birth. No disabilities or social impairment in childhood. Was gifted academically in high school. Identifies as gay but says she was never sexually active. Started having trouble concentrating and being motivated when she went to college. Reported memory and decision-making deficits. Lost a lot of her friends in college. She thought they were stalking her and she was sending them bizarre and excessive text messages.

TRAUMA/ABUSE HISTORY: Denies.

MENTAL STATUS EXAMINATION

Appearance: Casual attire. Appears younger than stated age. Is very thin and petite.

Behavior and psychomotor activity: Cooperative. Good eye contact. No abnormal movements.

Consciousness: Alert.

Orientation: Times 3.

Memory: Tended to have difficulty providing a clear history. Could not accurately identify the dates she attended college. Could not remember details of her medication history or menstrual history.

Concentration and attention: Generally attentive. Will formally assess attention and concentration on next visit as she seems very anxious and uncomfortable

	and is particularly worried about her medication being reordered. She reports that her concentration is decreased by ongoing auditory hallucinations that are distracting.
Visuospatial ability:	Not assessed.
Abstract thought:	Not assessed.
Intellectual functioning:	Average or above.
Speech and language:	Of normal rate and tone.
Perceptions:	She reports that she still hears voices most of the time but she knows not to trust them and tries to ignore them. She thinks they interfere with her ability to concentrate and attend college.
Thought processes:	Clear and logical.
Thought content:	No unusual content identified.
Suicidality or homicidality:	None.
Mood:	Good.
Affect:	Full range and appropriate to content of speech.
Impulse control:	Good.
Judgment/insight/reliability:	Good/good/good.

FORMULATING THE DIAGNOSIS

What diagnosis should be considered?

295.90 (F20.9) Schizophrenia; Multiple Episodes, Currently in Partial Remission

Diagnostic Criteria

A. Two (or more) of the following, each present for a significant portion of time during a 1-month period (or less if successfully treated). At least one of these must be (1), (2), or (3):
   1. Delusions.
   2. Hallucinations.

3. Disorganized speech (eg, frequent derailment or incoherence).
4. Grossly disorganized or catatonic behavior.
5. Negative symptoms (ie, diminished emotional expression or avolition).

B. For a significant portion of the time since the onset of the disturbance, level of functioning in one or more major areas, such as work, interpersonal relations, or self-care, is markedly below the level achieved prior to the onset (or when the onset is in childhood or adolescence, there is failure to achieve expected level of interpersonal, academic, or occupational functioning).

C. Continuous signs of the disturbance persist for at least 6 months. This 6-month period must include at least 1 month of symptoms (or less if successfully treated) that meet Criterion A (ie, active-phase symptoms) and may include periods of prodromal or residual symptoms. During these prodromal or residual periods, the signs of the disturbance may be manifested by only negative symptoms or by two or more symptoms listed in Criterion A present in an attenuated form (eg, odd beliefs, unusual perceptual experiences).

D. Schizoaffective disorder and depressive or bipolar disorder with psychotic features have been ruled out because either (1) no major depressive or manic episodes have occurred concurrently with the active-phase symptoms, or (2) if mood episodes have occurred during active-phase symptoms, they have been present for a minority of the total duration of the active and residual periods of the illness.

E. The disturbance is not attributable to the physiologic effects of a substance (eg, a drug of abuse, a medication) or another medical condition.

F. If there is a history of autism spectrum disorder or a communication disorder of childhood onset, the additional diagnosis of schizophrenia is made only if prominent delusions or hallucinations, in addition to the other required symptoms of schizophrenia, are also present for at least 1 month (or less if successfully treated).

Specify if:
The following course specifiers are only to be used after a 1-year duration of the disorder and if they are not in contradiction to the diagnostic course criteria.

- **First episode, currently in acute episode:** First manifestation of the disorder meeting the defining diagnostic symptom and time criteria. An *acute episode* is a time period in which the symptom criteria are fulfilled.
- **First episode, currently in partial remission:** *Partial remission* is a period of time during which an improvement after a previous episode is maintained and in which the defining criteria of the disorder are only partially fulfilled.

- **First episode, currently in full remission:** *Full remission* is a period of time after a previous episode during which no disorder-specific symptoms are present.
- **Multiple episodes, currently in acute episode:** Multiple episodes may be determined after a minimum of two episodes (ie, after a first episode, a remission, and a minimum of one relapse).
- **Multiple episodes, currently in partial remission**
- **Multiple episodes, currently in full remission**
- **Continuous:** Symptoms fulfilling the diagnostic symptom criteria of the disorder are remaining for the majority of the illness course, with subthreshold symptom periods being very brief relative to the overall course.
- **Unspecified**

Specify if:

- **With catatonia** (refer to the criteria for catatonia associated with another mental disorder, for definition).

Coding note: Use additional code 293.89 (F06.1) catatonia associated with schizophrenia to indicate the presence of the comorbid catatonia.

Specify current severity:

- Severity is rated by a quantitative assessment of the primary symptoms of psychosis, including delusions, hallucinations, disorganized speech, abnormal psychomotor behavior, and negative symptoms. Each of these symptoms may be rated for its current severity (most severe in the last 7 days) on a 5-point scale ranging from 0 (not present) to 4 (present and severe). **Note:** Diagnosis of schizophrenia can be made without using this severity specifier.

(Reprinted with permission from the *Diagnostic and Statistical Manual of Mental Disorders*. 5th ed. Arlington, VA: American Psychiatric Publication; 2013.)

What is your rationale for the diagnosis?

The patient reports a history of paranoid delusions and auditory hallucinations lasting for more than a 1-month period. She also has been experiencing avolition. Her level of functioning at school was significantly impaired. She continues to experience residual symptoms (auditory hallucinations, impairment of executive functioning) even with treatment with an antipsychotic. There is no indication of schizoaffective disorder and depressive or bipolar disorder with psychotic features. The disturbances are not attributable to substance use, medication, or another medical condition. There is no history of symptoms of autism spectrum disorder or a communication disorder. The patient has had repeated episodes and her symptoms are only partially remitted with antipsychotic medication. Therefore, the diagnosis of schizophrenia; multiple episodes, currently in partial remission is indicated.

What test or tools should be considered to help identify the correct diagnosis?

Previous psychiatric records should be obtained to confirm the symptoms and course of the illness.

What differential diagnosis should be considered?

None indicated.

FORMULATING THE TREATMENT PLAN

What treatment would you prescribe and what is the rationale?

Psychopharmacology: Olanzapine 15 mg daily was reordered. An increase in the olanzapine was recommended. The patient was fearful of developing diabetes because there is a family history of diabetes and refused an increase. The patient was informed that she would be monitored closely for any metabolic side effects and should reconsider an increase in the olanzapine.

Because the patient did not respond adequately to trials of multiple antipsychotic medications, clozapine should be considered. Clozapine is the gold standard for treatment-refractory patients and is recommended after adequate trials of other antipsychotic medications.

Once the positive symptoms are treated adequately, treatment of the patient's negative symptoms should be addressed. Treatment with antidepressants may be helpful.

Diagnostic Tests: Besides routine tests, an A1C test should be ordered to monitor glucose metabolism and screen for metabolic syndrome.

Abnormal Involuntary Movement Scale (AIMS) should be completed at a minimum of every 6 months to screen for antipsychotic-induced movement disorders, which can be accessed at http://www.cqaimh.org/pdf/tool_aims.pdf.

Referrals: Advise the patient and her family to connect with the National Alliance on Mental Illness, which can be located online at https://www.nami.org/Find-Your-Local-NAMI

Type of Psychotherapy: Supportive psychotherapy for the patient and her family is recommended to assist in identifying challenges and goals associated with having a severely and persistently mentally ill family member.

Psychoeducation: Literature about schizophrenia from the National Institute of Mental Health for the patient and her family can be obtained online at https://www.nimh.nih.gov/health/publications/schizophrenia-booklet-12-2015/index.shtml

What standard guidelines would you use to assess or treat the patient?

National Guideline Clearinghouse (NGC). Guideline summary: psychosis and schizophrenia in adults: treatment and management. Agency for Healthcare Research and Quality (AHRQ); 2014. Available at: https://www.guideline.gov/summaries/summary/47863/psychosis-and-schizophrenia-in-adults-treatment-and-management?q = schizophrenia

CLINICAL NOTE

- Although most guidelines recommend completing an AIMS every 6 to 12 months, patients can be assessed for movement abnormalities upon observation when they are sitting in the waiting area, walking into the office, and being interviewed.
- Written consent to communicate with the patient's aunt and uncle should be obtained. They should be advised to report any concerns or observations of unusual behavior so that the patient can be seen and her treatment adjusted accordingly.

REFERENCES/RECOMMENDED READINGS

American Psychiatric Association. *Diagnostic and Statistical Manual of Mental Disorders.* 5th ed. Arlington, VA: American Psychiatric Publishing; 2013.

Coltuc R-V, Stoica V. Metabolic syndrome—cardiovascular and metabolic, complex, difficult to quantify risk factor. *Modern Med.* 2016;23(1):54-59.

Riordan HJ, Antonini P, Murphy MF. Atypical antipsychotics and metabolic syndrome in patients with schizophrenia: risk factors, monitoring, and healthcare implications. *Am Health Drug Benefits.* 2011;4(5):292-302.

Stein DJ, Lerer B, Stahl SM. *Essential Evidence-Based Psychopharmacology.* 2nd ed. Cambridge: Cambridge University Press; 2012.

CASE 23 APPENDIX

Metabolic Monitoring

METABOLIC SYNDROME

Metabolic syndrome (MS) is the name given to the cluster of risk factors leading to cardiovascular disease. The criteria proposed by the National Cholesterol Education Program Adult Treatment Panel (ATP III)[1] are widely used as a reference.

According to the ATP III guidelines, a patient with any three of the risk factors in the chart (below) is considered to have MS.

TABLE 23-1 ATP III Criteria for Clinical Identification of Metabolic Syndrome

Risk Factor	Defining Level
Abdominal Obesity	Waist Circumference
• Men	• >102 cm (>40 inches)
• Women	• >88 cm (>35 inches)
Triglycerides	≥ 150/dL
HDL Cholesterol	
• Men	• <40 mg/dL
• Women	• <50 mg/dL
Blood Pressure	≥130/≥85 mm Hg
Fasting Glucose	≥ 10 mg/dL

(Appendix: Metabolic Monitoring. Reprinted with permission from Center for Quality Assessment and Improvement in Mental Health.)

[1]*National Cholesterol Education Program. Executive Summary of the Third Report of the National Cholesterol Education Program (NCEP) Expert Panel on Detection, Evaluation, and Treatment of High Blood Cholesterol in Adults (ATPIII). JAMA* 2001;285:2486-2497.

CORRELATION BETWEEN METABOLIC SYNDROME AND SECOND-GENERATION ANTIPSYCHOTICS (SGAs)[2]

Many studies suggest that prevalence of diabetes and obesity among individuals with schizophrenia and affective disorders is 1 to 2 times higher than in the general population.

Treatment with some SGAs has been found to cause an increase in body weight, which is associated with increased insulin resistance and concordant elevation of serum lipids.[3]

The currently available SGAs vary in liability for weight gain, risk for development of type II diabetes, and worsening lipid profiles. Because of the variability, the ADA/APA/ACE/NAASO consensus guidelines[4]:

- Recommended scheduled monitoring of metabolic risk factors.
    - Suggested clinicians switch the patient to a SGA medication with a lower weight-gaining liability if the patient experiences a weight gain of >5% of initial weight.

TABLE 23-2 Recommended Schedule for Monitoring Patients on SGAs

	Baseline	4 Weeks	8 Weeks	12 Weeks	Quarterly	Annually	Every 5 Years
Personal/Family History	×					×	
Weight (BMI)	×	×	×	×	×		
Waist Circumference	×					×	
Blood Pressure	×			×		×	
Fasting Plasma glucose[a]	×			×		×	
Fasting Lipid profile	×			×			×

[a]Per recommendations from The Mount Sinai Conference: measurement of fasting plasma glucose level is preferred, but measurement of hemoglobin A1C is acceptable if a fasting plasma glucose test is not feasible.[5]

[2]SGAs include: clozapine, olanzapine, ziprasidone, risperidone, olanzapine-fluoxetine (combination).

[3]Newcomer JW, Haupt D. The metabolic effects of antipsychotic medication. *Can J Psychiatry*. 2006;51:480-491.

[4]American Diabetes Association. Consensus development conference on antipsychotic drugs and obesity and diabetes. *Diabet Care*. 2004;27:596-601.

[5]*National Cholesterol Education Program. Executive Summary of the Third Report of the National Cholesterol Education Program (NCEP) Expert Panel on Detection, Evaluation, and Treatment of High Blood Cholesterol in Adults (ATPIII). JAMA* 2001;285:2486-2497.

TABLE 23-3 Metabolic Syndrome Monitoring Form

Patient Name ________________________________ Date of Visit ____________

Metabolic Syndrome[6] considered positive for MS if 3 or more risk criteria present

Measure	Risk Criteria	Baseline	_/_/_/	_/_/_/	_/_/_/	_/_/_/	_/_/_/
Abdominal Obesity	Men >40 inches						
	Women >35 inches						
Triglycerides	≥150 mg/dL						
HDL Cholesterol	Men <40 mg/dL						
	Women <50 mg/dL						
Blood Pressure	≥130/≥85 mm Hg						
Fasting Plasma Glucose[a]	≥100 mg/dL						

[a]Per recommendations from The Mount Sinai Conference: measurement of fasting plasma glucose level is preferred, but measurement of hemoglobin A1C is acceptable if a fasting plasma glucose test is not feasible.[7]

Weight/BMI[7]	BMI ≥ 30						

Lipid Monitoring Results

	Baseline	_/_/_/	_/_/_/	_/_/_/	_/_/_/	_/_/_/
Total						
LDL						
HDL						
TG						

Serum Lipid Levels Reference Ranges

	Optimal/Desired[1]	Near/Above Optimal	Borderline High	High	Very High
Total	<200		200–239	≥240	
LDL	<100	100–129	130–159		≥190
HDL	<40 men			≥60	
	<50 women				
TG	<150		150–199	200–499	≥500

[1]*National Cholesterol Education Program. Executive Summary of the Third Report of the National Cholesterol Education Program (NCEP) Expert Panel on Detection, Evaluation, and Treatment of High Blood Cholesterol in Adults (ATPIII). JAMA* 2001;285:2486-2497.

[6]Other obesity indicators not in the ATP III recommendations: Actual Weight or BMI (Weight/height in kg/m^2; overweight 25–29, obese ≥30).

[7]Marder SR, Essock SM, Miller AL, et al. Physical health monitoring of patients with schizophrenia. *Am J Psychiatry*. 2004;161:1334-1349.

CASE 24

Out of Control Eating with a History of Depression

IDENTIFICATION: The patient is a 27-year-old single Caucasian woman. She is a graduate student in her third year studying for a Master's degree in Divinity. She lives alone in graduate housing. She was referred by her psychotherapist for a medication evaluation.

CHIEF COMPLAINT: "I'm having terrible cravings for food, alcohol, and cigarettes. It's awful. I'm binging on sweets and chocolate three or four times a week. I'm going to AA, I've been abstinent for four months from alcohol and cigarettes, but it's been incredibly hard. I have a temporary sponsor and I'm seeing a therapist, but it's not enough. I need to do something. I can't stand this."

HISTORY OF CHIEF COMPLAINT: The patient reports that she was emotionally stable during graduate school until the last semester of her third year. At that time, she started drinking heavily. Instead of drinking wine and beer, she began drinking vodka. She started drinking three to four shots of vodka when alone and reported that she frequently would "black out" and have no memory of the evening. She never drank in the morning. After her boyfriend broke up with her because of her drinking, she tried multiple times to cut down. This pattern of drinking went on for 3 months and was affecting her academic work and her relationships with friends. She reported cravings for alcohol during the day. At that point, she decided see a psychotherapist. After several weeks she successfully cut down on alcohol and cigarettes. When interviewed for this evaluation she had been abstinent from alcohol and cigarettes for 4 months. She saw the psychotherapist weekly and was attending Alcoholics Anonymous (AA) several days each week. During the past 4 months she reported uncontrollable binging on large amounts of sweets and chocolate. She ate alone and experienced remorse and guilt. She had gained 15 lb. She denied purging or restricting.

PAST PSYCHIATRIC HISTORY: The patient had her first episode of depression in her junior year in college. She was a music performance major and hoped to be a professional musician. Her depression was characterized by anhedonia, tiredness, decreased motivation, decreased concentration, and increased appetite with weight gain, excessive sleeping, and suicidal ideation. She did not have intent or a plan and never made a suicide attempt. Her ideation was passive, "maybe it would be better if I would get cancer and die." There were no identifiable situational triggers. She engaged in cognitive-behavioral therapy (CBT) at the college counseling center that she described as "helpful." She was prescribed bupropion extended release 150 mg at the college Wellness Center by a psychiatric nurse practitioner. She has continued taking the same dose of bupropion since that time. Thereafter, she denied any episodes of depression or anxiety.

MEDICAL HISTORY: The patient denied any chronic or acute medical problems except monthly menstrual migraines since she was a teen. Her menstrual cycle was regular. She reported premenstrual symptoms including increased appetite, craving sweets, fatigue, and irritability. She had never been pregnant and used an etonogestrel/ethinyl estradiol vaginal ring for contraception. She reported seasonal allergies managed with loratadine. No known drug allergies. No history of sexually transmitted illnesses. No hospitalizations or surgeries.

She reported an increased appetite, craving sweets, and a 15-lb weight gain in the past 4 months after she stopped smoking cigarettes and drinking alcoholic beverages. Prior to this she had always made an effort to eat well and exercise regularly. She did not drink soda or sweetened beverages. She did not eat fast food. She did drink caffeinated coffee in the morning. She worked out at a gym four to five times a week. She ran on a treadmill for 30 minutes and did weight training throughout graduate school. She denied any difficulty initiating or maintaining her sleep. After she stopped drinking and smoking, there was a noticeable change in her eating habits, which included food cravings.

A review of systems was negative.

Vital signs at evaluation: BP, 100/68; P, 76; Ht, 5'6"; Wt, 165 lb; BMI, 26.6.

HISTORY OF DRUG OR ALCOHOL ABUSE: The patient reported that she started smoking cigarettes in high school and smoked consistently without any success when trying to quit. She smoked ¾ of a pack most days. She started to drink beer and wine in college socially on the weekends. She tried marijuana a few times but reported that she felt "out of control" and did not enjoy it. She denied drinking more than she intended to or irritating anyone with her drinking until her third and final semester of graduate school. Her social drinking escalated and she started drinking alone and frequently drinking until she blacked out. Her behavior upset her boyfriend who thought she was "an alcoholic." After the breakup, she decided to stop smoking cigarettes and drinking alcohol. She had not been drinking alcohol or smoking cigarettes for 4 months prior to this evaluation. She was attending AA meetings most days of the week, had a sponsor, and had a psychotherapist.

FAMILY HISTORY: The patient reported a "normal" upbringing in a religious family. Her parents are both college educated, are active in their church, and have stable employment. She reports a good relationship with both of her parents. She described her mother as a "heavy" drinker in the past. Her mother does not drink alcohol now, but does smoke cigarettes. Mother has no history of depression or anxiety. Mother's father was described as an "alcoholic."

The patient described her father as a stable person who is a social drinker. He smokes cigarettes. He has no significant family history of psychiatric or substance problems. The patient's brother has a history of anxiety starting in high school and polysubstance abuse. He made several suicide attempts while in college. He was never hospitalized. He failed out of college and is currently a heavy drinker, smokes marijuana daily, and smokes cigarettes. He is unemployed and has lost his driver's license after two Driving Under the Influence charges. He lives with his parents and is not receiving treatment for his anxiety or substance issues.

PERSONAL HISTORY

Perinatal: The patient had a full-term birth. Mother was not using alcohol or drugs, or smoking cigarettes while pregnant. The patient was breastfed until 6 months of age.

Childhood: She denied any developmental problems in childhood. No history of sleep disturbance, school phobia, or bedwetting.

Adolescence: She was quite successful academically in adolescence and active in the school band and church activities.

Adulthood: In college, she studied music and hoped to be a professional musician. She reported that she enjoyed college and has maintained college friendships. She worked for several years in a law office after college. She volunteered in her church in the young adult education program. She decided to get an advanced degree in Divinity and abandoned her plans to be a classical musician. She did very well in her graduate studies until her third and final year when her drinking escalated.

TRAUMA/ABUSE HISTORY: None reported.

MENTAL STATUS EVALUATION

Appearance: Well groomed. She was professionally dressed. Overweight. Normal gait and posture.

Behavior and psychomotor activity: Good eye contact. Normal psychomotor activity.

Consciousness:	Alert.
Orientation:	Oriented to person, place, and time.
Memory:	The patient denies any gaps in her memory except when she has "blacked out" after heavy drinking. When examined, exhibited normal recent and remote memory.
Concentration/attention:	Good.
Visuospatial ability:	Not assessed formally.
Abstract thought:	Not assessed formally.
Intellectual functioning:	Very bright and articulate.
Speech and language:	Mildly pressured speech initially during the interview.
Perceptions:	No abnormalities.
Thought process:	Logical and goal directed.
Thought content:	Anxious and very distressed about her cravings for alcohol and cigarettes. She was concerned that she would relapse and start drinking again given the stress of academic work.
Suicidality and homicidality:	Denies any desire to harm herself or others.
Mood:	Anxious.
Affect:	Congruent with mood.
Impulse control:	Good.
Judgment/insight/reliability:	Good.

FORMULATING THE DIAGNOSIS

Which diagnosis should be considered?

296.26 (F32.5) Major Depressive Disorder, Single Episode, in Remission

Diagnostic Criteria

A. Five (or more) of the following symptoms have been present during the same 2-week period and represent a change from previous functioning; at least one of the symptoms is either (1) depressed mood or (2) loss of interest or pleasure.
   - **Note:** Do not include symptoms that are clearly attributable to another medical condition.
     1. Depressed mood most of the day, nearly every day, as indicated by either subjective report (eg, feels sad, empty, hopeless) or observation made by others (eg, appears tearful). (**Note:** In children and adolescents, can be irritable mood.)
     2. Markedly diminished interest or pleasure in all, or almost all, activities most of the day, nearly every day (as indicated by either subjective account or observation).
     3. Significant weight loss when not dieting or weight gain (eg, a change of more than 5% of body weight in a month), or decrease or increase in appetite nearly every day. (**Note:** In children, consider failure to make expected weight gain.)
     4. Insomnia or hypersomnia nearly every day.
     5. Psychomotor agitation or retardation nearly every day (observable by others, not merely subjective feelings of restlessness or being slowed down).
     6. Fatigue or loss of energy nearly every day.
     7. Feelings of worthlessness or excessive or inappropriate guilt (which may be delusional) nearly every day (not merely self-reproach or guilt about being sick).
     8. Diminished ability to think or concentrate, or indecisiveness, nearly every day (either by subjective account or as observed by others).
     9. Recurrent thoughts of death (not just fear of dying), recurrent suicidal ideation without a specific plan, or a suicide attempt or a specific plan for committing suicide.

B. The symptoms cause clinically significant distress or impairment in social, occupational, or other important areas of functioning.

C. The episode is not attributable to the physiologic effects of a substance or another medical condition.

Note: Criteria A–C represent a major depressive episode (MDE).

Note: Responses to a significant loss (eg, bereavement, financial ruin, losses from a natural disaster, a serious medical illness or disability) may include the feelings of intense sadness, rumination about the loss, insomnia, poor appetite, and weight loss noted in Criterion A, which may resemble a depressive episode. Although such symptoms may be understandable or considered appropriate to the loss, the presence of an MDE in addition to the normal response to a significant loss should also be carefully considered. This decision inevitably requires the exercise of clinical judgment based on the individual's history and the cultural norms for the expression of distress in the context of loss.

In distinguishing grief from an MDE, it is useful to consider that in grief the predominant affect is feelings of emptiness and loss, while in an MDE it is persistent depressed mood and the inability to anticipate happiness or pleasure. The dysphoria in grief is likely to decrease in intensity over days to weeks and occurs in waves, the so-called pangs of grief. These waves tend to be associated with thoughts or reminders of the deceased. The depressed mood of an MDE is more persistent and not tied to specific thoughts or preoccupations. The pain of grief may be accompanied by positive emotions and humor that are uncharacteristic of the pervasive unhappiness and misery characteristic of an MDE. The thought content associated with grief generally features a preoccupation with thoughts and memories of the deceased, rather than the self-critical or pessimistic ruminations seen in an MDE. In grief, self-esteem is generally preserved, whereas in an MDE feelings of worthlessness and self-loathing are common. If self-derogatory ideation is present in grief, it typically involves perceived failings vis-à-vis the deceased (eg, not visiting frequently enough, not telling the deceased how much he or she was loved). If a bereaved individual thinks about death and dying, such thoughts are generally focused on the deceased and possibly about "joining" the deceased, whereas in an MDE such thoughts are focused on ending one's own life because of feeling worthless, undeserving of life, or unable to cope with the pain of depression.

D. The occurrence of the MDE is not better explained by schizoaffective disorder, schizophrenia, schizophreniform disorder, delusional disorder, or other specified and unspecified schizophrenia spectrum and other psychotic disorders.
E. There has never been a manic episode or a hypomanic episode.
    - **Note:** This exclusion does not apply if all of the manic-like or hypomanic-like episodes are substance-induced or are attributable to the physiologic effects of another medical condition.

(Reprinted with permission from the *Diagnostic and Statistical Manual of Mental Disorders*. 5th ed. Arlington, VA: American Psychiatric Publication; 2013.)

What is your rationale for the diagnosis?

The patient described a history consistent with major depressive disorder single episode, in remission. Her depression was characterized by anhedonia, tiredness, decreased motivation, decreased concentration, and increased appetite with weight gain, excessive sleeping, and passive suicidal ideation. Her symptoms have been in remission since starting treatment.

Which diagnosis should be considered?

305.90 (F10.20) Alcohol Use Disorder, Severe, in Early Remission

Diagnostic Criteria

A. A problematic pattern of alcohol use leading to clinically significant impairment or distress, as manifested by at least two of the following, occurring within a 12-month period:
   1. Alcohol is often taken in larger amounts or over a longer period than was intended.
   2. There is a persistent desire or unsuccessful efforts to cut down or control alcohol use.
   3. A great deal of time is spent in activities necessary to obtain alcohol, use alcohol, or recover from its effects.
   4. Craving, or a strong desire or urge to use alcohol.
   5. Recurrent alcohol use resulting in a failure to fulfill major role obligations at work, school, or home.
   6. Continued alcohol use despite having persistent or recurrent social or interpersonal problems caused or exacerbated by the effects of alcohol.
   7. Important social, occupational, or recreational activities are given up or reduced because of alcohol use.
   8. Recurrent alcohol use in situations in which it is physically hazardous.
   9. Alcohol use is continued despite knowledge of having a persistent or recurrent physical or psychological problem that is likely to have been caused or exacerbated by alcohol.
   10. Tolerance, as defined by either of the following:
       a. A need for markedly increased amounts of alcohol to achieve intoxication or desired effect.
       b. A markedly diminished effect with continued use of the same amount of alcohol.
   11. Withdrawal, as manifested by either of the following:
       a. The characteristic withdrawal syndrome for alcohol (refer to Criteria A and B of the criteria set for alcohol withdrawal).
       b. Alcohol (or a closely related substance, such as a benzodiazepine) is taken to relieve or avoid withdrawal symptoms.

Specify if:

- **In early remission:** After full criteria for alcohol use disorder were previously met, none of the criteria for alcohol use disorder have been met for at least 3 months but for less than 12 months (with the exception that Criterion A4, "Craving, or a strong desire or urge to use alcohol," may be met).
- **In sustained remission:** After full criteria for alcohol use disorder were previously met, none of the criteria for alcohol use disorder have been met at any time during a period of 12 months or longer (with the exception that Criterion A4, "Craving, or a strong desire or urge to use alcohol," may be met).

Specify if:

- **In a controlled environment:** This additional specifier is used if the individual is in an environment where access to alcohol is restricted.

Code based on current severity: Note for *ICD-10-CM* codes: If an alcohol intoxication, alcohol withdrawal, or another alcohol-induced mental disorder is also present, do not use the codes below for alcohol use disorder. Instead, the comorbid alcohol use disorder is indicated in the fourth character of the alcohol-induced disorder code (see the coding note for alcohol intoxication, alcohol withdrawal, or a specific alcohol-induced mental disorder). For example, if there is comorbid alcohol intoxication and alcohol use disorder, only the alcohol intoxication code is given, with the fourth character indicating whether the comorbid alcohol use disorder is mild, moderate, or severe: F10.129 for mild alcohol use disorder with alcohol intoxication or F10.229 for a moderate or severe alcohol use disorder with alcohol intoxication.

Specify **current severity:**

- **305.00 (F10.10) Mild:** Presence of 2–3 symptoms.
- **303.90 (F10.20) Moderate:** Presence of 4–5 symptoms.
- **303.90 (F10.20) Severe:** Presence of 6 or more symptoms.

(Reprinted with permission from the *Diagnostic and Statistical Manual of Mental Disorders*. 5th ed. Arlington, VA: American Psychiatric Publication; 2013.)

What is your rationale for the diagnosis?

The patient describes a pattern of alcohol use that led to significant distress. She consumed larger and larger amounts over time (switched from wine to vodka), started drinking alone, had craving for alcohol, started having problems at work and school related to her use, and had a breakup with her boyfriend. She tried unsuccessfully to cut down and had recurrent alcohol use, which was physically hazardous (blacking out). She met 9 out of the 11 diagnostic criteria (all the criteria except for tolerance or withdrawal). She has stopped drinking for more than 3 months and less than 12 months (4 months). Therefore, she meets the criteria for alcohol use disorder, severe, in early remission.

Which diagnosis should be considered?

307.51 (F50.81) Binge-Eating Disorder, Mild-Moderate

Diagnostic Criteria

A. Recurrent episodes of binge eating. An episode of binge eating is characterized by both of the following:
   1. Eating, in a discrete period of time (eg, within any 2-hour period), an amount of food that is definitely larger than what most people would eat in a similar period of time under similar circumstances.
   2. A sense of lack of control over eating during the episode (eg, a feeling that one cannot stop eating or control what or how much one is eating).

B. The binge-eating episodes are associated with three (or more) of the following:
   1. Eating much more rapidly than normal.
   2. Eating until feeling uncomfortably full.
   3. Eating large amounts of food when not feeling physically hungry.
   4. Eating alone because of feeling embarrassed by how much one is eating.
   5. Feeling disgusted with oneself, depressed, or very guilty afterward.

C. Marked distress regarding binge eating is present.

D. The binge eating occurs, on average, at least once a week for 3 months.

E. The binge eating is not associated with the recurrent use of inappropriate compensatory behavior as in bulimia nervosa and does not occur exclusively during the course of bulimia nervosa or anorexia nervosa.

Specify if:

- **In partial remission:** After full criteria for binge-eating disorder were previously met, binge eating occurs at an average frequency of less than one episode per week for a sustained period of time.
- **In full remission:** After full criteria for binge-eating disorder were previously met, none of the criteria have been met for a sustained period of time.

Specify current severity:
The minimum level of severity is based on the frequency of episodes of binge eating (see below). The level of severity may be increased to reflect other symptoms and the degree of functional disability.

- **Mild:** 1–3 binge-eating episodes per week.
- **Moderate:** 4–7 binge-eating episodes per week.
- **Severe:** 8–13 binge-eating episodes per week.
- **Extreme:** 14 or more binge-eating episodes per week.

(Reprinted with permission from the *Diagnostic and Statistical Manual of Mental Disorders*. 5th ed. Arlington, VA: American Psychiatric Publication; 2013.)

What is your rationale for the diagnosis?

The patient describes recurrent episodes of binge eating characterized by eating an amount of food larger than what is normally consumed and feeling out of control. The episodes are associated with eating when not hungry, being embarrassed by how much she is eating, and feeling disgusted with herself afterward. ("I'm having terrible cravings for food...It's awful. I'm binging on sweets and chocolate three or four times a week.") She is distressed about the binging, and the binge eating is not associated with the use of compensatory behavior such as bulimia. Therefore, the diagnosis of binge-eating disorder, mild-moderate is applicable.

What tests or tools should be considered to help identify the correct diagnosis?

Yale–Brown Obsessive Compulsive Scale Modified for Binge Eating (YBOCS-BE)
Beck Anxiety Index (BAI)
The Alcohol Use Disorder Identification Test (AUDIT)
Mood Disorder Questionnaire Screening Tool (MDQ)

What differential diagnosis should be considered?

300.02 (F41.1) Generalized anxiety disorder (GAD) often co-occurs with alcohol use disorder and binge-eating disorder. However, there are no identified symptoms or history consistent with GAD. Therefore, the diagnosis is not applicable.

FORMULATING THE TREATMENT STRATEGY

What treatment would you prescribe and what is the rationale?

Psychopharmacology: Increase bupropion extended release to 300 mg daily.

Although the patient has only had one depressive episode rather than the three or more that would justify maintenance therapy on an antidepressant, she has been on this maintenance dose for several years. Given her difficulties with alcohol, smoking cessation, and binge eating, a conservative and potentially helpful approach would be to increase the dosage of bupropion extended release to 300 mg daily. It is FDA approved for major depressive disorder and smoking cessation. It inhibits the uptake or norepinephrine and dopamine which may decrease her nicotine cravings. The patient should be screened for any history of seizure disorder or anorexia/bulimia as bupropion may lower the seizure threshold.

Naltrexone 50 mg daily.

Naltrexone is FDA approved for alcohol and opiate dependence. It is an opioid antagonist and decreases cravings for alcohol. Of note, naltrexone and bupropion together are FDA approved as Contrave for obesity and long-term weight loss treatment. It is thought that this formulation decreases food cravings. She has gained 15 lb since binge eating and this combination may help her lose the weight she gained.

If the patient's response to the addition of naltrexone and increased dose of bupropion is not satisfactory, other medications may need to be considered. Topiramate starting at 50 mg BID has been shown to reduce appetite. Another option is lisdexamfetamine dimesylate, which is the first FDA-approved medication to treat moderate to severe binge-eating disorder. It is a schedule II stimulant. The potential for abuse should be taken into consideration whenever prescribing a medication in this category. The dosage studied was 50 to 70 mg in the morning, however, starting at 30 mg and slowly titrating as necessary is prudent. Before prescribing lisdexamfetamine dimesylate, the patient should be screened for any cardiac history or family history of sudden death.

Diagnostic Tests: Routine labs that include creatinine are recommended before starting bupropion.

Monitor blood pressure at each visit because bupropion extended release can raise blood pressure.

Monitor weight monthly.

Referral: Continue psychotherapy and attending AA meetings regularly. Collaborate with psychotherapist.

Type of Psychotherapy: Whether in individual or group sessions, psychotherapy has been effective in reduce binging episodes and problem drinking. Examples include the following:

Cognitive Behavioral Therapy (CBT): This therapy focuses on modifying cognitions and behaviors. CBT may improve coping with issues that can trigger binge-eating episodes and drinking such as negative feelings, body image and self-esteem issues, or a depressed mood. It may also provide a better sense of control behavior and help regulate eating and drinking patterns.

Interpersonal Psychotherapy: This type of therapy focuses on relationships with people with the goal to improve interpersonal skills. This may help reduce binge eating and drinking that is triggered by poor relationships and unhealthy communication skills.

Dialectical Behavior Therapy: This form of therapy stresses behavioral skills to improve stress tolerance, emotional regulation, and relationships with others. Mindfulness is an essential component. Emotional regulation can reduce the desire to binge eat and drink alcohol excessively.

Psychoeducation: The patient should be advised to carry a medication card stating that she is taking naltrexone in case of emergency situations where pain management is needed.

Guided self-help that specifically addresses binge-eating disorder has been found to be helpful for many patients. One free booklet is "Binge Eating: Breaking the Cycle, A self-help guide towards recovery," which can be retrieved at http://www.bodywhys.ie/m/uploads/BEDBookletUpload.pdf

What standard guidelines would you use to treat or assess this patient?

There are limited recent guidelines for the treatment of binge-eating disorder despite the high prevalence of binge eating associated with obesity, which is a known serious health risk. The most recent guideline provided by the American Psychiatric Association was published in 2006 and is listed below.

Treatment of patients with eating disorders, 3rd ed. American Psychiatric Association. *Am J Psychiatry*. 2006;163:4.

REFERENCES/RECOMMENDED READINGS

American Psychiatric Association. *Diagnostic and Statistical Manual of Mental Disorders*. 5th ed. Arlington, VA: American Psychiatric Publishing; 2013.

Leahy L, Kohler CG, eds. *Manual of Clinical Psychopharmacology for Nurses*. Arlington, VA: American Psychiatric Publishing; 2013.

Marrazzi MA, Markham KM, Kinzie J, Luby ED. Binge eating disorder: response to naltrexone. *Int J Obes Relat Metab Disord*. 1995;19:143-145.

Stahl S. *The Prescriber's Guide: Stahl's Essential Psychopharmacology*. New York: Cambridge University Press; 2011.

Striegel-Moore RH, Wilson GT, DeBar L, et al. Cognitive behavioral guided self-help for the treatment of recurrent binge eating. *J Consult Clin Psychol*. 2010;78:312.

CASE 25

Depressed and Anxious Postpartum

IDENTIFICATION: The patient is a 28-year-old, married, African-American woman with a 4-month-old infant daughter and a 3-year-old stepson. She is enrolled in graduate school. She is seen for this evaluation in an outpatient setting. Her primary care provider recommended that she be evaluated for postpartum depression.

CHIEF COMPLAINT: "Sometimes I feel down. I have low motivation, and I can't concentrate."

HISTORY OF CHIEF COMPLAINT: She became concerned because she is not able to focus on her school assignments after returning to college this month. The patient is adamant that she does not want to take any medication because she is breastfeeding. Patient reports feeling fatigued all the time.

PAST PSYCHIATRIC HISTORY: The patient saw a counselor when she was 9 years old for anxiety. After a family friend died, she developed obsessive thinking and kept thinking that her mother would die. She became fearful every time she was separated from her parents. She wrote excessive checklists. She had social anxiety so her primary care provider prescribed citalopram 20 mg when she started college as an undergraduate. Also, she was treated with cognitive behavioral therapy (CBT) that she thought was very helpful for reducing her obsessive thinking and social anxiety. She stopped the citalopram prior to becoming pregnant. She thought her mood was fine without the citalopram until a few months postpartum. She told her primary care provider who recommended that she be seen by a psychiatric specialist and be evaluated for postpartum depression.

MEDICAL HISTORY

Had normal menses prior to her pregnancy. Not menstruating since.

Full-term vaginal birth 4 months ago.

Currently breastfeeding and wants to continue breastfeeding until the baby is at least a year old.

Average height and weight.

Sleep is only intermittent due to breastfeeding demands and raising a 3 year old. She reports sleeping for approximately five hours per night. She denies napping during the daytime. She reports feeling chronically tired due to lack of sleep.

HISTORY OF DRUG OR ALCOHOL ABUSE: Denied.

FAMILY HISTORY: The patient was raised in an intact family with an older sister. Her father has history of depression and her maternal grandmother is reported to have bipolar disorder. The patient lives with her husband, her 3-year-old stepson, and her 4-month-old infant. She describes her husband as being very supportive. They have a lot of friends and social activities. Her parents live far away and have only been able to visit once since the baby was born.

PERSONAL HISTORY

Perinatal: No complications reported.

Childhood: Developed obsessive fear that her mother would die after a family friend died. Developed significant separation anxiety. She had to compulsively hug her parents when they left the house; otherwise, she thought something bad would happen to them.

Adolescence: Experienced social anxiety but maintained some friendships. When sexually transmitted infections (STIs) were covered in her classroom lecture, she experienced panic attacks.

Adulthood: Her husband is supportive. She is raising her 3-year-old stepson and their 4-month-old son. She was academically successful until the current semester in which she is struggling to complete her work. She is a nonpracticing Baptist. No military or legal history.

The couple maintains an active social life, hosting parties, etc., in spite of the increased demands with the pregnancy and childcare. The patient is chronically tired and does not have any assistance with childcare, other than by her husband who is not home much due to his job demands. She feels compelled to maintain the same social activity regardless of how tired she is because she does not want to disappoint her husband.

TRAUMA/ABUSE HISTORY: Denied.

MENTAL STATUS EXAMINATION

Appearance: Arrived with her infant in a stroller. Casually dressed.

Behavior and psychomotor activity: No abnormal movements. Cooperative. Good eye contact. Has a positive attitude toward the baby. She shows a full range of expression and smiles appropriately when talking about the baby. She appears pleased when describing recent pleasurable social occasions with her husband and friends.

Consciousness:	Alert.
Orientation:	Times three.
Memory:	Not formally assessed but no gross memory deficits apparent. Was able to provide detailed history of her symptoms and treatment.
Concentration and attention:	Not formally assessed but reports having difficulty focusing in class and completing assignment. Denies any difficulty in child-care tasks.
Visuospatial ability:	Not formally assessed.
Abstract thought:	No deficits noted.
Intellectual functioning:	Average or above.
Speech and language:	Normal rate and volume.
Perceptions:	No abnormalities.
Thought processes:	Logical and coherent.
Thought content:	Significant obsessive and compulsive symptoms identified with Yale-Brown Obsessive Compulsive Scale (Y-BOCS) checklist; mainly somatic obsessions and checking and counting compulsions. No suicidal or homicidal thoughts.
Mood:	"Down." Anxious about falling behind in school.

Affect: Although the patient reports a low, anxious mood, her symptoms seem mild and her anxiety seems predominantly related to worrying about falling behind academically.

Impulse control: Good.

Judgment/insight/reliability: Good/good/good.

FORMULATING THE DIAGNOSIS

What diagnosis should be considered?

307.45 (G47.23) Circadian Rhythm Sleep-Wake Disorder; Irregular Sleep-Wake Type

Diagnostic Criteria

A. A persistent or recurrent pattern of sleep disruption that is primarily due to an alteration of the circadian system or to a misalignment between the endogenous circadian rhythm and the sleep-wake schedule required by an individual's physical environment or social or professional schedule.
B. The sleep disruption leads to excessive sleepiness or insomnia, or both.
C. The sleep disturbance causes clinically significant distress or impairment in social, occupational, and other important areas of functioning.

Coding note: For *ICD-9-CM*, code **307.45** for all subtypes. For *ICD-10-CM*, code is based on subtype.

Specify whether:

- **307.45 (G47.21) Delayed sleep phase type:** A pattern of delayed sleep onset and awakening times, with an inability to fall asleep and awaken at a desired or conventionally acceptable earlier time.
    1. *Specify* if:
        - **Familial:** A family history of delayed sleep phase is present.
    2. *Specify* if:
        - **Overlapping with non-24-hour sleep-wake type:** Delayed sleep phase type may overlap with another circadian rhythm sleep-wake disorder, non-24-hour sleep-wake type.
- **307.45 (G47.22) Advanced sleep phase type:** A pattern of advanced sleep onset and awakening times, with an inability to remain awake or asleep until the desired or conventionally acceptable later sleep or wake times.
    1. *Specify* if:
        - **Familial:** A family history of advanced sleep phase is present.

- **307.45 (G47.23) Irregular sleep-wake type:** A temporally disorganized sleep-wake pattern, such that the timing of sleep and wake periods is variable throughout the 24-hour period.
- **307.45 (G47.24) Non-24-hour sleep-wake type:** A pattern of sleep-wake cycles that is not synchronized to the 24-hour environment, with a consistent daily drift (usually to later and later times) of sleep onset and wake times.
- **307.45 (G47.26) Shift work type:** Insomnia during the major sleep period and/or excessive sleepiness (including inadvertent sleep) during the major awake period associated with a shift work schedule (ie, requiring unconventional work hours).
- **307.45 (G47.20) Unspecified type**

Specify if:

- **Episodic:** Symptoms last at least 1 month but less than 3 months.
- **Persistent:** Symptoms last 3 months or longer.
- **Recurrent:** Two or more episodes occur within the space of 1 year.

(Reprinted with permission from the *Diagnostic and Statistical Manual of Mental Disorders*. 5th ed. Arlington, VA: American Psychiatric Publication; 2013.)

What is your rationale for the diagnosis?

This patient is experiencing a consistent pattern of sleep disruption related to the demands of nightly breastfeeding. The sleep disruption has contributed to excessive fatigue. The sleep disturbance has contributed to significant distress and impaired functioning as evidenced by her decreased concentration and motivation to complete her academic work. These findings meet the criteria for a circadian rhythm sleep-wake disorder.

What diagnosis should be considered?

300.3 (F42.2) Obsessive-Compulsive Disorder; with Good Insight

Diagnostic Criteria

A. Presence of obsessions, compulsions, or both:
  - Obsessions are defined by (1) and (2):
    1. Recurrent and persistent thoughts, urges, or images that are experienced, at some time during the disturbance, as intrusive and unwanted, and that in most individuals cause marked anxiety or distress.
    2. The individual attempts to ignore or suppress such thoughts, urges, or images, or to neutralize them with some other thought or action (ie, by performing a compulsion).

- Compulsions are defined by (1) and (2):
  1. Repetitive behaviors (eg, hand washing, ordering, checking) or mental acts (eg, praying, counting, repeating words silently) that the individual feels driven to perform in response to an obsession or according to rules that must be applied rigidly.
  2. The behaviors or mental acts are aimed at preventing or reducing anxiety or distress, or preventing some dreaded event or situation; however, these behaviors or mental acts are not connected in a realistic way with what they are designed to neutralize or prevent, or are clearly excessive.
  - **Note:** Young children may not be able to articulate the aims of these behaviors or mental acts.

B. The obsessions or compulsions are time-consuming (eg, take more than 1 hour per day) or cause clinically significant distress or impairment in social, occupational, or other important areas of functioning.

C. The obsessive-compulsive symptoms are not attributable to the physiologic effects of a substance (eg, a drug of abuse, a medication) or another medical condition.

D. The disturbance is not better explained by the symptoms of another mental disorder (eg, excessive worries, as in generalized anxiety disorder; preoccupation with appearance, as in body dysmorphic disorder; difficulty discarding or parting with possessions, as in hoarding disorder; hair pulling, as in trichotillomania [hair-pulling disorder]; skin picking, as in excoriation [skin-picking] disorder; stereotypies, as in stereotypic movement disorder; ritualized eating behavior, as in eating disorders; preoccupation with substances or gambling, as in substance-related and addictive disorders; preoccupation with having an illness, as in illness anxiety disorder; sexual urges or fantasies, as in paraphilic disorders; impulses, as in disruptive, impulse-control, and conduct disorders; guilty ruminations, as in major depressive disorder; thought insertion or delusional preoccupations, as in schizophrenia spectrum and other psychotic disorders; or repetitive patterns of behavior, as in autism spectrum disorder).

Specify if:

- **With good or fair insight:** The individual recognizes that obsessive-compulsive disorder (OCD) beliefs are definitely or probably not true or that they may or may not be true.
- **With poor insight:** The individual thinks OCD beliefs are probably true.
- **With absent insight/delusional beliefs:** The individual is completely convinced that OCD beliefs are true.

(Reprinted with permission from the *Diagnostic and Statistical Manual of Mental Disorders*. 5th ed. Arlington, VA: American Psychiatric Publication; 2013.)

What is your rationale for the diagnosis?

The patient has a long history of recurrent and persistent thoughts (fear that harm will come to her loved ones) and has frequent checking behaviors to make sure that nothing terrible will happen. The obsessions and compulsions cause some distress but they are mitigated by her good insight. She is aware that her thoughts are irrational and usually is able to manage them with CBT skills that she learned. The obsessions and compulsions are not attributable to the use of substance or another medical condition and are not better explained by another mental disorder. Therefore, she meets the criteria for OCD.

What test or tools should be considered to help identify the correct diagnosis?

The Y-BOCS, which can be used to assess obsessive and compulsive symptoms, which can be accessed at: http://www.seinstitute.com/wp-content/uploads/2015/08/YBOC-Symptom-Checklist.pdf

What differential diagnosis should be considered?

296.21 (F32.0) Major Depressive Disorder, Mild, with Mixed Features with Peripartum Onset

This is a possible diagnosis as the patient is reporting depression and anxiety that has developed in the postpartum period. (The *DSM-5* refers to major depressive episodes beginning prior to or after delivery as having a peripartum onset.) However, her symptoms do not meet five or more of the nine criteria required for this diagnosis. Nonetheless, her symptoms should be monitored closely for any worsening that would indicate a diagnosis of major depressive disorder.

The Beck Depression Inventory should be used to evaluate any increasing severity of symptoms, particularly any suicidal or homicidal symptoms.

FORMULATING THE TREATMENT STRATEGY

What treatment would you prescribe and what is the rationale?

Psychopharmacology: No medications prescribed. Nonpharmacologic measures are encouraged, particularly measures to improve her sleep since her symptoms are not severe and may be predominantly related to her impaired sleep. It would be important to include the patient's husband in the treatment plan. The patient should be informed that if her mood does not improve significantly, she should consider resuming her antidepressant medication. A review of the risks and benefits, particularly related to the effects on the baby, would need to be clearly discussed and documented.

Diagnostic Tests: None indicated.

Referrals: CBT therapist.

Type of Psychotherapy: Because CBT was helpful in the past for managing her OCD symptoms, it is recommended at this time. Supportive individual or couples counseling may also be helpful to develop a realistic plan that promotes sufficient rest for the patient.

Psychoeducation: The patient's husband should be included in psychoeducation provided to the patient. Expectations about the level of the couples' social activity may need to be reevaluated. His input regarding the patient's level of functioning may be helpful in formulating the treatment plan. In general, it is important to treat the family as a unit especially when there is a change in the family structure such as the birth of a child.

What standard guidelines would you use to assess or treat the patient?

None.

CLINICAL NOTE

- The patient's obstetrician/midwife should be consulted regarding the prescription of any psychotropic medications when the patient is pregnant or breastfeeding.

REFERENCES/RECOMMENDED READINGS

American Psychiatric Association. *Diagnostic and Statistical Manual of Mental Disorders.* 5th ed. Arlington, VA: American Psychiatric Publishing; 2013.

Haig D. Troubled sleep: night waking, breastfeeding and parent–offspring conflict. *Evol Med Public Health.* 2014;2014:32-39.

Lee KA, Zaffke ME, McEnany G. Parity and sleep patterns during and after pregnancy. *Obstet Gynecol.* 2000;95:14-18.

Massachusetts General Hospital. Breastfeeding & Psychiatric Medications; 2015. Available at: https://womensmentalhealth.org/specialty-clinics/breastfeeding-and-psychiatric-medication/?doing_wp_cron=1480445812.3832159042358398437500

National Institutes of Health, National Heart, Lung, and Blood Institute (2017). How Much Sleep Is Enough? Available at https://www.nhlbi.nih.gov/health/health-topics/topics/sdd/howmuch#

CASE 26

Opiates Are Ruining My Life

IDENTIFICATION: The patient is a 28-year-old single white male, who lives with his biologic parents. He is seen for psychiatric evaluation at a private psychiatric outpatient practice.

CHIEF COMPLAINT: "I need serious help to stop using [heroin/opiates]. . .it's ruining my life."

HISTORY OF CHIEF COMPLAINT: Patient returned from 9 months in a rehab and halfway house program in Florida. Within 4 months of returning, he ran into an old female acquaintance and "I ended up in my old haunts and started using again." He reports using four to five bags of heroin intravenously on a daily basis. His last use was 2 hours prior to the appointment.

PAST PSYCHIATRIC HISTORY: Patient reports being diagnosed with attention deficit hyperactivity disorder (ADHD) in fifth grade. He believes that he was prescribed mixed amphetamine salts, extended-release methylphenidate, and possibly atomoxetine between fifth and eighth grade. He reports, "I didn't like taking them, they made me spacey, I used to hide them." He never had any inpatient or outpatient psychiatric treatment and his medications were prescribed by his family practitioner. When in his first rehabilitation program at the age of 25, he was diagnosed with depression and started on fluoxetine, but stopped it shortly after discharge: "I just never got it refilled again." He reports, "I was depressed since the break-up of my engagement...I don't think I've really gotten over it and maybe the drugs help to numb the feelings." During his rehab in Florida, he was diagnosed with opioid use disorder and major depressive disorder. He was prescribed mirtazapine for depression and "off-label" for insomnia and quetiapine "off-label" for insomnia. These medications continued upon his discharge and return home, and despite his relapse, the patient reports continuing the medications. "They really helped me sleep and I feel better with them. I've just gotta stop using."

MEDICAL HISTORY: Patient suffered a concussion at the age of 17 in an ice hockey game. He believes he lost consciousness for about 2 minutes. He was evaluated in the emergency department of a local hospital and given a computerized tomography (CT) scan. The CT was negative, and he was discharged home. He denies any history of seizures or recurrent headaches or visual disturbances. He has no chronic illnesses. He has never had surgery or been medically or psychiatrically hospitalized. He has no known medication, food, or environmental allergies.

His present medications include mirtazapine 45 mg at bedtime and quetiapine 200 mg at bedtime. He reports adherence to his medications and this was confirmed by the pharmacy's prescription fill record.

Limited Physical Examination: As patient reports his last use of IV heroin was 2 hours prior to the appointment, a Clinical Opioid Withdrawal Scale (COWS) was administered (see Appendix). COWS=0.

Vital signs: HR, 68; Resp, 16; Temp, 98.4°F; BP, 108/62

Patient presents as calm, cooperative, without restlessness or tremors, pupils are constricted, skin is smooth with "track marks" on forearms and hands bilaterally; patient denies any pain, cramping, or nausea and exhibits no congestion or lacrimation.

HISTORY OF DRUG OR ALCOHOL ABUSE: Patient reports smoking marijuana "a couple times in high school and my early 20s, but smoking weed and drinking was never my thing." Around the age of 24, patient reports being given "Oxys" at a party and "I found my thing. . .I felt relaxed, I could be social." His use of oxycodone escalated to 15 to 20 30-mg tablets per day and when without the drug, he reports experiencing "nausea, shakes, and chills." By the age of 25 and having had withdrawal symptoms at least 4 to 5 times in the prior year, he entered his first detoxification and rehabilitation program, which lasted 28 days. He remained "clean" for 8 months and then started using oxycodone again. "I realized that the pills were expensive and heroin was cheaper. At first I started snorting it, but once I injected, the high was like nothing I ever experienced. . .I needed more." The patient reports increased use from three bags per day to a "bundle" [10 bags] or more over the course of the next 6 months. "By the age of 27, I was a mess, I couldn't hold a job, I had fights with my parents and never saw my friends. I checked into rehab and begged them to send me for long-term." The patient completed a local 30-day rehab program and then went to Florida for a 90-day program followed by a halfway house for 6 months. The patient was abstinent for 4 months, then began using four to five bags of intravenous heroin again 2 weeks prior to this appointment.

FAMILY HISTORY: The patient was raised by his biologic parents with whom he currently resides. His mother, age 56, smokes cigarettes and is diagnosed with "anxiety" for which she is prescribed citalopram 20 mg daily. She works in a manufacturing company. His father is 64 years old and retired from his teaching position of 35 years. Two years ago, his father was diagnosed with early-onset dementia, but has been refusing treatment. The patient reports, "I'm scared to drive with him. He gets lost and has no reflexes and doesn't pay any attention when there's a red light or stop sign." The patient also reports, "He would drive me to the city to get my fix, so I guess it wasn't that bad, but my mom would just yell at both of us, and I can't take it anymore." The patient has an older sister, age 34. "She's a heavy drinker. Every time we have a family get together, she's drunk!" She lives with her boyfriend of 10 years. The patient also has a 30-year-old brother who is married and has two children, a daughter age 5 and a son age 3. "He's the only normal one in the family."

The patient's relationships with family members are strained since he began using opiates and then heroin. "Sometimes they're supportive and seem like they want to help me, but most of the time, they just tell me I'm a junkie and better get over it." None of his family members attend Nar-Anon or other family support meetings.

PERSONAL HISTORY

Perinatal/childhood: No known abnormalities or complications.

Adolescence: Patient is a high school graduate and averaged B's throughout high school. He was active in playing ice hockey until his concussion at the age of 17.

Adulthood: At the age of 24, patient was engaged to his girlfriend of 3 years. The relationship ended when she "cheated" with one of the patient's good friends. The patient reports he suffered from depression since that time, but has not sought treatment other than through the substance use programs. He is presently single and not involved in any relationships. He identifies as heterosexual.

At the time of his engagement, patient was completing courses for certification as a massage therapist. He completed the program, but never took the certifications/licensure examination. He averaged B's through his massage therapy program. He is currently unemployed, but works "odd jobs that my friends get me, under the table."

The patient has had three legal charges over the years. He was charged with loitering, solicitation of controlled dangerous substances, and reckless driving. All of the charges occurred while the patient was intoxicated, though drug screening was never done at the times of his arrest. The patient completed his community service hours and has paid his fines. He has 6 months of probation remaining and must remain abstinent to avoid incarceration.

He has state-based medical insurance and is not on disability.

TRAUMA/ABUSE HISTORY: He denies any history of physical, sexual, or emotional abuse.

MENTAL STATUS EXAMINATION

Appearance: Neatly groomed 28-year-old single male who appears his stated age.

Behavior and psychomotor activity: Cooperative, easily engaged, no restlessness or abnormal movements, good eye contact throughout exam.

Consciousness:	Awake and alert.
Orientation:	Oriented to person, place, time, and situation.
Memory:	Short- and long-term memory grossly intact without deficits.
Concentration and attention:	Adequate for purposes of examination, some questions needed to be repeated.
Visuospatial ability:	Not assessed.
Abstract thought:	Able to interpret "Don't cry over spilled milk" as "no sense in crying once something's over."
Intellectual functioning:	Appears to be of average intellect, good vocabulary, and sentence structure.
Speech and language:	Speech is of normal tone and rate with occasional brief (1 to 2 seconds) delays in responses.
Perceptions:	No evidence of responding to internal stimulation or altered perceptions. Patient denies hallucinatory experiences both while intoxicated and while "clean."

Thought processes: Logical, goal, and future oriented.

Thought content: Patient focused on wanting to recover and remain abstinent from drugs.

Suicidality or homicidality: He denies any current or past suicidal or homicidal ideations, plans, or intent. Patient denies past and current aggressive and self-injurious behaviors as well. He denies that his use of drugs is in any way an attempt to kill himself.

Mood: Mood is dysphoric and anxious.

Affect: Affect is congruent with his mood.

Impulse control: Adequate, except when trying to avoid using drugs.

Judgment/insight/reliability: Patient is a good historian, he presents as genuine and honest.

FORMULATING THE DIAGNOSIS

Which diagnosis (or diagnoses) should be considered?

292.89 (F11.229) Opioid Intoxication, without Perceptual Disturbances, with Comorbid Opioid Use Disorder, Severe

Diagnostic Criteria

A. Recent use of an opioid.
B. Clinically significant problematic behavioral or psychological changes (eg, initial euphoria followed by apathy, dysphoria, psychomotor agitation or retardation, impaired judgment) that developed during, or shortly after, opioid use.
C. Pupillary constriction (or pupillary dilation due to anoxia from severe overdose) and one (or more) of the following signs or symptoms developing during, or shortly after, opioid use:
   1. Drowsiness or coma.
   2. Slurred speech.
   3. Impairment in attention or memory.
D. The signs or symptoms are not attributable to another medical condition and are not better explained by another mental disorder, including intoxication with another substance.

Specify if:

- **With perceptual disturbances:** This specifier may be noted in the rare instance in which hallucinations with intact reality testing or auditory, visual, or tactile illusions occur in the absence of a delirium.

Coding note: The *ICD-9-CM* code is **292.89.** The *ICD-10-CM* code depends on whether or not there is a comorbid opioid use disorder and whether or not there are perceptual disturbances.

- **For opioid intoxication without perceptual disturbances:** If a mild opioid use disorder is comorbid, the *ICD-10-CM* code is **F11.129,** and if a moderate or severe opioid use disorder is comorbid, the *ICD-10-CM* code is **F11.229.** If there is no comorbid opioid use disorder, then the *ICD-10-CM* code is **F11.929.**
- **For opioid intoxication with perceptual disturbances:** If a mild opioid use disorder is comorbid, the *ICD-10-CM* code is **F11.122,** and if a moderate or severe opioid use disorder is comorbid, the *ICD-10-CM* code is **F11.222.** If there is no comorbid opioid use disorder, then the *ICD-10-CM* code is **F11.922.**

(Reprinted with permission from the *Diagnostic and Statistical Manual of Mental Disorders.* 5th ed. Arlington, VA: American Psychiatric Publishing; 2013.)

Which diagnosis (or diagnoses) should be considered?

304.00 (F11.20) Opioid Use Disorder, Severe

Diagnostic Criteria

A. A problematic pattern of opioid use leading to clinically significant impairment or distress, as manifested by at least two of the following, occurring within a 12-month period:
   1. Opioids are often taken in larger amounts or over a longer period than was intended.
   2. There is a persistent desire or unsuccessful efforts to cut down or control opioid use.
   3. A great deal of time is spent in activities necessary to obtain the opioid, use the opioid, or recover from its effects.
   4. Craving, or a strong desire or urge to use opioids.
   5. Recurrent opioid use resulting in a failure to fulfill major role obligations at work, school, or home.
   6. Continued opioid use despite having persistent or recurrent social or interpersonal problems caused or exacerbated by the effects of opioids.
   7. Important social, occupational, or recreational activities are given up or reduced because of opioid use.
   8. Recurrent opioid use in situations in which it is physically hazardous.

9. Continued opioid use despite knowledge of having a persistent or recurrent physical or psychological problem that is likely to have been caused or exacerbated by the substance.
10. Tolerance, as defined by either of the following:
    a. A need for markedly increased amounts of opioids to achieve intoxication or desired effect.
    b. A markedly diminished effect with continued use of the same amount of an opioid.
        - **Note:** This criterion is not considered to be met for those taking opioids solely under appropriate medical supervision.

    Withdrawal, as manifested by either of the following:
    a. The characteristic opioid withdrawal syndrome (refer to Criteria A and B of the criteria set for opioid withdrawal).
    b. Opioids (or a closely related substance) are taken to relieve or avoid withdrawal symptoms.
        - **Note:** This criterion is not considered to be met for those individuals taking opioids solely under appropriate medical supervision.

Specify if:

- **In early remission:** After full criteria for opioid use disorder were previously met, none of the criteria for opioid use disorder have been met for at least 3 months but for less than 12 months (with the exception that Criterion A4, "Craving, or a strong desire or urge to use opioids," may be met).
- **In sustained remission:** After full criteria for opioid use disorder were previously met, none of the criteria for opioid use disorder have been met at any time during a period of 12 months or longer (with the exception that Criterion A4, "Craving, or a strong desire or urge to use opioids," may be met).

Specify if:

- **On maintenance therapy:** This additional specifier is used if the individual is taking a prescribed agonist medication such as methadone or buprenorphine and none of the criteria for opioid use disorder have been met for that class of medication (except tolerance to, or withdrawal from, the agonist). This category also applies to those individuals being maintained on a partial agonist, an agonist/antagonist, or a full antagonist such as oral naltrexone or depot naltrexone.
- **In a controlled environment:** This additional specifier is used if the individual is in an environment where access to opioids is restricted.

Coding based on current severity: Note for *ICD-10-CM* codes: If an opioid intoxication, opioid withdrawal, or another opioid-induced mental disorder is also present, do not use the codes below for opioid use disorder. Instead, the comorbid opioid use disorder is indicated in the fourth character of the opioid-induced disorder code (see the coding note for opioid intoxication, opioid withdrawal, or a specific opioid-induced mental disorder).

For example, if there is comorbid opioid-induced depressive disorder and opioid use disorder, only the opioid-induced depressive disorder code is given, with the fourth character indicating whether the comorbid opioid use disorder is mild, moderate, or severe: F11.14 for mild opioid use disorder with opioid-induced depressive disorder or F11.24 for a moderate or severe opioid use disorder with opioid-induced depressive disorder.

Specify current severity:

- **305.50 (F11.10) Mild:** Presence of two to three symptoms.
- **304.00 (F11.20) Moderate:** Presence of four to five symptoms.
- **304.00 (F11.20) Severe:** Presence of six or more symptoms.

(Reprinted with permission from the *Diagnostic and Statistical Manual of Mental Disorders*. 5th ed. Arlington, VA: American Psychiatric Publishing; 2013.)

What is the rationale for the diagnoses?

Opioid Intoxication and Opioid Use Disorder

Patient reports last use of IV heroin 2 hours prior to appointment, pupils are pinpoint/constricted with no associated withdrawal symptoms. Patient has struggled with heroin addiction over the past 4 years and has been unsuccessful with abstinence for greater than 8 months. His use has escalated over time and interfered with family, relationships, and work. His use is associated with legal consequences. Opioids have been taken to relieve withdrawal symptoms.

Which diagnosis (or diagnoses) should be considered?

300.4 (F34.1) Persistent Depressive Disorder (Dysthymia) with Anxious Distress, Late Onset, Moderate (in remission on medications)

Diagnostic Criteria

This disorder represents a consolidation of *DSM-IV*-defined chronic major depressive disorder and dysthymic disorder.

A. Depressed mood for most of the day, for more days than not, as indicated by either subjective account or observation by others, for at least 2 years.

Note: In children and adolescents, mood can be irritable and duration must be at least 1 year.

B. Presence, while depressed, of two (or more) of the following:
   1. Poor appetite or overeating.
   2. Insomnia or hypersomnia.
   3. Low energy or fatigue.
   4. Low self-esteem.
   5. Poor concentration or difficulty making decisions.
   6. Feelings of hopelessness.

C. During the 2-year period (1 year for children or adolescents) of the disturbance, the individual has never been without the symptoms in Criteria A and B for more than 2 months at a time.
D. Criteria for a major depressive disorder may be continuously present for 2 years.
E. There has never been a manic episode or a hypomanic episode, and criteria have never been met for cyclothymic disorder.
F. The disturbance is not better explained by a persistent schizoaffective disorder, schizophrenia, delusional disorder, or other specified or unspecified schizophrenia spectrum and other psychotic disorder.
G. The symptoms are not attributable to the physiologic effects of a substance (eg, a drug of abuse, a medication) or another medical condition (eg, hypothyroidism).
H. The symptoms cause clinically significant distress or impairment in social, occupational, or other important areas of functioning.

Note: Because the criteria for a major depressive episode include four symptoms that are absent from the symptom list for persistent depressive disorder (dysthymia), a very limited number of individuals will have depressive symptoms that have persisted longer than 2 years but will not meet criteria for persistent depressive disorder. If full criteria for a major depressive episode have been met at some point during the current episode of illness, they should be given a diagnosis of major depressive disorder. Otherwise, a diagnosis of other specified depressive disorder or unspecified depressive disorder is warranted.

Specify if:

- **With anxious distress**
- **With mixed features**
- **With melancholic features**
- **With atypical features**
- **With mood-congruent psychotic features**
- **With mood-incongruent psychotic features**
- **With peripartum onset**

Specify if:

- **In partial remission**
- **In full remission**

Specify if:

- **Early onset:** If onset is before age 21 years.
- **Late onset:** If onset is at age 21 years or older.

Specify if (for most recent 2 years of persistent depressive disorder):

- **With pure dysthymic syndrome:** Full criteria for a major depressive episode have not been met in at least the preceding 2 years.

- **With persistent major depressive episode:** Full criteria for a major depressive episode have been met throughout the preceding 2-year period.
- **With intermittent major depressive episodes, with current episode:** Full criteria for a major depressive episode are currently met, but there have been periods of at least 8 weeks in at least the preceding 2 years with symptoms below the threshold for a full major depressive episode.
- **With intermittent major depressive episodes, without current episode:** Full criteria for a major depressive episode are not currently met, but there has been one or more major depressive episodes in at least the preceding 2 years.

Specify current severity:

- **Mild**
- **Moderate**
- **Severe**

(Reprinted with permission from the *Diagnostic and Statistical Manual of Mental Disorders*. 5th ed. Arlington, VA: American Psychiatric Publishing; 2013.)

What is the rationale for the diagnosis?

Persistent Depressive Disorder with Anxious Distress

This disorder is presently in remission due to psychopharmacotherapy, which has continued despite patient's heroin use. The depressive symptoms have been less severe and without suicidality. The symptoms have persisted for longer than 2 years. Prior to beginning medications the symptoms included: fatigue, insomnia, poor appetite, anxiety, and feeling hopeless. They have interfered with work, family, and relationships. The symptoms returned after the patient's first use of an antidepressant was discontinued.

What test or tools should be considered to help identify the correct diagnosis?

COWS was used to rule out opioid withdrawal versus intoxication.

Hamilton Depression Scale.

What differential diagnosis (or diagnoses) should be considered?

(F11.24) Substance-Induced Depressive Disorder, with Opioid Use Disorder, Severe

This disorder is characterized by the depressive symptoms developing during or shortly after substance intoxication or withdrawal from the opioids. For this patient, the depressive symptoms historically occurred separate from the substance use.

FORMULATING THE TREATMENT STRATEGY

What treatment would you prescribe and what is the rationale?

Psychopharmacology: Since the patient has never had a trial of medication-assisted treatment for opiod use disorder, he is a good candidate for this treatment. The risks and benefits of naltrexone extended-release injectable suspension (Vivitrol) versus buprenorphine/naloxone (Suboxone) should be discussed with the patient to determine which medication-assisted treatment option is best for this individual. In this case, the patient chose naltrexone extended-release injectable suspension.

To prepare patient for outpatient medication-assisted therapy using naltrexone extended-release injectable suspension for opioid use disorder, patient must be opioid free for 7 to 10 days to avoid precipitous withdrawal. An at-home "detox" using prescription and over-the-counter medications to reduce the discomfort of withdrawal will be offered. The patient's mother is willing to supervise an at-home detoxification and patient is willing to commit to this in-home protocol.

The following combination of medications can be used to relieve the discomfort of withdrawal symptoms over a 5- to 10-day period with a progressive decrease in the frequency of dosing. Patient should be encouraged to rest and drink plenty of clear liquids, eat as tolerated, and be out of bed as tolerated (Leahy and Kohler, 2013, p. 445):

Clonidine 0.1 mg one tablet every 4 hours as needed for elevated blood pressure/flushing
Hydroxyzine 50 mg 1 capsule every 4 hours as needed for anxiety/agitation/insomnia
Ibuprofen 600 mg one tablet every 6 hours as needed for aches/pain
Dicyclomine 20 mg one tablet every 6 hours as needed for abdominal cramping/nausea
Diphenoxylate 2.5 mg/Atropine 0.25 mg one to two tablets every 6 hours as needed for diarrhea

Once patient has been opioid free for a period of 7 to 10 days, the next phase of pharmacotherapy can begin:

Naltrexone for extended-release injectable suspension (Vivitrol) 380 mg IM every 4 weeks.

Patient MUST be opioid free for 7 to 10 days prior to receiving his first injection to avoid precipitous withdrawal, which may be severe enough to require hospitalization. A urine drug screen should completed to determine that the patient is opiate-free prior to initiating treatment with naltrexone extended-release injectable suspension. Naltrexone for extended-release injectable suspension will be administered as an intramuscular (IM) gluteal injection, alternating buttocks with each subsequent monthly injection.

Additionally, the patient will continue on the previously prescribed medications to maintain remission of his depression and insomnia:

Quetiapine 200 mg one tablet at bedtime for insomnia
Mirtazapine 45 mg one tablet at bedtime for depression and insomnia

As patient has a history of relapse, the following should also be included in the treatment plan:

Naloxone 0.4 mg auto-injector or NARCAN (naloxone) 4 mg/0.1 mL nasal spray
Administer 1 auto-injector to the thigh or 1 spray to each nostril as needed for suspected opioid overdose (patient is unresponsive, respirations are markedly slowed) and immediately contact emergency response (Dial 911).

Diagnostic Tests: Routine laboratory tests, including liver function tests, should be drawn, as liver dysfunction has been associated with naltrexone for extended-release injectable suspension. Thyroid function tests (triiodothyronine, thyroxine, and thyroid-stimulating hormone) should be included to continue to monitor for potential medical etiology underlying the depression. A lipid panel and hemoglobin A1C should be monitored given the use of quetiapine.

A supervised urine drug screen should be conducted on to ensure patient's abstinence from opioids and other drugs/alcohol.

During the patient's in-home detox, the patient and family members can use the COWS to monitor patient's withdrawal symptoms.

Referrals: If abnormalities appear in the laboratory studies, the patient should be referred to the primary care practitioner or associated medical specialist to treat the medical condition.

Patient should also be referred to a 12-step facilitation program (Narcotics Anonymous or Alcoholics Anonymous) to support his recovery.

Types of Psychotherapy

Motivational interviewing (MI): MI is a psychotherapy technique, which has utility in the treatment of opioid use disorders. The engaging, nonjudgmental approach and meeting the patient at their level allows for the therapeutic relationship to develop and the treatment to be a collaboration between patient and practitioner.

Cognitive behavioral therapy (CBT): Individual therapy utilizing techniques found in CBT will be helpful in challenging the patient to explore the thoughts leading to the emotional distress and ultimately the self-destructive behaviors associated with opioid use disorders. The focus of any therapies for the patient with an opioid use disorder should be on maintaining abstinence while simultaneously developing healthy coping and life skills.

Psychoeducation

The patient and his mother will be educated about the side effects, risks, and benefits of all the medications utilized in the in-home detoxification. They will also be educated on the use of the COWS to monitor the withdrawal symptoms.

Once the patient has been opioid free for over 7 days, he will be scheduled an appointment for the naltrexone injection and informed of the side effects, risks, and benefits of this medication-assisted therapy for opioid use disorder. He will be advised to carry a wallet card and/or wear a medical alert bracelet to inform others that he is prescribed and taking extended-release naltrexone. He will be given patient education materials regarding naltrexone for extended-release injectable suspension.

Additionally, the patient and family will be given instructions on the use of naloxone should the patient relapse and appear to be overdosing. The signs and symptoms of opioid overdose will be discussed with the patient and family and the instructions for use of both the naloxone auto-injector and nasal spray will be provided. It will be emphasized that naloxone is only a temporary measure to allow time for the overdosed patient to be transferred to an emergency department for further care. Naloxone is NOT a cure for opioid overdose. Patient education materials will also be provided for this drug.

What standard guidelines would you use to treat or assess this patient?

- MATx (Medication-Assisted Treatment of Opioid Use Disorders)

MATx is a free smartphone app to support practitioners who use or plan to use Medication-Assisted Treatments with their patients diagnosed with an Opioid Use Disorder. It also offers evidence-based treatment guidelines, *ICD-10* codes, clinical support tools, and the Substance Abuse Mental Health Service Association's (SAMHSA) treatment locators.

Available through the app Store and through SAMHSA at http://store.samhsa.gov/apps/mat/

- Medication-Assisted Treatment for Opioid Use Disorder: Pocket Guide

A FREE publication offering guidelines for practitioners using medication-assisted treatments for patients with opioid use disorders.

Available through SAMHSA at http://store.samhsa.gov/product/Medication-Assisted-Treatment-of-Opioid-Use-Disorder-Pocket-Guide/SMA16-4892PG

- Clinical Use of Extended-Release Injectable Naltrexone in the Treatment of Opioid Use Disorder: A Brief Guide

This FREE guide offers clinicians information regarding assessment, initiating and monitoring treatment, and deciding when to discontinue treatment.

Available through SAMHSA at http://store.samhsa.gov/product/Clinical-Use-of-Extended-Release-Injectable-Naltrexone-in-the-Treatment-of-Opioid-Use-Disorder-A-Brief-Guide/SMA14-4892R

- SAMHSA's Opioid Overdose Toolkit

This FREE publication is a comprehensive guide for the community, first responders, prescribers, patients, and family members regarding the opioid epidemic, opioid overdose, and treatments.

Available through SAMHSA at: https://store.samhsa.gov/shin/content/SMA13-4742/Overdose_Toolkit_2014_Jan.pdf

- The ASAM National Practice Guideline for the Use of Medications in the Treatment of Addiction Involving Opioid Use

This publication is available from the American Society of Addiction Medicine at https://www.asam.org/resources/guidelines-and-consensus-documents/npg

CLINICAL NOTE

- Addiction is a disease of the brain. It is not a moral failing.
- Approach patients suspected of opioid use disorders in a nonjudgmental, compassionate manner. Focus on the patient's interest in becoming physically and mentally healthy. Partner with the patient and their family to support the patient's recovery.
- Individuals with opioid use disorders often relapse. It is imperative that the patient and family be educated that once a patient has remained abstinent for even a brief period of time, a relapse on a previously used amount of opiates may lead to overdose. Use of naloxone for opioid overdose will only offer a brief period of time to allow the patient to obtain emergency treatment through a local hospital.
- Medication-assisted treatments for opioid use disorders should occur as part of a comprehensive treatment plan including psychotherapies, 12-step facilitation programs, and medical oversight.
- Originally prescription of buprenorphine treatment was limited to physicians. However, nurse practitioners and physician assistants can now obtain waivers to prescribe buprenorphine. Information can be obtained at: https://www.samhsa.gov/medication-assisted-treatment/qualify-nps-pas-waivers. Practitioners should be knowledgeable about buprenorphine as a treatment option whether or not they are prescribing it.

REFERENCES/RECOMMENDED READINGS

American Psychiatric Association. *The Diagnostic and Statistical Manual of Mental Disorders (DSM 5)*. 5th ed. Washington, DC: American Psychiatric Publishing; 2013.

Leahy LG, Kohler C, eds. *The Clinical Manual of Psychopharmacology for Nurses*. Arlington, VA: American Psychiatric Publishing; 2013.

U.S Food and Drug Administration. (2010). Highlights of Prescribing Information (Vivitrol). Available at: https://www.accessdata.fda.gov/drugsatfda_docs/label/2010/021897s015lbl.pdf. Accessed on October 10, 2017.

Wesson DR, Ling W. The Clinical Opiate Withdrawal Scale (COWS). *J Psychoactive Drugs*. 2003;35(2):253-259. Available at: https://www.drugabuse.gov/sites/default/files/files/ClinicalOpiateWithdrawalScale.pdf

Wheeler K. *Psychotherapy for the Advanced Practice Psychiatric Nurse: A How-to Guide for Evidence-Based Practice*. 2nd ed. New York, NY: Springer Publishing; 2013.

CASE 26 APPENDIX

Wesson and Ling Clinical Opiate Withdrawal Scale (COWS)

INTRODUCTION

The Clinical Opiate Withdrawal Scale (COWS) (Table 26-1) is an 11-item scale designed to be administered by a clinician. This tool can be used in both inpatient and outpatient settings to reproducibly rate common signs and symptoms of opiate withdrawal and monitor these symptoms over time.

The summed score for the complete scale can be used to help clinicians determine the stage or severity of opiate withdrawal and assess the level of physical dependence on opioids.

Practitioners sometimes express concern about the objectivity of the items in the COWS; however, the symptoms of opioid withdrawal have been likened to a severe influenza infection (e.g., nausea, vomiting, sweating, joint aches, agitation, tremor), and patients should not exceed the lowest score in most categories without exhibiting some observable sign or symptom of withdrawal.

CLINICAL OPIATE WITHDRAWAL SCALE

For each item, circle the number that best describes the patient's signs or symptoms. Rate on just the apparent relationship to opiate withdrawal. For example, if heart rate is increased because the patient was jogging just prior to assessment, the increase pulse rate would not add to the score.

Source: Wesson DR, Ling W. The Clinical Opiate Withdrawal Scale (COWS). *J Psychoactive Drugs.* 2003;35(2):253-259.

TABLE 26-1 Clinical Opiate Withdrawal Scale

For each item, circle the number that best describes the patient's signs or symptoms. Rate on just the apparent relationship to opiate withdrawal. For example, if heart rate is increased because the patient was jogging just prior to assessment, the increased pulse rate would not add to the score.

Patient's Name: ______________________ Date and Time __/__/__:______

Reason for this assessment: ________________________________

Resting Pulse Rate: _______ beats/minute

Measured after patient is sitting or lying for one minute

0 pulse rate 80 or below

1 pulse rate 81–100

2 pulse rate 101–120

4 pulse rate greater than 120

GI Upset: *over last 1/2 hour*

0 no GI symptoms

1 stomach cramps

2 nausea or loose stool

3 vomiting or diarrhea

5 multiple episodes of diarrhea or vomiting

Sweating: *over past 1/2 hour not accounted for by room temperature or patient activity.*

0 no report of chills or flushing

1 subjective report of chills or flushing

2 flushed or observable moistness on face

3 beads of sweat on brow or face

4 sweat streaming off face

Tremor *observation of outstretched hands*

0 no tremor

1 tremor can be felt, but not observed

2 slight tremor observable

4 gross tremor or muscle twitching

Restlessness *Observation during assessment*

0 able to sit still

1 reports difficulty sitting still, but is able to do so

3 frequent shifting or extraneous movements of legs/arms

5 unable to sit still for more than a few seconds

Yawning *Observation during assessment*

0 no yawning

1 yawning once or twice during assessment

2 yawning three or more times during assessment

4 yawning several times/minute

Pupil Size

0 pupils pinned or normal size for room light

1 pupils possibly larger than normal for room light

2 pupils moderately dilated

5 pupils so dilated that only the rim of the iris is visible

Anxiety or Irritability

0 none

1 patient reports increasing irritability or anxiousness

2 patient obviously irritable or anxious

4 patient so irritable or anxious that participation in the assessment is difficult

TABLE 26-1 Clinical Opiate Withdrawal Scale (*continued*)

Bone or joint aches *If patient was having pain previously, only the additional component attributed to opiates withdrawal is scored* 0 not present 1 mild diffuse discomfort 2 patient reports severe diffuse aching of joints/muscles 4 patient is rubbing joints or muscles and is unable to sit still because of discomfort	**Gooseflesh skin** 0 skin is smooth 3 piloerection of skin can be felt or hairs standing up on arms 5 prominent piloerection
Runny nose or tearing *Not accounted for by cold symptoms or allergies* 0 not present 1 nasal stuffiness or unusually moist eyes 2 nose running or tearing 4 nose constantly running or tears streaming down cheeks	Total Score_______ The total score is the sum of all 11 items Initials of person completing assessment: _________

Score 5–12 = mild; 13–24 = moderate; 25–36 = moderately severe; more than 36 = severe withdrawal
Journal of PSV

(Reprinted with permission from Wesson DR, Ling W. The Clinical Opiate Withdrawal Scale (COWS). *J Psychoactive Drugs*. 2003;35(2):253-259.)

CASE 27

Blacking Out

IDENTIFICATION: The patient is a 28-year-old, single, white female in a monogamous relationship, residing with her boyfriend. She experienced a seizure-like episode while at her primary care physician's office, and was brought to the Emergency Department by EMS shortly thereafter. She is seen for the psychiatric evaluation while hospitalized on a medical floor by the consult liaison psychiatric nurse practitioner.

CHIEF COMPLAINT: "I feel sick to my stomach and my anxiety and flashbacks are so bad that my whole body starts shaking and then I black out."

HISTORY OF CHIEF COMPLAINT: The following information was obtained from an interview with the patient, an interview with her family, a review of her medical records, and collateral information from the medical team and nursing staff.

The patient reportedly had severe anxiety while in the waiting room at her primary care doctor's office earlier this morning. She began to experience "shakiness" and started having a flashback to an episode of sexual abuse after which she does not recollect any further details of the incident. Her primary care physician reports that the episode lasted about 3 to 4 minutes during which the patient's whole body was rhythmically shaking while she was staring off into space; she was also incontinent of urine. She did not fall or hit her head during the episode. The patient denies biting her tongue. She reports feeling physically exhausted afterward for a few hours, but did not exhibit any postictal signs or symptoms such as lethargy or confusion; she does not have any recollection of the event occurring.

She reports that she has been experiencing nausea and stomach cramps for the past few weeks, which led her to schedule the medical appointment. The seizure-like episodes first started about 4 years ago and have increased in frequency over the past week, occurring several times per day.

The patient has a history of bipolar II disorder but denies current signs and symptoms of mania or hypomania. She reports difficulty sleeping, poor concentration, poor appetite, low energy level, and nightmares that have worsened over the last several weeks. She denies depressed mood or diminished interest in activities or social isolation. She was fired from her job as a waitress 1 month ago due to tardiness and too many sick calls. She reports a 10-lb weight loss over the past month.

Urine toxicology is positive for cannabinoids and negative for opiates. No recent or past head injuries. Patient denies chest pain or respiratory difficulties. No reports of fever. Muscle tone is adequate. She does complain of some moderate nausea and stomach upset, although no reported vomiting.

Current medications prior to this hospitalization: lamotrigine 200 mg daily, gabapentin 300 mg TID, trazodone 50 mg nightly, sertraline 100 mg daily, lithium 300 mg BID, and melatonin.

PAST PSYCHIATRIC HISTORY: The patient was voluntarily hospitalized in January 2012 for suicidal ideation. She denies a history of actual suicide attempts. Posthospitalization, she started seeing a psychiatrist on an outpatient basis with a diagnosis of bipolar II disorder and posttraumatic stress disorder (PTSD) secondary to sexual abuse. She has also had multiple outpatient treatments at trauma specialty facilities.

MEDICAL HISTORY: No known drug allergies. Height 5′ 5″, weight 145 lb. Denies head injuries. Multiple hospitalizations for pseudoseizures and gastrointestinal complaints (nausea and stomach aches) since 2012. She was never placed on antiepileptic medication because all past video EEG findings were normal.

History of a treated STI. History of bipolar II disorder and PTSD.

Denies any other medical or surgical history.

HISTORY OF DRUG OR ALCOHOL ABUSE: Reports cannabis and heroin use starting at age 23.

The patient reports that she smokes one blunt approximately 3 times per week with the last use 1 day prior to admission. She had attended several inpatient treatment facilities and intensive out-patient (IOP) programs for her polysubstance abuse with the last admission 3 years ago. She denies any heroin use since that time.

FAMILY HISTORY: The patient reports an unremarkable family upbringing. She is the second oldest of three girls. Her mother, older sister, aunts, and grandmother have anxiety and depression. She currently lives with her boyfriend of 2 years in an apartment. She reports he is very supportive.

PERSONAL HISTORY

Perinatal: Uncomplicated pregnancy and vaginal birth. Indicates that her mother did not use drugs or alcohol during her pregnancy. She was breastfed for approximately 6 months and then formula fed.

Childhood: The patient achieved all developmental milestones within appropriate time frames. No history of harmful behaviors to self, other individuals, or cruelty to animals.

No reported history of head banging, rocking behavior, attachment issues, separation anxiety, gender identity issues, sleep disturbances including nightmares, or bed wetting. No report of any academic or social issues. Learning disabilities or Child Study team evaluations were denied.

Adolescence: The patient reports always having low self-esteem. Indicates that she was "always hard on myself," but despite this report indicated that she was able to establish close relationships throughout school. She denies any binging, purging, or restricting her caloric intake to the point where she was severely underweight. She denied issues regarding her body image, bullying, or a history of abuse. She was involved in soccer and field hockey.

She was sexually active at age 17.

Adulthood: The patient is currently unemployed. Denies service in the military. Denies any prior arrests or legal issues. The patient completed high school and some college, but dropped out because it "became too much financially and emotionally." She has worked in retail as a sales associate and as a waitress at several different restaurants. She reports difficulty holding a job due to her hospitalizations and low frustration tolerance. She reports Catholicism as her faith, although she is not active in the church and sees herself as more of a spiritual person than traditionally religious.

TRAUMA/ABUSE HISTORY: The patient reports that she was raped at age 19, after which she reports being severely depressed and isolating herself. Her family reports she would often stare off into space in the middle of a conversation, and it would be difficult to snap her out of it. About several weeks after the severe sexual abuse, she started experiencing flashbacks, nightmares, and hypervigilance. She was unable to concentrate and began illicit drug use to cope with her anxiety and fear. The drugs helped her escape the anxiety triggered by the traumatic memories.

MENTAL STATUS EXAMINATION

Appearance: Casually groomed with short brown hair and brown eyes. Dressed in casual attire. She is cooperative and pleasant throughout the interview.

Behavior and psychomotor activity: Difficulty maintaining eye contact as she scans her surroundings repeatedly. Constantly twirling hair and shaking foot restlessly.

Consciousness:	Alert.
Orientation:	Oriented to person, place, and time.
Memory:	Recent and remote memory intact. Able to recall her own phone number and the content of her last meal. Able to recall the last three presidents and address where she grew up.
Immediate retention impaired:	Able to recall two of three objects. Repeated two of six digits forward correctly.
Concentration and attention:	Easily distracted, although able to answer questions with redirection. Spelled the word WORLD correctly forward and backward, serial 7's could not be completed, and serial 3's were also unable to be completed.
Visuospatial ability:	Intact. Able to correctly draw a clock face and copy assigned figure.
Abstract thought:	Intact. Similarities and proverbs were correctly answered.
Intellectual functioning:	Fund of knowledge and vocabulary are age-appropriate.
Speech and language:	Speech is quiet volume, but clear, with English as the primary language.
Perceptions:	Denies auditory, visual, or tactile hallucinations. Denies derealization or depersonalization.
Thought processes:	Thoughts are logical and goal directed.
Thought content:	Reports that since the sexual trauma, she is constantly "paranoid" and afraid that someone is going to hurt her.

Suicidality or homicidality: Denies SI or HI.

Mood: "Anxious and scared."

Affect: Mood congruent.

Impulsive control: Describes a history of being highly impulsive, but exhibited good impulse control during the interview.

Judgment/insight/reliability: Minimal insight with fair judgment. The patient seems to be a reliable historian.

FORMULATING THE DIAGNOSIS

Which diagnosis (or diagnoses) should be considered?

(F44.5) Conversion Disorder (Functional Neurological Symptom Disorder) with Attacks or Seizures, Persistent, with Psychological Stressor

Diagnostic Criteria

A. One or more symptoms of altered voluntary motor or sensory function.
B. Clinical findings provide evidence of incompatibility between the symptom and recognized neurologic or medical conditions.
C. The symptom or deficit is not better explained by another medical or mental disorder.
D. The symptom or deficit causes clinically significant distress or impairment in social, occupational, or other important areas of functioning or warrants medical evaluation.

Coding note: The *ICD-9-CM* code for conversion disorder is **300.11,** which is assigned regardless of the symptom type. The *ICD-10-CM* code depends on the symptom type (see below).

Specify symptom type:

- **(F44.4) With weakness or paralysis**
- **(F44.4) With abnormal movement** (eg, tremor, dystonic movement, myoclonus, gait disorder)
- **(F44.4) With swallowing symptoms**
- **(F44.4) With speech symptom** (eg, dysphonia, slurred speech)
- **(F44.5) With attacks or seizures**
- **(F44.6) With anesthesia or sensory loss**

- **(F44.6) With special sensory symptom** (eg, visual, olfactory, or hearing disturbance)
- **(F44.7) With mixed symptoms**

Specify if:

- **Acute episode:** Symptoms present for less than 6 months.
- **Persistent:** Symptoms occurring for 6 months or more.

Specify if:

- **With psychological stressor** *(specify stressor)*
- **Without psychological stressor**

(Reprinted with permission from the *Diagnostic and Statistical Manual of Mental Disorders*. 5th ed. Arlington, VA: American Psychiatric Publication; 2013.)

What is the rationale for the diagnosis?

The patient exhibits the signs and symptoms that meet the criteria for the diagnosis of conversion disorder. Her persistent seizure-like episodes with altered motor (rhythmic movements) and sensory functioning (urinary incontinence) meet component A of the diagnostic criteria. Unremarkable EEG results meet Criterion B of the diagnostic criteria. A comprehensive medical workup with unremarkable findings meets Criterion C of the diagnosis. Finally, the pseudoseizures cause significant clinical distress with multiple hospitalizations and impairment in occupational functioning, meeting the fourth component D of diagnosis criteria for conversion disorder. The rationale for the diagnostic specifier "persistent" is justified because the psychogenic seizures have been occurring for greater than 6 months. Finally, the specifier "with psychological stressor" was included because she suffers from PTSD as well as the recent loss of her job which is creating financial pressure.

Which diagnosis (or diagnoses) should be considered?

309.81 (F43.10) Posttraumatic Stress Disorder

Diagnostic Criteria

Note: The following criteria apply to adults, adolescents, and children older than 6 years.

A. Exposure to actual or threatened death, serious injury, or sexual violence in one (or more) of the following ways:
    1. Directly experiencing the traumatic event(s).
    2. Witnessing, in person, the event(s) as it occurred to others.
    3. Learning that the traumatic event(s) occurred to a close family member or a close friend. In cases of actual or threatened death of a family member or friend, the event(s) must have been violent or accidental.

4. Experiencing repeated or extreme exposure to aversive details of the traumatic event(s) (eg, first responders collecting human remains; police officers repeatedly exposed to details of child abuse).
    - **Note:** Criterion A4 does not apply to exposure through electronic media, television, movies, or pictures, unless this exposure is work related.

B. Presence of one (or more) of the following intrusion symptoms associated with the traumatic event(s), beginning after the traumatic event(s) occurred:
1. Recurrent, involuntary, and intrusive distressing memories of the traumatic event(s).
    - **Note:** In children older than 6 years, repetitive play may occur in which themes or aspects of the traumatic event(s) are expressed.
2. Recurrent distressing dreams in which the content and/or affect of the dream is related to the traumatic event(s).
    - **Note:** In children, there may be frightening dreams without recognizable content.
3. Dissociative reactions (eg, flashbacks) in which the individual feels or acts as if the traumatic event(s) were recurring. (Such reactions may occur on a continuum, with the most extreme expression being a complete loss of awareness of present surroundings.)
    - **Note:** In children, trauma-specific reenactment may occur in play.
4. Intense or prolonged psychological distress at exposure to internal or external cues that symbolize or resemble an aspect of the traumatic event(s).
5. Marked physiologic reactions to internal or external cues that symbolize or resemble an aspect of the traumatic event(s).

C. Persistent avoidance of stimuli associated with the traumatic event(s), beginning after the traumatic event(s) occurred, as evidenced by one or both of the following:
1. Avoidance of or efforts to avoid distressing memories, thoughts, or feelings about or closely associated with the traumatic event(s).
2. Avoidance of or efforts to avoid external reminders (people, places, conversations, activities, objects, situations) that arouse distressing memories, thoughts, or feelings about or closely associated with the traumatic event(s).

D. Negative alterations in cognitions and mood associated with the traumatic event(s), beginning or worsening after the traumatic event(s) occurred, as evidenced by two (or more) of the following:
1. Inability to remember an important aspect of the traumatic event(s) (typically due to dissociative amnesia and not to other factors such as head injury, alcohol, or drugs).
2. Persistent and exaggerated negative beliefs or expectations about oneself, others, or the world (eg, "I am bad," "No one can be

trusted," "The world is completely dangerous," "My whole nervous system is permanently ruined").

3. Persistent, distorted cognitions about the cause or consequences of the traumatic event(s) that lead the individual to blame himself/herself or others.
4. Persistent negative emotional state (eg, fear, horror, anger, guilt, or shame).
5. Markedly diminished interest or participation in significant activities.
6. Feelings of detachment or estrangement from others.
7. Persistent inability to experience positive emotions (eg, inability to experience happiness, satisfaction, or loving feelings).

E. Marked alterations in arousal and reactivity associated with the traumatic event(s), beginning or worsening after the traumatic event(s) occurred, as evidenced by two (or more) of the following:
   1. Irritable behavior and angry outbursts (with little or no provocation) typically expressed as verbal or physical aggression toward people or objects.
   2. Reckless or self-destructive behavior.
   3. Hypervigilance.
   4. Exaggerated startle response.
   5. Problems with concentration.
   6. Sleep disturbance (eg, difficulty falling or staying asleep or restless sleep).

F. Duration of the disturbance (Criteria B to E) is more than 1 month.

G. The disturbance causes clinically significant distress or impairment in social, occupational, or other important areas of functioning.

H. The disturbance is not attributable to the physiologic effects of a substance (eg, medication, alcohol) or another medical condition.

Specify whether:

- With dissociative symptoms: The individual's symptoms meet the criteria for PTSD, and in addition, in response to the stressor, the individual experiences persistent or recurrent symptoms of either of the following:
  1. Depersonalization: Persistent or recurrent experiences of feeling detached from, and as if one were an outside observer of, one's mental processes or body (eg, feeling as though one were in a dream; feeling a sense of unreality of self or body or of time moving slowly).
  2. Derealization: Persistent or recurrent experiences of unreality of surroundings (eg, the world around the individual is experienced as unreal, dream-like, distant, or distorted).
     - **Note:** To use this subtype, the dissociative symptoms must not be attributable to the physiologic effects of a substance (eg, blackouts, behavior during alcohol intoxication) or another medical condition (eg, complex partial seizures).

Specify if:

- With delayed expression: If the full diagnostic criteria are not met until at least 6 months after the event (although the onset and expression of some symptoms may be immediate).

(Reprinted with permission from the *Diagnostic and Statistical Manual of Mental Disorders*. 5th ed. Arlington, VA: American Psychiatric Publication; 2013.)

What is the rationale for the diagnosis?

The patient was exposed to sexual violence when she was raped at the age of 19. She has since experienced intrusive symptoms in the form of flashbacks. She subsequently attempts to avoid traumatic memories by trying to "escape with drugs." She experienced significant fear following the event and described feeling "paranoid." She developed negative beliefs (thinking people were going to hurt her). She developed a marked alteration in arousal with a poor concentration and difficulty sleeping. Therefore, the patient's symptoms meet the criteria for PTSD.

Which diagnosis (or diagnoses) should be considered?

304.00 (F11.20) Opioid Use Disorder, in Sustained Remission

Diagnostic Criteria

A. A problematic pattern of opioid use leading to clinically significant impairment or distress, as manifested by at least two of the following, occurring within a 12-month period:
   1. Opioids are often taken in larger amounts or over a longer period than was intended.
   2. There is a persistent desire or unsuccessful efforts to cut down or control opioid use.
   3. A great deal of time is spent in activities necessary to obtain the opioid, use the opioid, or recover from its effects.
   4. Craving, or a strong desire or urge to use opioids.
   5. Recurrent opioid use resulting in a failure to fulfill major role obligations at work, school, or home.
   6. Continued opioid use despite having persistent or recurrent social or interpersonal problems caused or exacerbated by the effects of opioids.
   7. Important social, occupational, or recreational activities are given up or reduced because of opioid use.
   8. Recurrent opioid use in situations in which it is physically hazardous.
   9. Continued opioid use despite knowledge of having a persistent or recurrent physical or psychological problem that is likely to have been caused or exacerbated by the substance.

10. Tolerance, as defined by either of the following:
    a. A need for markedly increased amounts of opioids to achieve intoxication or desired effect.
    b. A markedly diminished effect with continued use of the same amount of an opioid.
        - **Note:** This criterion is not considered to be met for those taking opioids solely under appropriate medical supervision.
11. Withdrawal, as manifested by either of the following:
    a. The characteristic opioid withdrawal syndrome (refer to Criteria A and B of the criteria set for opioid withdrawal, pp. 547–548).
    b. Opioids (or a closely related substance) are taken to relieve or avoid withdrawal symptoms.
        - **Note:** This criterion is not considered to be met for those individuals taking opioids solely under appropriate medical supervision.

Specify if:

- **In early remission:** After full criteria for opioid use disorder were previously met, none of the criteria for opioid use disorder have been met for at least 3 months but for less than 12 months (with the exception that Criterion A4, "Craving, or a strong desire or urge to use opioids," may be met).
- **In sustained remission:** After full criteria for opioid use disorder were previously met, none of the criteria for opioid use disorder have been met at any time during a period of 12 months or longer (with the exception that Criterion A4, "Craving, or a strong desire or urge to use opioids," may be met).

Specify if:

- **On maintenance therapy:** This additional specifier is used if the individual is taking a prescribed agonist medication such as methadone or buprenorphine and none of the criteria for opioid use disorder have been met for that class of medication (except tolerance to, or withdrawal from, the agonist). This category also applies to those individuals being maintained on a partial agonist, an agonist/antagonist, or a full antagonist such as oral naltrexone or depot naltrexone.
- **In a controlled environment:** This additional specifier is used if the individual is in an environment where access to opioids is restricted.

Coding based on current severity: Note for *ICD-10-CM* codes: If an opioid intoxication, opioid withdrawal, or another opioid-induced mental disorder is also present, do not use the codes below for opioid use disorder. Instead, the comorbid opioid use disorder is indicated in the 4th character of the opioid-induced disorder code (see the coding note for opioid intoxication, opioid withdrawal, or a specific opioid-induced mental disorder). For example, if there is comorbid opioid-induced depressive disorder and opioid use disorder, only the opioid-induced depressive disorder code is given, with the 4th character indicating whether the comorbid opioid use disorder is mild, moderate, or severe: F11.14 for mild opioid use disorder with opioid-induced depressive disorder or F11.24 for a moderate or severe opioid use disorder with opioid-induced depressive disorder.

Specify current severity:

- **305.50 (F11.10) Mild:** Presence of two to three symptoms.
- **304.00 (F11.20) Moderate:** Presence of four to five symptoms.
- **304.00 (F11.20) Severe:** Presence of six or more symptoms.

(Reprinted with permission from the *Diagnostic and Statistical Manual of Mental Disorders*. 5th ed. Arlington, VA: American Psychiatric Publication; 2013.)

What is the rationale for the diagnosis?

The patient had a pattern of opioid use that led to significant impairment as evidenced by multiple hospital admissions and IOP programs for treatment. She has subsequently avoided any relapse for the past 3 years and therefore, the diagnosis also includes the specifier, in sustained remission.

Which diagnosis (or diagnoses) should be considered?

296.89 (F31.81) Bipolar II (Provisional).

Diagnostic Criteria
For a diagnosis of bipolar II disorder, it is necessary to meet the following criteria for a current or past hypomanic episode *and* the following criteria for a current or past major depressive episode (MDE):

Hypomanic Episode

A. A distinct period of abnormally and persistently elevated, expansive, or irritable mood and abnormally and persistently increased activity or energy, lasting at least 4 consecutive days and present most of the day, nearly every day.
B. During the period of mood disturbance and increased energy and activity, three (or more) of the following symptoms have persisted (four if the mood is only irritable), represent a noticeable change from usual behavior, and have been present to a significant degree:
   1. Inflated self-esteem or grandiosity.
   2. Decreased need for sleep (eg, feels rested after only 3 hours of sleep).
   3. More talkative than usual or pressure to keep talking.
   4. Flight of ideas or subjective experience that thoughts are racing.
   5. Distractibility (ie, attention too easily drawn to unimportant or irrelevant external stimuli), as reported or observed.

6. Increase in goal-directed activity (either socially, at work or school, or sexually) or psychomotor agitation.
7. Excessive involvement in activities that have a high potential for painful consequences (eg, engaging in unrestrained buying sprees, sexual indiscretions, or foolish business investments).

C. The episode is associated with an unequivocal change in functioning that is uncharacteristic of the individual when not symptomatic.

D. The disturbance in mood and the change in functioning are observable by others.

E. The episode is not severe enough to cause marked impairment in social or occupational functioning or to necessitate hospitalization. If there are psychotic features, the episode is, by definition, manic.

F. The episode is not attributable to the physiologic effects of a substance (eg, a drug of abuse, a medication, other treatment) or another medical condition.
   - **Note:** A full hypomanic episode that emerges during antidepressant treatment (eg, medication, electroconvulsive therapy) but persists at a fully syndromal level beyond the physiologic effect of that treatment is sufficient evidence for a hypomanic episode diagnosis. However, caution is indicated so that one or two symptoms (particularly increased irritability, edginess, or agitation following antidepressant use) are not taken as sufficient for diagnosis of a hypomanic episode, nor necessarily indicative of a bipolar diathesis.

Major Depressive Episode

A. Five (or more) of the following symptoms have been present during the same 2-week period and represent a change from previous functioning; at least one of the symptoms is either (1) depressed mood or (2) loss of interest or pleasure.
   - **Note:** Do not include symptoms that are clearly attributable to a medical condition.
     1. Depressed mood most of the day, nearly every day, as indicated by either subjective report (eg, feels sad, empty, or hopeless) or observation made by others (eg, appears tearful). (Note: In children and adolescents, can be irritable mood.)
     2. Markedly diminished interest or pleasure in all, or almost all, activities most of the day, nearly every day (as indicated by either subjective account or observation).
     3. Significant weight loss when not dieting or weight gain (eg, a change of more than 5% of body weight in a month), or decrease or increase in appetite nearly every day. (Note: In children, consider failure to make expected weight gain.)
     4. Insomnia or hypersomnia nearly every day.
     5. Psychomotor agitation or retardation nearly every day (observable by others; not merely subjective feelings of restlessness or being slowed down).

6. Fatigue or loss of energy nearly every day.
7. Feelings of worthlessness or excessive or inappropriate guilt (which may be delusional) nearly every day (not merely self-reproach or guilt about being sick).
8. Diminished ability to think or concentrate, or indecisiveness, nearly every day (either by subjective account or as observed by others).
9. Recurrent thoughts of death (not just fear of dying), recurrent suicidal ideation without a specific plan, a suicide attempt, or a specific plan for committing suicide.

B. The symptoms cause clinically significant distress or impairment in social, occupational, or other important areas of functioning.
C. The episode is not attributable to the physiologic effects of a substance or another medical condition.

Note: Criteria A to C above constitute an MDE.

Note: Responses to a significant loss (eg, bereavement, financial ruin, losses from a natural disaster, a serious medical illness or disability) may include the feelings of intense sadness, rumination about the loss, insomnia, poor appetite, and weight loss noted in Criterion A, which may resemble a depressive episode. Although such symptoms may be understandable or considered appropriate to the loss, the presence of an MDE in addition to the normal response to a significant loss should be carefully considered. This decision inevitably requires the exercise of clinical judgment based on the individual's history and the cultural norms for the expression of distress in the context of loss.

In distinguishing grief from an MDE, it is useful to consider that in grief the predominant affect is feelings of emptiness and loss, whereas in an MDE it is persistent depressed mood and the inability to anticipate happiness or pleasure. The dysphoria in grief is likely to decrease in intensity over days to weeks and occurs in waves, the so-called pangs of grief. These waves tend to be associated with thoughts or reminders of the deceased. The depressed mood of an MDE is more persistent and not tied to specific thoughts or preoccupations. The pain of grief may be accompanied by positive emotions and humor that are uncharacteristic of the pervasive unhappiness and misery characteristic of an MDE. The thought content associated with grief generally features a preoccupation with thoughts and memories of the deceased, rather than the self-critical or pessimistic ruminations seen in an MDE. In grief, self-esteem is generally preserved, whereas in an MDE feelings of worthlessness and self-loathing are common. If self-derogatory ideation is present in grief, it typically involves perceived failings vis-à-vis the deceased (eg, not visiting frequently enough, not telling the deceased how much he or she was loved). If a bereaved individual thinks about death and dying, such thoughts are generally focused on the deceased and possibly about "joining" the deceased, whereas in an MDE such thoughts are focused on ending one's own life because of feeling worthless, undeserving of life, or unable to cope with the pain of depression.

Bipolar II Disorder

A. Criteria have been met for at least one hypomanic episode (Criteria A to F under "Hypomanic Episode") and at least one MDE (Criteria A to C under "Major Depressive Episode").
B. There has never been a manic episode.
C. The occurrence of the hypomanic episode(s) and MDE(s) is not better explained by schizoaffective disorder, schizophrenia, schizophreniform disorder, delusional disorder, or other specified or unspecified schizophrenia spectrum and other psychotic disorder.
D. The symptoms of depression or the unpredictability caused by frequent alternation between periods of depression and hypomania cause clinically significant distress or impairment in social, occupational, or other important areas of functioning.

Coding and Recording Procedures

- Bipolar II disorder has one diagnostic code: 296.89 (F31.81). Its status with respect to current severity, presence of psychotic features, course, and other specifiers cannot be coded but should be indicated in writing (eg, 296.89 [F31.81] bipolar II disorder, current episode depressed, moderate severity, with mixed features; 296.89 [F31.81] bipolar II disorder, most recent episode depressed, in partial remission).

Specify **current or most recent episode:**

- **Hypomanic**
- **Depressed**

(Reprinted with permission from the *Diagnostic and Statistical Manual of Mental Disorders*. 5th ed. Arlington, VA: American Psychiatric Publication; 2013.)

What is the rationale for the diagnosis?

Although the patient does not currently exhibit any hypomanic/manic or depressive symptoms, she reports being diagnosed with bipolar II disorder and is treated with medications that would support this diagnosis.

What test or tools should be considered to help identify the correct diagnosis?

Video electroencephalogram (EEG) to R/O seizure activity.

Head computerized tomography (CT) to R/O any intracranial mass or bleeding possibly causing seizures (not always captured on video EEG).

Assess the context in which the seizure-like episode occurs (High stress? Precipitating factors?)

What differential diagnosis (or diagnoses) should be considered?

The following differentials should continue to be considered, but with the current clinical information, they do not meet the diagnostic criteria required.

ICD-10 (G40.909) Epilepsy, unspecified, not intractable, without status epilepticus
300.82 (F45.1) Somatic symptom disorder
300.19 (F68.10) Factitious disorder and malingering
300.14 (F44.81) Dissociative identity disorder
305.20 (F12.10) Cannabis use disorder, mild

FORMULATING THE TREATMENT STRATEGY

What treatment would you prescribe and what is the rationale?

Psychopharmacology: Verification of current medications can be completed by contacting the patient's pharmacy and accessing the prescription monitoring online system.

The patient should be continued on the medications she was prescribed prior to her hospitalization, which include lamotrigine 200 mg daily, gabapentin 300 mg TID, trazodone 50 mg nightly, sertraline 100 mg daily, lithium 300 mg BID and melatonin.

Sertraline (and venlafaxine) have been identified as helpful in the management of depression associated with psychogenic seizures. Lamotrigine and lithium are FDA approved to treat bipolar disorders. Gabapentin is used off-label to treat anxiety. Trazodone is used off-label to treat insomnia. Melatonin, which is available over-the-counter, is recommended for insomnia.

As the patient continues to be psychiatrically reassessed, adjustments to the medication regimen can be considered. However, as a rule, anticonvulsants such as lamotrigine and gabapentin should not be discontinued abruptly.

Diagnostic tests:

Video EEG
Head CT
Additional testing that may be recommended following neurology consult to rule out underlying neurologic disorder.

Referrals: Continued neurologic evaluation because 5% to 10% of adults with psychogenic seizures also have epilepsy.

Individual psychotherapy should be recommended.

Type of psychotherapy: Psychodynamic psychotherapy

This therapy is focused on developing insight and reducing symptoms associated with anxiety and unresolved interpersonal conflict. The goal is to relieve emotional distress and assist in the development of coping skills to deal with current and future stressful events.

Eye movement desensitization and reprocessing (EMDR) should be recommended since the patient's symptoms started with the trauma of sexual assault. EMDR is indicated for treatment of individual's who have PTSD.

Psychoeducation: Information about conversion disorder can be found at: https://medlineplus.gov/ency/article/000954.htm.

What standard guidelines would you use to treat or assess this patient?

None.

CLINICAL NOTE

- There is some controversy about whether conversion disorder is a form of dissociative disorder. Since dissociative disorder is generally viewed as a response to previous trauma, a thorough trauma history should be taken with any individual who presents with a conversion disorder.

REFERENCES/RECOMMENDED READINGS

American Psychiatric Association. *Diagnostic and Statistical Manual of Mental Disorders.* 5th ed. Arlington, VA: American Psychiatric Publishing; 2013.

Brown RJ, Cardeña E, Nijenhuis E, Sar V, van der Hart O. Should conversion disorder be reclassified as a dissociative disorder in DSM–V? *Psychosomatics*. 2007;48(5):369-378.

Gates J, Rowan AJ, eds. *Non-epileptic Seizures*. 2nd ed. Boston, MA: Butterworth-Heinemann; 2000.

Saddock BJ, Saddock VA. *Synopsis of Psychiatry: Behavioral Sciences/Clinical Psychiatry*. Philadelphia, PA: Lippincott Williams & Wilkins; 2007.

Smith BJ. Closing the major gap in PNES research: finding a home for a borderland disorder. *Epilepsy Currents*. 2014;14(2):63-67.

Stahl S. *The Prescriber's Guide: Essential Psychopharmacology*. New York, NY: Cambridge University Press; 2011.

Trauma-Informed Approach and Trauma-Specific Interventions. 2015. Available at: https://www.samhsa.gov/nctic/trauma-interventions.

CASE 28

Back in School and Cannot Focus

IDENTIFICATION: The patient is a 28-year-old single Hispanic female who is self-referred for a psychiatric evaluation at an outpatient psychiatric office.

CHIEF COMPLAINT: "I can't concentrate. I cry when I think I won't be able to graduate."

HISTORY OF CHIEF COMPLAINT: The patient is planning to enroll in nursing school and is struggling academically. She is attending prerequisite courses for nursing school at a community college. She delayed going to college because she thought she would not be able to graduate. She says she cannot manage more than one class at a time. She reports that she has a bad memory and cannot remember anything. When she reads assignments, she cannot comprehend the information initially and has to read it over many times. She says she loses keys and other items very frequently. She says she has a "bad temper." The patient reports that she procrastinates and is always tired. She has always had a hard time focusing in school and is easily bored. The patient is constantly worried about whether she will be able to graduate from college.

PAST PSYCHIATRIC HISTORY: The patient says she has felt tired for "as long as I can remember." Reports always feeling emotional over everything but more so after the birth of her daughter. After her daughter was born, the patient cried excessively and felt like her daughter was in constant danger. She realized later that she probably had postpartum depression.

She has flashbacks to sexual abuse she experienced when she was 12 years old. She worries about her daughter being exposed to a similar situation. She is hypervigilant about whoever her daughter is with. She feels like she has to constantly look over her shoulder.

No history of psychiatric treatment, other than seeing a school counselor because she felt under a lot of stress due to her home environment. No psychiatric medication or suicide attempts.

MEDICAL HISTORY: No known drug allergies. History of hepatitis A. Regular menses and has an intrauterine device for contraception. Had one full-term pregnancy 6 years ago. No surgeries. Appetite is good. Reports long-standing difficulty getting to sleep.

HISTORY OF DRUG OR ALCOHOL ABUSE: Denies.

FAMILY HISTORY: The patient's father was an "alcoholic." She repeatedly witnessed domestic violence toward her mother by her father. The domestic violence stopped 10 years ago when her father stopped drinking alcohol. At age 10 the patient became the caretaker of her younger sister due to her mother's long hours at work. The patient lives near her parents and has frequent contact with them.

PERSONAL HISTORY

Perinatal: Full-term vaginal birth. No known complications.

Childhood: Had trouble focusing in school. Never evaluated for any learning disorders.

Adolescence: Saw a school counselor because she felt under a lot of stress due to her home environment. Made friends easily at school. Barely passed most of her classes in high school. Identifies as heterosexual.

Adulthood: Has a boyfriend who is very supportive. Is currently enrolled in a community college and struggling academically even though she is quite motivated. She identifies as Hispanic and Catholic. She does not currently attend mass but considers herself a spiritual person. Was working recently as a sales associate. Had some traffic violations for speeding and careless driving in the past.

TRAUMA/ABUSE HISTORY: Was sexually abused on two occasions by an older male cousin when she was 12 years old. Sometimes has flashbacks about it, especially when she has to leave her daughter with a caretaker.

MENTAL STATUS EXAMINATION

Appearance: Casual, neat, and clean. Cooperative.

Behavior and psychomotor activity: Good eye contact.

Consciousness: Alert.

Orientation: Oriented to person, place, and time.

Memory: Recent, intact, remote: able to name the past four presidents.

Concentration and attention: When subtracting serial 3′s from 100 said "98, 96, 93, 80." Then she was asked to do the calculations on paper and was able to do them accurately. Her handwriting was very neat and organized.

Visuospatial ability: Not assessed.

Abstract thought: Able to interpret simple proverb "What goes around comes around." When asked to describe similarities between an orange and a grapefruit, she said they have seeds and grow on trees, which reflects a more concrete interpretation.

Intellectual functioning: Average.

Speech and language: Articulate. Normal rate and volume.

Perceptions: No hallucinations, delusions, depersonalization, or derealization.

Thought processes: Logical and coherent.

Thought content: Worries about failing classes at school.

Suicidality or homicidality: Denied.

Mood: "Anxious."

Affect: Although the patient reported that she cries a lot at home and is weepy and emotional, her mood was stable during the interview. She was able to laugh appropriately. No sign of depression. Her affect seemed in the normal range.

Impulse control: Good.

Judgment/insight/reliability: Good/good/good.

FORMULATING THE DIAGNOSIS

Which diagnosis (or diagnoses) should be considered?

314.00 (F90.0) Attention-Deficit/Hyperactivity Disorder, Predominantly Inattentive Presentation, Moderate

Diagnostic Criteria

A. A persistent pattern of inattention and/or hyperactivity–impulsivity that interferes with functioning or development, as characterized by (1) and/or (2):
   1. **Inattention:** Six (or more) of the following symptoms have persisted for at least 6 months to a degree that is inconsistent with developmental level and that negatively impacts directly on social and academic/occupational activities:
      - **Note:** The symptoms are not solely a manifestation of oppositional behavior, defiance, hostility, or failure to understand tasks or instructions. For older adolescents and adults (age 17 and older), at least five symptoms are required.
        a. Often fails to give close attention to details or makes careless mistakes in schoolwork, at work, or during other activities (eg, overlooks or misses details, work is inaccurate).
        b. Often has difficulty sustaining attention in tasks or play activities (eg, has difficulty remaining focused during lectures, conversations, or lengthy reading).
        c. Often does not seem to listen when spoken to directly (eg, mind seems elsewhere, even in the absence of any obvious distraction).
        d. Often does not follow through on instructions and fails to finish schoolwork, chores, or duties in the workplace (eg, starts tasks but quickly loses focus and is easily sidetracked).
        e. Often has difficulty organizing tasks and activities (eg, difficulty managing sequential tasks; difficulty keeping materials and belongings in order; messy, disorganized work; has poor time management; fails to meet deadlines).

f. Often avoids, dislikes, or is reluctant to engage in tasks that require sustained mental effort (eg, schoolwork or homework; for older adolescents and adults, preparing reports, completing forms, reviewing lengthy papers).
g. Often loses things necessary for tasks or activities (eg, school materials, pencils, books, tools, wallets, keys, paperwork, eyeglasses, mobile phones).
h. Is often easily distracted by extraneous stimuli (for older adolescents and adults, may include unrelated thoughts).
i. Is often forgetful in daily activities (eg, doing chores, running errands; for older adolescents and adults, returning calls, paying bills, keeping appointments).

2. **Hyperactivity and impulsivity:** Six (or more) of the following symptoms have persisted for at least 6 months to a degree that is inconsistent with developmental level and that negatively impacts directly on social and academic/occupational activities:
   - **Note:** The symptoms are not solely a manifestation of oppositional behavior, defiance, hostility, or a failure to understand tasks or instructions. For older adolescents and adults (age 17 and older), at least five symptoms are required.

     a. Often fidgets with or taps hands or feet or squirms in seat.
     b. Often leaves seat in situations when remaining seated is expected (eg, leaves his or her place in the classroom, in the office or other workplace, or in other situations that require remaining in place).
     c. Often runs about or climbs in situations where it is inappropriate. (**Note:** In adolescents or adults, may be limited to feeling restless.)
     d. Often unable to play or engage in leisure activities quietly.
     e. Is often "on the go," acting as if "driven by a motor" (eg, is unable to be or uncomfortable being still for extended time, as in restaurants, meetings; may be experienced by others as being restless or difficult to keep up with).
     f. Often talks excessively.
     g. Often blurts out an answer before a question has been completed (eg, completes people's sentences; cannot wait for turn in conversation).
     h. Often has difficulty waiting his or her turn (eg, while waiting in line).
     i. Often interrupts or intrudes on others (eg, butts into conversations, games, or activities; may start using other people's things without asking or receiving permission; for adolescents and adults, may intrude into or take over what others are doing).

B. Several inattentive or hyperactive–impulsive symptoms were present prior to age 12 years.

C. Several inattentive or hyperactive–impulsive symptoms are present in two or more settings (eg, at home, school, or work; with friends or relatives; in other activities).
D. There is clear evidence that the symptoms interfere with, or reduce the quality of, social, academic, or occupational functioning.
E. The symptoms do not occur exclusively during the course of schizophrenia or another psychotic disorder and are not better explained by another mental disorder (eg, mood disorder, anxiety disorder, dissociative disorder, personality disorder, substance intoxication, or withdrawal).

Specify whether:

- **314.01 (F90.2) Combined presentation:** If both Criterion A1 (inattention) and Criterion A2 (hyperactivity–impulsivity) are met for the past 6 months.
- **314.00 (F90.0) Predominantly inattentive presentation:** If Criterion A1 (inattention) is met but Criterion A2 (hyperactivity–impulsivity) is not met for the past 6 months.
- **314.01 (F90.1) Predominantly hyperactive/impulsive presentation:** If Criterion A2 (hyperactivity–impulsivity) is met and Criterion A1 (inattention) is not met for the past 6 months.

Specify if:

- **In partial remission:** When full criteria were previously met, fewer than the full criteria have been met for the past 6 months, and the symptoms still result in impairment in social, academic, or occupational functioning.

Specify current severity:

- **Mild:** Few, if any, symptoms in excess of those required to make the diagnosis are present, and symptoms result in no more than minor impairments in social or occupational functioning.
- **Moderate:** Symptoms or functional impairment between "mild" and "severe" are present.
- **Severe:** Many symptoms in excess of those required to make the diagnosis, or several symptoms that are particularly severe, are present, or the symptoms result in marked impairment in social or occupational functioning.

(Reprinted with permission from the *Diagnostic and Statistical Manual of Mental Disorders*. 5th ed. Arlington, VA: American Psychiatric Publishing; 2013.)

What is the rationale for the diagnosis?

The patient reported a pattern of inattention characterized by the following: not able to give close attention to details (has to read over and over to understand), had difficulty sustaining attention ("I get bored easily"), loses things necessary for tasks ("lose my keys and other items"), has difficulty finishing schoolwork, is often forgetful ("I have trouble remembering things"), and avoids tasks that require sustained attention (avoided going to college because she did not think she could manage the assignments). The symptoms were present prior to the age of 12. The inattention is present at home and school. The symptoms clearly interfere with her ability to function academically. The symptoms are not better explained by another mental disorder. The patient did have sexual abuse at the age of 12, which may have contributed to symptoms associated with posttraumatic stress disorder (PTSD) and which could impact concentration and memory. However, according to her history, she experienced difficulty academically prior to that time. Therefore, the diagnosis of Attention Deficit Hyperactivity Disorder, Predominantly inattentive presentation is applicable.

Which diagnosis (or diagnoses) should be considered?

309.81 (F43.10) Posttraumatic Stress Disorder

Diagnostic Criteria

Note: The following criteria apply to adults, adolescents, and children older than 6 years. For children 6 years and younger, see corresponding criteria below.

A. Exposure to actual or threatened death, serious injury, or sexual violence in one (or more) of the following ways:
   1. Directly experiencing the traumatic event(s).
   2. Witnessing, in person, the event(s) as it occurred to others.
   3. Learning that the traumatic event(s) occurred to a close family member or close friend. In cases of actual or threatened death of a family member or friend, the event(s) must have been violent or accidental.
   4. Experiencing repeated or extreme exposure to aversive details of the traumatic event(s) (eg, first responders collecting human remains; police officers repeatedly exposed to details of child abuse).
      - **Note:** Criterion A4 does not apply to exposure through electronic media, television, movies, or pictures, unless this exposure is work related.

B. Presence of one (or more) of the following intrusion symptoms associated with the traumatic event(s), beginning after the traumatic event(s) occurred:
   1. Recurrent, involuntary, and intrusive distressing memories of the traumatic event(s).
      - **Note:** In children older than 6 years, repetitive play may occur in which themes or aspects of the traumatic event(s) are expressed.
   2. Recurrent distressing dreams in which the content and/or affect of the dream is related to the traumatic event(s).
      - **Note:** In children, there may be frightening dreams without recognizable content.

3. Dissociative reactions (eg, flashbacks) in which the individual feels or acts as if the traumatic event(s) were recurring. (Such reactions may occur on a continuum, with the most extreme expression being a complete loss of awareness of present surroundings.)
   - **Note:** In children, trauma-specific reenactment may occur in play.
4. Intense or prolonged psychological distress at exposure to internal or external cues that symbolize or resemble an aspect of the traumatic event(s).
5. Marked physiologic reactions to internal or external cues that symbolize or resemble an aspect of the traumatic event(s).

C. Persistent avoidance of stimuli associated with the traumatic event(s), beginning after the traumatic event(s) occurred, as evidenced by one or both of the following:
   1. Avoidance of or efforts to avoid distressing memories, thoughts, or feelings about or closely associated with the traumatic event(s).
   2. Avoidance of or efforts to avoid external reminders (people, places, conversations, activities, objects, situations) that arouse distressing memories, thoughts, or feelings about or closely associated with the traumatic event(s).

D. Negative alterations in cognitions and mood associated with the traumatic event(s), beginning or worsening after the traumatic event(s) occurred, as evidenced by two (or more) of the following:
   1. Inability to remember an important aspect of the traumatic event(s) (typically due to dissociative amnesia and not to other factors such as head injury, alcohol, or drugs).
   2. Persistent and exaggerated negative beliefs or expectations about oneself, others, or the world (eg, "I am bad," "No one can be trusted," "The world is completely dangerous," "My whole nervous system is permanently ruined").
   3. Persistent, distorted cognitions about the cause or consequences of the traumatic event(s) that lead the individual to blame himself/herself or others.
   4. Persistent negative emotional state (eg, fear, horror, anger, guilt, or shame).
   5. Markedly diminished interest or participation in significant activities.
   6. Feelings of detachment or estrangement from others.
   7. Persistent inability to experience positive emotions (eg, inability to experience happiness, satisfaction, or loving feelings).

E. Marked alterations in arousal and reactivity associated with the traumatic event(s), beginning or worsening after the traumatic event(s) occurred, as evidenced by two (or more) of the following:
   1. Irritable behavior and angry outbursts (with little or no provocation) typically expressed as verbal or physical aggression toward people or objects.
   2. Reckless or self-destructive behavior.

3. Hypervigilance.
4. Exaggerated startle response.
5. Problems with concentration.
6. Sleep disturbance (eg, difficulty falling or staying asleep or restless sleep).

F. Duration of the disturbance (Criteria B to E) is more than 1 month.

G. The disturbance causes clinically significant distress or impairment in social, occupational, or other important areas of functioning.

H. The disturbance is not attributable to the physiologic effects of a substance (eg, medication, alcohol) or another medical condition.

Specify whether:

- **With dissociative symptoms:** The individual's symptoms meet the criteria for PTSD, and the individual experiences persistent or recurrent symptoms of either of the following:
  1. **Depersonalization:** Persistent or recurrent experiences of feeling detached from, and as if one were an outside observer of, one's mental processes or body (eg, feeling as though one were in a dream; feeling a sense of unreality of self or body or of time moving slowly).
  2. **Derealization:** Persistent or recurrent experiences of unreality of surroundings (eg, the world around the individual is experienced as unreal, dream-like, distant, or distorted).
     - **Note:** To use this subtype, the dissociative symptoms must not be attributable to the physiologic effects of a substance (eg, blackouts) or another medical condition (eg, complex partial seizures).

Specify if:

- **With delayed expression:** If the full diagnostic criteria are not met until at least 6 months after the event (although the onset and expression of some symptoms may be immediate).

(Reprinted with permission from the *Diagnostic and Statistical Manual of Mental Disorders*. 5th ed. Arlington, VA: American Psychiatric Publishing; 2013.)

What is the rationale for the diagnosis?

The patient witnessed physical abuse by her father to her mother. There are probably residual disturbances related to this trauma, but the patient mainly reports symptoms related to the sexual abuse she experienced at the age of 12. She experiences intrusive memories of the event and dissociative reactions (flashbacks), persistent avoidance of stimuli (tries to avoid having her daughter be under someone else's care), negative alteration in cognition or mood associated with the event (does not believe her daughter will be safe without her), is hypervigilant (feels like she always has to look over her shoulder and has sleep disturbance). These disturbances have occurred for more than 1 month and cause clinically significant distress. The disturbance is not attributable to the physiologic effects of a substance. Therefore, the criteria for the diagnosis of PTSD are met.

What test or tools should be considered to help identify the correct diagnosis?

Adult ADHD Tool Kit: Assessment Tools.
Available at: http://naceonline.com/AdultADHDtoolkit/assessmenttools/assessmenttoolssection-1.pdf

What differential diagnosis (or diagnoses) should be considered?

None indicated.

FORMULATING THE TREATMENT STRATEGY

What treatment would you prescribe and what is the rationale?

Psychopharmacology: Lisdexamfetamine dimesylate 30 mg in AM.

Lisdexamfetamine dimesylate is a CNS stimulant that is FDA approved to treat attention deficit hyperactivity disorder (ADHD) in children (6 years and older) and adults. The typical starting dose is 30 mg in the AM.

Prazosin 1 mg HS. The dose can be titrated to 4 mg HS. Prazosin antagonizes peripheral alpha-1 adrenergic receptors. It is FDA approved as an antihypertensive. However, it is also used off-label to treat nightmares and sleep disturbances associated with PTSD.

Diagnostic Tests: None indicated as the patient had recently had a complete medical workup and results were WNL. The patient denied any history of cardiac conditions and denied incidents of sudden deaths with any of her relatives. If the patient had any history of cardiac conditions or any family history of sudden deaths, an EKG would be ordered along with a consultation with her primary care provider and/or cardiologist regarding the safety of prescribing a psychostimulant.

Monitor blood pressure because stimulants can increase blood pressure and heart rate, whereas prazosin may decrease blood pressure.

Observe the patient for any numbness, skin color changes, or sensitivity to temperature in her hands and feet as it may indicate Raynaud's phenomenon, which is a potential adverse effect of lisdexamfetamine dimesylate. These signs would indicate the need for a medical referral.

Referrals: Refer to trauma-focused psychotherapist because the patient experiences disturbances related to the history of sexual abuse. Therefore, therapy to address these symptoms is indicated.

Type of Psychotherapy: Trauma-focused psychotherapy. Trauma-focused therapy uses a variety of techniques to help dispel feelings experienced due to trauma mainly through cognitive restructuring techniques.

Psychoeducation: The patient should be educated about ADHD. She can be referred to CHADD at: http://www.chadd.org/understanding-adhd/for-adults.aspx

Techniques to improve organization and increase retention of new information should be reviewed with the patient (eg, making lists, avoid distractions when studying, using apps on phone as reminders).

The patient should be informed of the risks/benefits of lisdexamfetamine dimesylate. She should be advised to take it in the AM because the medication may contribute to insomnia if taken later in the day. Advise the patient to take adequate nutrition and fluids as this medication may suppress appetite.

The patient should be advised to use contraceptives as lisdexamfetamine dimesylate is not recommended for use during pregnancy.

What standard guidelines would you use to treat or assess this patient?

Clinician's Guide to Medications for PTSD from the U.S. Department of Veterans Affairs can be accessed at: http://www.ptsd.va.gov/professional/treatment/overview/clinicians-guide-to-medications-for-ptsd.asp

CLINICAL NOTE

- Adult ADHD can contribute to other disorders such as depression and anxiety. Individuals with ADHD may experience a lot of frustration if they cannot understand why they are not functioning as well as their peers. They may frequently be told that they are not living up to their potential or they need to try harder.

REFERENCES/RECOMMENDED READINGS

American Psychiatric Association. *Diagnostic and Statistical Manual of Mental Disorders.* 5th ed. Arlington, VA: American Psychiatric Publishing; 2013.

Koola MM, Varghese SP, Fawcett JA. High-dose prazosin for the treatment of post-traumatic stress disorder. *Ther Adv Psychopharmacol.* 2014;4(1):43-47. doi:10.1177/2045125313500982

Paloyelis Y, Mehta MA, Kuntsi J, Asherson P. Functional magnetic resonance imaging in attention deficit hyperactivity disorder (ADHD): a systematic literature review. *Exp Rev Neurotherapeut.* 2007;7(10):1337-1356. doi:10.1586/14737175.7.10.1337

CASE 29

Feeling more Anxious and Obsessive-Compulsive Disorder Is Worse

IDENTIFICATION: The patient is a 29-year-old, single, white female who works as a registered nurse and lives with her family. The patient is self-referred to a private psychiatric outpatient office.

CHIEF COMPLAINT: "Increasing anxiety and obsessive-compulsive disorder (OCD)."

HISTORY OF CHIEF COMPLAINT: The patient reports feeling overwhelmed and "lost," has lack of energy, and a lack of interest in things she used to enjoy. She is tired all the time. She has been dealing with OCD for most of her life, but it has become increasingly harder to manage. She is checking the stove and the doors more compulsively. Whenever she drives over a bump in the road she has to go around the block and return to the site to make sure she did not run over someone. Subsequently, she has been getting to work late. Other than driving to work she has been avoiding driving. This has contributed to her becoming socially isolated. Additionally, she has obsessional fears that someone she loves is going to die.

PAST PSYCHIATRIC HISTORY: The patient reports that she was anxious as a child and used to engage in compulsive behaviors. She would repeatedly check the doors at night to make sure they were locked. She saw a counselor while in high school because she was extremely anxious. She was seen by a psychiatrist who prescribed sertraline. The sertraline made her feel "uncomfortable" so she was switched to fluvoxamine and then later to fluoxetine. She does not know the reason the medication was switched. She thought she was doing fine so last year she stopped the medication. She was never hospitalized and denies any suicidal or self-injurious behaviors.

MEDICAL HISTORY: History of a tonsillectomy at 9 years. History of multiple strep throat infections. Menses is regular. No birth control. Denies being sexually active.

HISTORY OF DRUG OR ALCOHOL ABUSE: Denied.

FAMILY HISTORY: The patient was raised in an intact family and reports a close relationship with all her family members. Her older sister was treated for depression. She describes her grandmother repeatedly waking her up to make sure she was OK whenever she stayed at her house. The patient thought this behavior probably represented some form of compulsivity, although the grandmother was never treated. No other known psychiatric or medical conditions in the family.

PERSONAL HISTORY

Perinatal: Full-term vaginal birth. No complications.

Childhood: Anxious as a child. Engaged in frequent compulsive behaviors, including repeated checking.

Adolescence: Started seeing a counselor when she was in high school because of excessive anxiety.

Adulthood: The patient identifies as heterosexual. She reports having many friends. She likes her work in the hospital. Until recently when she began isolating herself, she saw many of her coworkers socially. No military or legal history.

TRAUMA/ABUSE HISTORY: Denied.

MENTAL STATUS EXAMINATION

Appearance: Well groomed. Average height and weight.

Behavior and psychomotor activity: Good eye contact. Cooperative. No motor abnormalities.

Consciousness:	Alert.
Orientation:	Times three.
Memory:	Intact.

Concentration and attention: Good.

Visuospatial ability: Not assessed.

Abstract thought: Present.

Intellectual functioning: Average or above.

Speech and language: Normal rate and volume.

Perceptions: No abnormalities apparent.

Thought processes: Goal directed.

Thought content: Obsesses about fear that people she loves are going to die. Obsessive thoughts about running over people when driving. Denies any suicidal or homicidal ideation.

Mood: Anxious.

Affect: Congruent to mood.

Impulse control: Good.

Judgment/insight/reliability: Good.

FORMULATING THE DIAGNOSIS

Which diagnosis should be considered?

300.3 (F42.2) Obsessive-Compulsive Disorder, with Good Insight.

Diagnostic Criteria

A. Presence of obsessions, compulsions, or both:
- Obsessions are defined by (1) and (2):
  1. Recurrent and persistent thoughts, urges, or images that are experienced, at some time during the disturbance, as intrusive and unwanted, and that in most individuals cause marked anxiety or distress.
  2. The individual attempts to ignore or suppress such thoughts, urges, or images, or to neutralize them with some other thought or action (ie, by performing a compulsion).

- Compulsions are defined by (1) and (2):
  3. Repetitive behaviors (eg, hand washing, ordering, checking) or mental acts (eg, praying, counting, repeating words silently) that the individual feels driven to perform in response to an obsession or according to rules that must be applied rigidly.
  4. The behaviors or mental acts are aimed at preventing or reducing anxiety or distress, or preventing some dreaded event or situation; however, these behaviors or mental acts are not connected in a realistic way with what they are designed to neutralize or prevent, or are clearly excessive.
     - **Note:** Young children may not be able to articulate the aims of these behaviors or mental acts.

B. The obsessions or compulsions are time-consuming (eg, take more than 1 hour per day) or cause clinically significant distress or impairment in social, occupational, or other important areas of functioning.

C. The obsessive-compulsive symptoms are not attributable to the physiologic effects of a substance (eg, a drug of abuse, a medication) or another medical condition.

D. The disturbance is not better explained by the symptoms of another mental disorder (eg, excessive worries, as in generalized anxiety disorder; preoccupation with appearance, as in body dysmorphic disorder; difficulty discarding or parting with possessions, as in hoarding disorder; hair pulling, as in trichotillomania [hair-pulling disorder]; skin picking, as in excoriation [skin-picking] disorder; stereotypies, as in stereotypic movement disorder; ritualized eating behavior, as in eating disorders; preoccupation with substances or gambling, as in substance-related and addictive disorders; preoccupation with having an illness, as in illness anxiety disorder; sexual urges or fantasies, as in paraphilic disorders; impulses, as in disruptive, impulse-control, and conduct disorders; guilty ruminations, as in major depressive disorder; thought insertion or delusional preoccupations, as in schizophrenia spectrum and other psychotic disorders; or repetitive patterns of behavior, as in autism spectrum disorder).

Specify if:

- **With good or fair insight:** The individual recognizes that OCD beliefs are definitely or probably not true or that they may or may not be true.
- **With poor insight:** The individual thinks OCD beliefs are probably true.
- **With absent insight/delusional beliefs:** The individual is completely convinced that OCD beliefs are true.

Specify if:

- **Tic-related:** The individual has a current or past history of a tic disorder.

(Reprinted with permission from the *Diagnostic and Statistical Manual of Mental Disorders*. 5th ed. Arlington, VA: American Psychiatric Publishing; 2013.)

What is your rationale for the diagnosis?

This patient has persistent thoughts of running over someone in her car which she tries to ignore. The thoughts are intrusive and are causing marked anxiety. She compulsively keeps driving over the same spot to make sure she did not run over someone. These repetitive behaviors are aimed at reducing anxiety or preventing or identifying a dreaded event. The obsessions and compulsions are time consuming and interfering with her ability to get to work and other events on time. She recognizes that her compulsions are part of her OCD and she is seeking treatment for them. Therefore, she meets the criteria for OCD with good insight.

What tests or tools should be considered to help identify the correct diagnosis?

The Florida Obsessive-Compulsive Inventory can be used to identify obsessive-compulsive symptoms. Follow-up evaluations using the Florida Obsessive-Compulsive Inventory can help evaluate the effectiveness of treatment (see Appendix).

What differential diagnosis should be considered?

None indicated.

FORMULATING THE TREATMENT STRATEGY

What treatment would you prescribe and what is the rationale?

Psychopharmacology: Fluvoxamine 50 mg daily. If tolerated increase by 50 mg every 2 weeks until asymptomatic or symptoms are manageable. The dose may need to be as high as 200 to 300 mg daily.

Fluvoxamine is FDA approved for the treatment of OCD. The gold standard for the treatment of OCD is either clomipramine or selective serotonin reuptake inhibitors. Doses for OCD usually need to be higher than for treatment of depression.

Diagnostic Tests: In addition to the routine laboratory tests, a Lyme titer, an Epstein-Barr virus antibody test, erythrocyte sedimentation rate (ESR), and an antinuclear antibody test (ANA) were are ordered.

These laboratory tests are ordered to rule out any medical comorbidity that may be contributing to her complaint of excessive tiredness.

Referral: Referral to a cognitive behavioral therapy (CBT) specialist may be helpful. Referral to a primary care provider may be indicated if patient's fatigue continues.

Psychotherapy: The combination of CBT with medication to treat OCD is more effective than medication alone. Identifying stressors and developing better coping skills may also help reduce OCD symptoms.

Psychoeducation Tools: The patient should be provided with literature available from the NIMH or another educational source about OCD. Understanding that OCD is more common than generally realized can possibly help reduce stigma and promote better understanding of treatment and expectations.

Using workbooks about OCD may be valuable with this population for understanding symptoms and treatment.

What standard guidelines would you use to treat or assess this patient?

"Practice guideline for the Treatment of Patient with Obsessive-compulsive Disorder" can be retrieved at: http://psychiatryonline.org/pb/assets/raw/sitewide/practice_guidelines/guidelines/ocd.pdf

CLINICAL NOTE

- If acute OCD symptoms are noted in a young child, the possibility of Pediatric Acute-onset Neuropsychiatric Syndrome (PANS) should be considered and a specialist should be consulted.

REFERENCES/RECOMMENDED READINGS

American Psychiatric Association. *Diagnostic and Statistical Manual of Mental Disorders.* 5th ed. Arlington, VA: American Psychiatric Publishing; 2013.

Hesser TS. *Kissing Doorknobs*: New York, NY: Laurel Leaf; 2010.

Hyman BM, Pedrick C. *The OCD Workbook: Your Guide to Breaking Free from Obsessive-Compulsive Disorder*. Oakland, CA: New Harbinger Publications; 2010.

Swedo SE, Leckman JF, Rose NR. From research subgroup to clinical syndrome: modifying the PANDAS criteria to describe PANS (Pediatric Acute-Onset Neuropsychiatric Syndrome). *Pediatr Ther.* 2012.

CASE 30

Unsteady after Being on Risperidone

IDENTIFICATION: The patient is a 29-year-old, single, African-American female accompanied by her middle-aged adoptive brother who is her guardian. Her previous psychiatric prescriber has retired. She is being evaluated in an outpatient mental health clinic. This is the third time she is being seen by this practitioner.

CHIEF COMPLAINT: The guardian explains that the patient needs risperidone to be reordered. He also reports that she is very unsteady on her feet.

HISTORY OF CHIEF COMPLAINT: The patient was started on risperidone 0.5 mg BID 6 months ago by her previous psychiatric provider for aggressive behavior, scratching and biting workers at her day program. After starting the risperidone, she was able to interact more appropriately at her day program without any aggressive behavior. Her guardian is concerned now because she is unsteady when walking; he reports that she has to hold onto the walls.

PAST PSYCHIATRIC HISTORY: No known history of hospitalizations, or suicidal attempts. She was diagnosed with CHARGE syndrome and has had a series of guardians. She is currently in a supervised day and work program. Limited history was obtained due to the guardian's lack of information and the patient's inability to communicate effectively.

MEDICAL HISTORY

Diagnosed with CHARGE syndrome according to the patient's guardian.

Prescribed metformin, unknown dosage. Her caretaker reports that her blood sugar is within normal limits.

Height 4′8″, weight, 120 lb.

HISTORY OF DRUG OR ALCOHOL ABUSE: None.

FAMILY HISTORY: The patient was adopted as an infant by an African-American family. The adoptive mother died when the patient was 16 years old. An adoptive sibling took care of the patient until 3 years ago when the sibling passed away. The patient is now under the care of her other adoptive sibling who is her guardian.

PERSONAL HISTORY

Perinatal: Information not known as patient was adopted as an infant.

Childhood: Information not known by the guardian.

Adolescence: The patient's adoptive mother died, and the patient was taken care of by her sibling.

Adulthood: The patient has limited intellectual capacity and requires full assistance with activities of daily living (ADLs).

TRAUMA/ABUSE HISTORY: None known.

MENTAL STATUS EXAMINATION

Appearance: Well groomed, small stature, tilts her head to the left. Smiling.

Behavior and psychomotor activity: Cooperative. Leans forward when walking with short shuffling steps. At the previous two visits, the patient's gait was normal.

Consciousness: Alert.

Orientation: Not oriented to time or place but responds to her name. Knows that it is the Christmas season and that it is raining outside. Repeats comments in a perseverative manner.

Memory: Remembers this writer's name. Able to state the name of limited objects in the room.

Concentration and attention: The patient is easily distracted by objects in the room.

Visuospatial ability:	Not assessed.
Abstract thought:	Not evident.
Intellectual functioning:	Severe to moderate intellectual impairment. Able to follow simple commands.
Speech and language:	Spontaneous. Able to form short sentences but most responses are only one word. Slightly loud.
Perception:	No evidence of any abnormalities.
Thought processes:	Perseverative about raining outside.
Thought content:	Says repeatedly "It's raining outside."
Suicidality and homicidality:	None.
Mood:	Euthymic.
Affect:	Congruent.
Impulsive control:	Interrupts when others are speaking but responds to redirection.
Judgment/Insight/Reliability:	All are limited by her intellectual capacity.

FORMULATING THE DIAGNOSIS

Which diagnosis should be considered?

318.1 (F72) Intellectual Disability (Intellectual Developmental Disorder), Severe

Diagnostic Criteria

Intellectual disability (intellectual developmental disorder) is a disorder with onset during the developmental period that includes both intellectual and adaptive functioning deficits in conceptual, social, and practical domains. The following three criteria must be met:

A. Deficits in intellectual functions, such as reasoning, problem solving, planning, abstract thinking, judgment, academic learning, and learning from experience, confirmed by both clinical assessment and individualized, standardized intelligence testing.

B. Deficits in adaptive functioning that result in failure to meet developmental and sociocultural standards for personal independence and social responsibility. Without ongoing support, the adaptive deficits limit functioning in one or more activities of daily life, such as communication, social participation, and independent living, across multiple environments, such as home, school, work, and community.
C. Onset of intellectual and adaptive deficits during the developmental period.

Note: The diagnostic term *intellectual disability* is the equivalent term for the *ICD-11* diagnosis of *intellectual developmental disorders.* Although the term *intellectual disability* is used throughout this manual, both terms are used in the title to clarify relationships with other classification systems. Moreover, a federal statute in the United States (Public Law 111-256, Rosa's Law) replaces the term *mental retardation* with *intellectual disability,* and research journals use the term *intellectual disability.* Thus, *intellectual disability* is the term in common use by medical, educational, and other professions and by the lay public and advocacy groups.

Specify current severity:
- **317 (F70) Mild**
- **318.0 (F71) Moderate**
- **318.1 (F72) Severe**
- **318.2 (F73) Profound**

(Reprinted with permission from the *Diagnostic and Statistical Manual of Mental Disorders.* 5th ed. Arlington, VA: American Psychiatric Publishing; 2013.)

What is your rationale for the diagnosis?

The levels of severity of intellectual disability are not defined by IQ scores but by the individual's adaptive functioning. This patient meets the criteria for severe impairment because of the following: In the conceptual domain she has little understanding of written language, numbers, quantity of time, or money and her caretaker provides most support for any problem solving for her. In the social domain, her language is limited and her speech includes predominantly one-word or one-phrase responses. She finds pleasure engaging with others. In the practical domain she requires support for all her ADLs and requires supervision at all times.

Concurrent diagnosis: Q89.8 CHARGE syndrome is reported by caretaker. It is presumed that genetic testing was completed in order to specifically identify this genetic disorder. Previous medical records would need to be obtained to verify this diagnosis. This condition has significant implications for cognitive functioning and physical health.

What tests or tools should be considered to help identify the correct diagnosis?

A thorough psychiatric examination with a Mental Status Exam was sufficient to diagnose this patient with Intellectual Disability. If the patient was higher functioning and there was some question about her intellectual abilities, a Montreal Cognitive Assessment (MoCA) could be completed. She would not be able to complete this assessment due to her low cognitive functioning.

Which diagnosis should be considered?

312.9 (F91.9) Unspecified Disruptive, Impulse-Control and Conduct Disorder

This category applies to presentations in which symptoms characteristic of a disruptive, impulse-control, and conduct disorder that causes clinically significant distress or impairment in social, occupational, or other important areas of functioning predominate but do not meet the full criteria for any of the disorders in the disruptive, impulse-control, and conduct disorders diagnostic class. The unspecified disruptive, impulse-control, and conduct disorder category is used in situations in which the clinician chooses *not* to specify the reason that the criteria are not met for a specific disruptive, impulse-control, and conduct disorder, and includes presentations in which there is insufficient information to make a more specific diagnosis (eg, in emergency room settings).

(Reprinted with permission from the *Diagnostic and Statistical Manual of Mental Disorders*. 5th ed. Arlington, VA: American Psychiatric Publishing; 2013.)

What is your rationale for the diagnosis?

The patient's history indicates an impulse control disorder, because her symptoms of scratching and biting the workers at her day care center have caused clinically significant distress in this important area of functioning and her symptoms do not meet the criteria for any of the other disorders in this category. It is not possible to specify the reasons that this patient does not meet the criteria for the other disorders in this category due to the limited information available; therefore, the diagnosis of unspecified disruptive, impulse-control and conduct disorder is chosen. Impulse control disorders are a common comorbidity for individuals with intellectual disability who may exhibit aggressive or self-injurious behaviors. It should be noted, however, that poor communication skills may be a major factor contributing to aggressive behavior in individuals with intellectual disability.

Which diagnosis should be considered?

332.1 (G21.11) Neuroleptic-Induced Parkinsonism

Parkinsonian tremor, muscular rigidity, akinesia (ie, loss of movement or difficulty initiating movement), or bradykinesia (ie, slowing movement) developing within a few weeks of starting or raising the dosage of a medication (eg, a neuroleptic) or after reducing the dosage of a medication used to treat extrapyramidal symptoms.

(Reprinted with permission from the *Diagnostic and Statistical Manual of Mental Disorders*. 5th ed. Arlington, VA: American Psychiatric Publishing; 2013.)

What is your rationale for the diagnosis?

The development of the slow shuffling gait and poor balance with the tendency to lean forward are symptoms resembling Parkinsonism that developed after taking risperidone for several months. Neuroleptics with their dopaminergic lowering effect have been known to cause pseudo-Parkinson symptoms.

What tests or tools should be considered to help identify the correct diagnosis?

Abnormal Involuntary Movement Scale (AIMS): The test is used to detect movement abnormalities, particularly tardive dyskinesia in patients taking neuroleptic medications.

What differential diagnosis should be considered?

Parkinsonism: If the patient's movement symptoms do not decrease with lowering the risperidone, Parkinsonism should be considered. A referral to a neurologist would then be indicated.

Possible medical comorbidities should be ruled out as certain conditions may contribute to behavioral issues.

FORMULATING THE TREATMENT PLAN

What treatment would you prescribe and what is the rationale?

Psychopharmacology: Reduce risperidone to 0.25 mg BID. Risperidone is indicated for the impulse control problems but the dose should be reduced due to the Parkinson-type symptoms.

Referrals: A full medical workup should be conducted to evaluate for any medical comorbidities that may contribute to mood or impulse control issues.

Additionally, a full cardiovascular workup should be conducted because individuals with CHARGE syndrome have a high incidence of cardiovascular abnormalities.

Type of Psychotherapy: Supportive therapy for the family member guardian may be indicated.

Psychoeducation: The guardian should be referred to the CHARGE Syndrome Foundation which can be accessed at:

http://www.chargesyndrome.org/about-charge.asp

The caretaker should be educated about preventing falls until the patient's gait is steady. For instance, showering without assistance, walking up or down stairs, or walking for long distances should be avoided.

What standard guidelines would you use to treat or assess this patient?

Guidelines for Understanding and Serving People with Intellectual Disabilities and Mental, Emotional, and Behavioral Disorders (see References section for citation).

CLINICAL NOTE

- Individuals with intellectual disabilities may have difficulty adjusting to changes in their environment including changes in staff at their day programs. Therefore, inquiries should be made to assess for any of these changes.

REFERENCES/RECOMMENDED READINGS

American Psychiatric Association. *Diagnostic and Statistical Manual of Mental Disorders*. 5th ed. Arlington, VA: American Psychiatric Publishing; 2013.

Putnam C. *Guidelines for Understanding and Serving People with Intellectual Disabilities and Mental, Emotional, and Behavioral Disorders*. Alexandria, VA: Florida Developmental Disabilities Council, Inc; 2009:1-30.

Shin H-W, Chung SJ. Drug-induced parkinsonism. *J Clin Neurol.* 2012;8(1):15-21.

CASE 31

Thinks He May Be Depressed

IDENTIFICATION: The patient is a 29-year-old, Latino, single male with no children, domiciled alone in an independent residence, referred by his primary care physician for a psychiatric evaluation. He is seen in an outpatient psychiatric clinic.

CHIEF COMPLAINT: "I think I may be depressed."

HISTORY OF CHIEF COMPLAINT: The patient reports increasingly depressive symptoms with onset 5 months ago in the context of stress from the impending short sale of his home, potential for homelessness, current unemployment, and financial strain. He reports depressive symptoms of depressed mood, low energy, low motivation, anhedonia, poor concentration, loneliness, low self-esteem, hopelessness, and decreased appetite with 2 to 3 lb weight loss over the past month. He reports difficulty falling and staying asleep due to anxious ruminations and restlessness, difficulty making decisions, intermittent irritability occurring at least once daily, and self-isolation. He endorses anxiety related to the stressors reported above, as manifested by restlessness, worry, and muscle tension. He reports that his current mental state interferes with his social functioning and ability to find better employment.

PAST PSYCHIATRIC HISTORY: This evaluation is the patient's first psychiatric treatment contact. He denies a history of prior psychotherapy, use of medication to treat psychiatric symptoms, or psychiatric hospitalization. Patient states that he previously felt depressive symptoms similar to those of the current episode. That depressive episode occurred 2 years ago after the patient lost his job; however, it remitted 8 to 9 months later without psychiatric intervention. Patient endorses a "lower mood" in the winter months, though denies any related impairment in functioning. Sleep dysfunction reportedly began four years ago without any known trigger and has persisted to the present. Although he reports moderate anxiety related to stressors, depressive symptoms preceded anxiety and are reported to be most distressing. No history of suicidal ideation, intent, plan, or attempt.

No current medications.

MEDICAL HISTORY: Patient was hospitalized multiple times as a child due to bronchitis and asthma. He was diagnosed with asthma at a young age, prescribed "a pump" that he does not use and cannot recall the name of.

Patient has allergies to shellfish, grass, perennial trees, dust mites, and cockroaches.

Height: 5'7". Weight: 180 lbs.

Impaired sleep secondary to anxious ruminations and restlessness.

Decreased appetite with 2 to 3 lb weight loss in the past month.

HISTORY OF DRUG OR ALCOHOL ABUSE: Alcohol use socially (2 to 4 times per month).

FAMILY HISTORY: The patient was born in Peru and is the first child of two siblings. His brother is 4 years younger and has a different biologic father. The patient immigrated to the United States as a child with his mother, stepfather, and brother. Patient did not have a relationship with his biologic father, who lives in Peru, until he was 18. At present the relationship is cordial though not close. Patient reports his mother is overbearing; therefore, he distances himself both physically and emotionally from her.

PERSONAL HISTORY

Perinatal: The patient was not aware of any birth complication or developmental delays.

Childhood: The patient completed elementary school with ease while living in South America. However, upon moving to the United States he initially found school difficult due to the Spanish/English language barrier. He was shy growing up and had few friends.

Adolescence: Was ridiculed for his poor English when in middle school. Eventually the patient adjusted and became a "B" student in high school, though received poorer grades in English. He graduated from high school.

Adulthood: Attended one semester of college until he decided to drop out and become a salesman. He initially did well in this position but was eventually laid off. Soon after, he worked as a waiter for a few months but disliked the job so he quit. He has always had an interest in pursuing a career in real estate but lacks motivation to move forward at this time. He has few friends currently. He states that he keeps friends at a distance because he has difficulty trusting others.

TRAUMA/ABUSE HISTORY: Patient was bullied in middle school due to his difficulty learning English.

MENTAL STATUS EXAMINATION

Appearance: Slumped posture with head angled down throughout majority of interview, casual dress, adequate hygiene.

Behavior and psychomotor activity: Generally cooperative and engaged; however, demonstrated guarded body language at times (arms crossed over chest), fair eye contact.

Consciousness:	Alert.
Orientation:	Oriented times 3.
Memory:	No impairment in recent or remote memory evident.
Concentration and attention:	Attention intact, able to follow questioning.
Visuospatial ability:	Not assessed.
Abstract thought:	Intact.
Intellectual functioning:	Average or above.
Speech and language:	Normal rate, rhythm, tone, and volume, spontaneous speech.
Perceptions:	No perceptual disturbance evident.
Thought processes:	Linear flow, logical.
Thought content:	Self-defeating thoughts, endorses thoughts suggestive of low self-worth. No obsessions or compulsions evident.
Suicidality and homicidality:	Denied.

Mood:	"Probably depressed."
Affect:	Constricted, congruent with stated mood.
Impulse control:	Good.
Judgment/insight/reliability:	Fair/fair/no evidence to suggest that patient is unreliable historian.

FORMULATING THE DIAGNOSIS

Which diagnosis should be considered?

296.32 (F33.1) Major Depressive Disorder, Recurrent Episode, Moderate with Anxious Distress

Diagnostic Criteria

A. Five (or more) of the following symptoms have been present during the same 2-week period and represent a change from previous functioning; at least one of the symptoms is either (1) depressed mood or (2) loss of interest or pleasure.
- **Note:** Do not include symptoms that are clearly attributable to another medical condition.
  1. Depressed mood most of the day, nearly every day, as indicated by either subjective report (eg, feels sad, empty, hopeless) or observation made by others (eg, appears tearful). (**Note:** In children and adolescents, can be irritable mood.)
  2. Markedly diminished interest or pleasure in all, or almost all, activities most of the day, nearly every day (as indicated by either subjective account or observation).
  3. Significant weight loss when not dieting or weight gain (eg, a change of more than 5% of body weight in a month), or decrease or increase in appetite nearly every day. (**Note:** In children, consider failure to make expected weight gain.)
  4. Insomnia or hypersomnia nearly every day.
  5. Psychomotor agitation or retardation nearly every day (observable by others, not merely subjective feelings of restlessness or being slowed down).
  6. Fatigue or loss of energy nearly every day.
  7. Feelings of worthlessness or excessive or inappropriate guilt (which may be delusional) nearly every day (not merely self-reproach or guilt about being sick).

8. Diminished ability to think or concentrate, or indecisiveness, nearly every day (either by subjective account or as observed by others).
9. Recurrent thoughts of death (not just fear of dying), recurrent suicidal ideation without a specific plan, or a suicide attempt or a specific plan for committing suicide.

B. The symptoms cause clinically significant distress or impairment in social, occupational, or other important areas of functioning.
C. The episode is not attributable to the physiologic effects of a substance or another medical condition.

Note: Criteria A to C represent a major depressive episode (MDE).

Note: Responses to a significant loss (eg, bereavement, financial ruin, losses from a natural disaster, a serious medical illness or disability) may include the feelings of intense sadness, rumination about the loss, insomnia, poor appetite, and weight loss noted in Criterion A, which may resemble a depressive episode. Although such symptoms may be understandable or considered appropriate to the loss, the presence of an MDE in addition to the normal response to a significant loss should also be carefully considered. This decision inevitably requires the exercise of clinical judgment based on the individual's history and the cultural norms for the expression of distress in the context of loss.

In distinguishing grief from an MDE, it is useful to consider that in grief the predominant affect is feelings of emptiness and loss, while in an MDE it is persistent depressed mood and the inability to anticipate happiness or pleasure. The dysphoria in grief is likely to decrease in intensity over days to weeks and occurs in waves, the so-called pangs of grief. These waves tend to be associated with thoughts or reminders of the deceased. The depressed mood of an MDE is more persistent and not tied to specific thoughts or preoccupations. The pain of grief may be accompanied by positive emotions and humor that are uncharacteristic of the pervasive unhappiness and misery characteristic of an MDE. The thought content associated with grief generally features a preoccupation with thoughts and memories of the deceased, rather than the self-critical or pessimistic ruminations seen in an MDE. In grief, self-esteem is generally preserved, whereas in an MDE feelings of worthlessness and self-loathing are common. If self-derogatory ideation is present in grief, it typically involves perceived failings vis-à-vis the deceased (eg, not visiting frequently enough, not telling the deceased how much he or she was loved). If a bereaved individual thinks about death and dying, such thoughts are generally focused on the deceased and possibly about "joining" the deceased, whereas in an MDE such thoughts are focused on ending one's own life because of feeling worthless, undeserving of life, or unable to cope with the pain of depression.

D. The occurrence of the MDE is not better explained by schizoaffective disorder, schizophrenia, schizophreniform disorder, delusional disorder, or other specified and unspecified schizophrenia spectrum and other psychotic disorders.
E. There has never been a manic episode or a hypomanic episode.
   - **Note:** This exclusion does not apply if all of the manic-like or hypomanic-like episodes are substance-induced or are attributable to the physiologic effects of another medical condition.

(Reprinted with permission from the *Diagnostic and Statistical Manual of Mental Disorders*. 5th ed. Arlington, VA: American Psychiatric Publishing; 2013.)

What is your rationale for the diagnosis?

The patient meets at least five of the criteria for major depressive disorder, present during the same 2-week period, and at least one of the symptoms is depressed mood or loss of interest or pleasure. The patient's depressive symptoms are not clearly attributable to another medical condition. The specifier anxious distress is applied as patient meets at least two of the five criteria for this specifier since he feels keyed up or tense and feels unusually restless, during the majority of days of the MDE.

What tests or tools should be considered to help identify the correct diagnosis?

The Beck Depression Inventory (BDI) questionnaire should be used to monitor the patient's depressive symptoms and to evaluate the need for treatment (see Appendix).

All potential medical comorbidities that may contribute to depressive symptoms should be ruled out, such as anemia, hypothyroidism, or vitamin deficiencies. A complete metabolic panel, thyroid panel, vitamin D, B-12, folic acid, and urinalysis should be obtained.

What differential diagnosis should be considered?

300.00 (F41.9) Unspecified Anxiety Disorder

Although the patient endorses anxiety symptoms, including worry, sleep disturbance, restlessness, irritability, difficulty concentrating, and muscle tension, these symptoms have not been present for at least 6 months (criteria for diagnosis of generalized anxiety disorder). The patient's anxiety symptoms do not clearly fit into any anxiety disorder diagnostic class. Therefore, a differential of unspecified anxiety disorder is considered. This diagnosis "...includes presentations in which symptoms characteristic of an anxiety disorder that cause clinically significant distress or impairment in social, occupational, or other important areas of functioning predominate but do not meet full criteria for any of the disorders in the anxiety disorders diagnostic class ..." (American Psychiatric Association, 2013). If the anxiety symptoms indicated above persist for at least 6 months and are present on more days than not, criteria for generalized anxiety disorder will be met and this diagnosis may be assigned.

309.28 (F43.23) Adjustment disorder, With mixed anxiety and depressed mood.

Although the onset of depressive symptoms occurred within 3 months of the onset of a stressor, the patient's symptoms meet criteria for an MDE. Therefore, a diagnosis of adjustment disorder is not applicable.

FORMULATING THE TREATMENT STRATEGY

What treatment would you prescribe and what is the rationale?

Psychopharmacology: Escitalopram 10 mg QD. A selective serotonin reuptake inhibitor (SSRI) is the first-line treatment option for major depression. Escitalopram is FDA-approved to treat both major depressive disorder and generalized anxiety disorder. Recommended treatment with escitalopram includes an initial dose of 10 mg per day, with single-dose administration in the morning or evening. The goal of pharmacologic treatment is remission of the depressive episode and prevention of relapse. If an adequate trial of 10 mg for 6 to 8 weeks is tolerable but results in only partial response, maximizing therapy by increasing the dose to 15 or 20 mg QD may be considered. Augmenting therapy or switching to alternative agents may also be considered if there is only partial remission of symptoms.

Referrals: Refer for individual cognitive therapy.

Psychotherapy: Cognitive therapy is a short-term psychotherapeutic modality indicated for the treatment of major depressive disorder. Cognitive therapy will enable the patient to identify and challenge cognitive distortions, such as persistent self-defeating thoughts, and replace negative thoughts with alternative, positive thoughts. In treating major depression, the combination of cognitive therapy and psychopharmacology is shown to be more effective than either therapy alone. Therefore, initiation of this therapy in combination with medication is recommended for this patient.

Psychoeducation: Advise the patient of the importance of ongoing therapy and medication management to promote remission of depressive episode and prevention of future relapses. Advise the patient to report symptoms of worsening depression or suicidality.

National Institute of Mental Health online patient education source about depression: http://www.nimh.nih.gov/health/topics/depression/index.shtml

CLINICAL NOTE

- Patients who are started for the first on antidepressant medication should be closely monitored for emergence of suicidality and/or manic or hypomanic symptoms. It is often difficult to differentiate between unipolar and bipolar depression. Antidepressants can contribute to mania if the patient is on the bipolar spectrum.

REFERENCES/RECOMMENDED READINGS

American Psychiatric Association. *Diagnostic and Statistical Manual of Mental Disorders*. 5th ed. Arlington, VA: American Psychiatric Publishing; 2013.

National Institute of Mental Health. Depression. Available at: http://www.nimh.nih.gov/health/topics/depression/index.shtml

Sadock BJ, Sadock VA, Ruiz P. *Kaplan & Sadock's Synopsis of Psychiatry: Behavioral/Sciences/Clinical Psychiatry*. 11th ed. Philadelphia, PA: Wolters Kluwer; 2015.

Stahl SM. *Stahl's Essential Psychopharmacology: Prescriber's Guide*. 5th ed. New York, NY: Cambridge University Press; 2014.

CASE 31 APPENDIX

Beck's Depression Inventory

This depression inventory can be self-scored. The scoring scale is at the end of the questionnaire.

1.
   - **0** I do not feel sad.
   - **1** I feel sad.
   - **2** I am sad all the time and I can't snap out of it.
   - **3** I am so sad and unhappy that I can't stand it.

2.
   - **0** I am not particularly discouraged about the future.
   - **1** I feel discouraged about the future.
   - **2** I feel I have nothing to look forward to.
   - **3** I feel the future is hopeless and that things cannot improve.

3.
   - **0** I do not feel like a failure.
   - **1** I feel I have failed more than the average person.
   - **2** As I look back on my life, all I can see is a lot of failures.
   - **3** I feel I am a complete failure as a person.

4.
   - **0** I get as much satisfaction out of things as I used to.
   - **1** I don't enjoy things the way I used to.
   - **2** I don't get real satisfaction out of anything anymore.
   - **3** I am dissatisfied or bored with everything.

5.
   - **0** I don't feel particularly guilty.
   - **1** I feel guilty a good part of the time.
   - **2** I feel quite guilty most of the time.
   - **3** I feel guilty all of the time.

6.
- **0** I don't feel I am being punished.
- **1** I feel I may be punished.
- **2** I expect to be punished.
- **3** I feel I am being punished.

7.
- **0** I don't feel disappointed in myself.
- **1** I am disappointed in myself.
- **2** I am disgusted with myself.
- **3** I hate myself.

8.
- **0** I don't feel I am any worse than anybody else.
- **1** I am critical of myself for my weaknesses or mistakes.
- **2** I blame myself all the time for my faults.
- **3** I blame myself for everything bad that happens.

9.
- **0** I don't have any thoughts of killing myself.
- **1** I have thoughts of killing myself, but I would not carry them out.
- **2** I would like to kill myself.
- **3** I would kill myself if I had the chance.

10.
- **0** I don't cry any more than usual.
- **1** I cry more now than I used to.
- **2** I cry all the time now.
- **3** I used to be able to cry, but now I can't cry even though I want to.

11.
- **0** I am no more irritated by things than I ever was.
- **1** I am slightly more irritated now than usual.
- **2** I am quite annoyed or irritated a good deal of the time.
- **3** I feel irritated all the time.

12.
- **0** I have not lost interest in other people.
- **1** I am less interested in other people than I used to be.
- **2** I have lost most of my interest in other people.
- **3** I have lost all of my interest in other people.

13.
- **0** I make decisions about as well as I ever could.
- **1** I put off making decisions more than I used to.
- **2** I have greater difficulty in making decisions more than I used to.
- **3** I can't make decisions at all anymore.

14.
- **0** I don't feel that I look any worse than I used to.
- **1** I am worried that I am looking old or unattractive.
- **2** I feel there are permanent changes in my appearance that make me look unattractive.
- **3** I believe that I look ugly.

15.

0 I can work about as well as before.
1 It takes an extra effort to get started at doing something.
2 I have to push myself very hard to do anything.
3 I can't do any work at all.

16.

0 I can sleep as well as usual.
1 I don't sleep as well as I used to.
2 I wake up 1–2 hours earlier than usual and find it hard to get back to sleep.
3 I wake up several hours earlier than I used to and cannot get back to sleep.

17.

0 I don't get more tired than usual.
1 I get tired more easily than I used to.
2 I get tired from doing almost anything.
3 I am too tired to do anything.

18.

0 My appetite is no worse than usual.
1 My appetite is not as good as it used to be.
2 My appetite is much worse now.
3 I have no appetite at all anymore.

19.

0 I haven't lost much weight, if any, lately.
1 I have lost more than five pounds.
2 I have lost more than ten pounds.
3 I have lost more than fifteen pounds.

20.

0 I am no more worried about my health than usual.
1 I am worried about physical problems like aches, pains, upset stomach, or constipation.
2 I am very worried about physical problems and it's hard to think of much else.
3 I am so worried about my physical problems that I cannot think of anything else.

21.

0 I have not noticed any recent change in my interest in sex.
1 I am less interested in sex than I used to be.
2 I have almost no interest in sex.
3 I have lost interest in sex completely.

INTERPRETING THE BECK'S DEPRESSION INVENTORY

Now that you have completed the questionnaire, add up the score for each of the 21 questions by counting the number to the left of each response you marked. The highest possible total for the whole test would be 63. This would mean you circled number 3 on all 21 questions. As the lowest possible score for each question is 0, the lowest possible score for the test would be 0. This would mean you circled 0 on each question. You can evaluate your depression according to the following table.

Total Score	Levels of Depression
1–10	These ups and downs are considered normal
11–16	Mild mood disturbance
17–20	Borderline clinical depression
21–30	Severe depression
Over 40	Extreme depression

CASE 32

Manic with Psychotic Features

IDENTIFICATION: The patient is a 29-year-old single unemployed Hispanic male who was admitted to a voluntary inpatient psychiatric unit.

CHIEF COMPLAINT: "I was just trying to find the truth so that I can save the world."

HISTORY OF CHIEF COMPLAINT: Prior to being admitted to the inpatient psychiatric unit, the patient was taken to the emergency room by police. The police were called when he was observed wandering for hours in a parking lot. Approximately 1 month prior to his admission, the patient had been fired from a job he had only had for 3 weeks for inappropriate behavior. According to his mother, the police had to be called to escort him from the premises because he refused to leave. Since that time, the patient has barely been sleeping and the family heard him laughing and talking to himself in the night. The patient said that his appetite has been nonexistent for the past 2 to 3 weeks. The mother said that although the patient is usually frugal, he has recently spent excessive amounts of money buying expensive business suits, which he has been charging to a credit card because he has no source of income. The patient said he is working on creative projects that will save the world, but is not at liberty to talk about them. He is religiously preoccupied and speaks of his special relationship with God. He is sexually preoccupied, and had been making sexually inappropriate comments to female nurses in the Emergency Department.

PAST PSYCHIATRIC HISTORY: The patient had no previous hospitalizations and had never been prescribed psychiatric medications. The only outpatient treatment he had was some counseling the previous spring at the university he had been attending. He said he did not find the counseling helpful. Even in his current mental state, the patient had some insight into what was occurring and said he thought he had bipolar disorder. He reports that for the past 4 years, he has been having episodes which could be described as hypomanic a couple of times a year in the spring and fall, increasing in intensity to the point that he failed his graduate program last spring. He said he also had periods of extreme depression when he was not even able to get out of bed. The family said that because the patient had been living away from home, they had not been aware of his problems until this current episode during which they had been trying to get him to seek help.

MEDICAL HISTORY: The patient has no known drug allergies. He does not have any current medical issues but in 2008 he had a bleeding stomach ulcer that required 3 or 4 days hospitalization and three blood transfusions. He is currently in good physical health, of normal height and weight, and stable vital signs. Labs on admission that included complete blood count (CBC), comprehensive metabolic panel, thyroid-stimulating hormone, and thyroxine were all within normal limits.

HISTORY OF DRUG OR ALCOHOL ABUSE: The patient says he began drinking alcohol and smoking marijuana at the age of 17. He considers himself a binge user of both substances. He says months will go by without him smoking marijuana and then he will have a period of "incessant" use. He said the same is true of drinking and he has experienced blackouts during alcohol use. The most recent episode was of binge drinking about a month prior to his hospitalization. His blood alcohol level and urine drug screen were both negative on admission.

FAMILY HISTORY: The patient's older brother and paternal aunt have bipolar disorder. The brother's illness is well-managed. He lives independently, has completed his education, and is a gainfully employed professional. A maternal cousin has schizophrenia.

The patient was raised in a family where the parents have an intact marriage and are both employed and are financially secure. The patient is the second oldest of four children, having an older brother, younger sister, and younger brother. He is currently living with his parents and younger siblings. He describes himself as being close to his mother and having a more contentious relationship with his father. He says he gets along with his siblings.

PERSONAL HISTORY

Perinatal: Information not known.

Childhood: He had no identified problems during childhood. He did well in school.

Adolescence: He did well academically in high school.

Adulthood: After college, he was accepted into a master's program in which he struggled until dropping out this past spring at which time he returned home to live with his family. During the first year of the master's program, the patient was arrested for trespassing and resisting arrest. He said he was intoxicated with alcohol at the time and that the charges were dropped. Initially after returning home, the patient was able to function in a job as a sports coach to adolescents; however, he left that job to take the one from which he was subsequently fired.

TRAUMA/ABUSE HISTORY: The patient denies any history of trauma or abuse saying he had a "wonderful" childhood.

MENTAL STATUS EXAMINATION

Appearance: The patient appears his stated age. He is impeccably groomed and wearing a business suit. He is cooperative with the interview and makes appropriate eye contact.

Behavior and psychomotor activity: The patient is very energetic and animated.

Consciousness:	Alert.
Orientation:	The patient is oriented to time, place, and person.
Memory:	The patient was not formally tested for memory. He was able to recall events in his life giving exact dates.
Concentration and attention:	The patient was easily distracted by things in the environment. For example, in the middle of a sentence, he was distracted by a small detail in a painting in the room and he spoke about it at great length. He needed frequent redirection back to the topic at hand.
Abstract thought:	Patient's responses indicate that he is able to understand concepts and generalizations.

Intellectual functioning:	Above average in intelligence as evidenced by vocabulary and fund of knowledge.
Speech and language:	Speech is spontaneous, overproductive, and somewhat pressured.
Perceptions:	The patient denied hallucinations and did not appear to be experiencing any perceptual distortions.
Thought processes:	Tangential with flight of ideas.
Thought content:	The patient displayed grandiosity, religious and sexual preoccupation, and some mild paranoia. The patient complained of having intrusive thoughts about other people and fearing that they could read his mind and know what he was thinking.
Suicidality or homicidality:	The patient denies any suicide plan or intent but says he sometimes wants to end it all. His family says that he has threatened suicide when intoxicated. He has never attempted suicide. He denies homicidal ideation but says he often gets very angry with people. Family says he becomes quite angry when intoxicated but denies that he has ever become physically aggressive.
Mood:	Elevated and expansive.
Affect:	Overanimated and congruent with his elevated mood.
Impulse control:	Impaired as evidenced by his excessive spending and inappropriate sexual comments.
Judgment/insight/reliability:	Although the patient has impaired judgment, he has considerable insight into the fact that he has an illness and needs medication and treatment to manage it.

FORMULATING THE DIAGNOSIS

What diagnosis should be considered?

296.44 (F31.2) Bipolar I Disorder with Mood Congruent Psychotic Features, Current Episode Manic

Diagnostic Criteria

For a diagnosis of bipolar I disorder, it is necessary to meet the following criteria for a manic episode. The manic episode may have been preceded by and may be followed by hypomanic or major depressive episodes (MDEs).

Manic Episode

A. A distinct period of abnormally and persistently elevated, expansive, or irritable mood and abnormally and persistently increased activity or energy, lasting at least 1 week and present most of the day, nearly every day (or any duration if hospitalization is necessary).
B. During the period of mood disturbance and increased energy or activity, three (or more) of the following symptoms (four if the mood is only irritable) are present to a significant degree and represent a noticeable change from usual behavior:
   1. Inflated self-esteem or grandiosity.
   2. Decreased need for sleep (eg, feels rested after only 3 hours of sleep).
   3. More talkative than usual or pressure to keep talking.
   4. Flight of ideas or subjective experience that thoughts are racing.
   5. Distractibility (ie, attention too easily drawn to unimportant or irrelevant external stimuli), as reported or observed.
   6. Increase in goal-directed activity (either socially, at work or school, or sexually) or psychomotor agitation (ie, purposeless non–goal-directed activity).
   7. Excessive involvement in activities that have a high potential for painful consequences (eg, engaging in unrestrained buying sprees, sexual indiscretions, or foolish business investments).
C. The mood disturbance is sufficiently severe to cause marked impairment in social or occupational functioning or to necessitate hospitalization to prevent harm to self or others, or there are psychotic features.
D. The episode is not attributable to the physiologic effects of a substance (eg, a drug of abuse, a medication, other treatment) or another medical condition.
   - **Note:** A full manic episode that emerges during antidepressant treatment (eg, medication, electroconvulsive therapy) but persists at a fully syndromal level beyond the physiologic effect of that treatment is sufficient evidence for a manic episode and, therefore, a bipolar I diagnosis.

Note: Criteria A to D constitute a manic episode. At least one lifetime manic episode is required for the diagnosis of bipolar I disorder.

Hypomanic Episode

A. A distinct period of abnormally and persistently elevated, expansive, or irritable mood and abnormally and persistently increased activity or energy, lasting at least 4 consecutive days and present most of the day, nearly every day.
B. During the period of mood disturbance and increased energy and activity, three (or more) of the following symptoms (four if the mood is only irritable) have persisted, represent a noticeable change from usual behavior, and have been present to a significant degree:
   1. Inflated self-esteem or grandiosity.
   2. Decreased need for sleep (eg, feels rested after only 3 hours of sleep).
   3. More talkative than usual or pressure to keep talking.
   4. Flight of ideas or subjective experience that thoughts are racing.
   5. Distractibility (ie, attention too easily drawn to unimportant or irrelevant external stimuli), as reported or observed.
   6. Increase in goal-directed activity (either socially, at work or school, or sexually) or psychomotor agitation.
   7. Excessive involvement in activities that have a high potential for painful consequences (eg, engaging in unrestrained buying sprees, sexual indiscretions, or foolish business investments).
C. The episode is associated with an unequivocal change in functioning that is uncharacteristic of the individual when not symptomatic.
D. The disturbance in mood and the change in functioning are observable by others.
E. The episode is not severe enough to cause marked impairment in social or occupational functioning or to necessitate hospitalization. If there are psychotic features, the episode is, by definition, manic.
F. The episode is not attributable to the physiologic effects of a substance (eg, a drug of abuse, a medication, other treatment) or another medical condition.
   - **Note:** A full hypomanic episode that emerges during antidepressant treatment (eg, medication, electroconvulsive therapy) but persists at a fully syndromal level beyond the physiologic effect of that treatment is sufficient evidence for a hypomanic episode diagnosis. However, caution is indicated so that one or two symptoms (particularly increased irritability, edginess, or agitation following antidepressant use) are not taken as sufficient for diagnosis of a hypomanic episode, nor necessarily indicative of a bipolar diathesis.

Note: Criteria A to F constitute a hypomanic episode. Hypomanic episodes are common in bipolar I disorder but are not required for the diagnosis of bipolar I disorder.

Major Depressive Episode

A. Five (or more) of the following symptoms have been present during the same 2-week period and represent a change from previous functioning; at least one of the symptoms is either (1) depressed mood or (2) loss of interest or pleasure.
   - **Note:** Do not include symptoms that are clearly attributable to another medical condition.
     1. Depressed mood most of the day, nearly every day, as indicated by either subjective report (eg, feels sad, empty, or hopeless) or observation made by others (eg, appears tearful). (Note: In children and adolescents, can be irritable mood.)
     2. Markedly diminished interest or pleasure in all, or almost all, activities most of the day, nearly every day (as indicated by either subjective account or observation).
     3. Significant weight loss when not dieting or weight gain (eg, a change of more than 5% of body weight in a month), or decrease or increase in appetite nearly every day. (Note: In children, consider failure to make expected weight gain.)
     4. Insomnia or hypersomnia nearly every day.
     5. Psychomotor agitation or retardation nearly every day (observable by others; not merely subjective feelings of restlessness or being slowed down).
     6. Fatigue or loss of energy nearly every day.
     7. Feelings of worthlessness or excessive or inappropriate guilt (which may be delusional) nearly every day (not merely self-reproach or guilt about being sick).
     8. Diminished ability to think or concentrate, or indecisiveness, nearly every day (either by subjective account or as observed by others).
     9. Recurrent thoughts of death (not just fear of dying), recurrent suicidal ideation without a specific plan, or a suicide attempt or a specific plan for committing suicide.

B. The symptoms cause clinically significant distress or impairment in social, occupational, or other important areas of functioning.

C. The episode is not attributable to the physiologic effects of a substance or another medical condition.

Note: Criteria A to C constitute an MDE. MDEs are common in bipolar I disorder but are not required for the diagnosis of bipolar I disorder.

Note: Responses to a significant loss (eg, bereavement, financial ruin, losses from a natural disaster, a serious medical illness or disability) may include the feelings of intense sadness, rumination about the loss, insomnia, poor appetite, and weight loss noted in Criterion A, which may resemble a depressive episode. Although such symptoms may be understandable or considered appropriate to the loss, the presence of an MDE in addition to the normal response to a significant loss should also be carefully considered. This decision inevitably requires the exercise of clinical judgment based on the individual's history and the cultural norms for the expression of distress in the context of loss.

In distinguishing grief from an MDE, it is useful to consider that in grief the predominant affect is feelings of emptiness and loss, while in an MDE it is persistent depressed mood and the inability to anticipate happiness or pleasure. The dysphoria in grief is likely to decrease in intensity over days to weeks and occurs in waves, the so-called pangs of grief. These waves tend to be associated with thoughts or reminders of the deceased. The depressed mood of an MDE is more persistent and not tied to specific thoughts or preoccupations. The pain of grief may be accompanied by positive emotions and humor that are uncharacteristic of the pervasive unhappiness and misery characteristic of an MDE. The thought content associated with grief generally features a preoccupation with thoughts and memories of the deceased, rather than the self-critical or pessimistic ruminations seen in an MDE. In grief, self-esteem is generally preserved, whereas in an MDE, feelings of worthlessness and self-loathing are common. If self-derogatory ideation is present in grief, it typically involves perceived failings vis-à-vis the deceased (eg, not visiting frequently enough, not telling the deceased how much he or she was loved). If a bereaved individual thinks about death and dying, such thoughts are generally focused on the deceased and possibly about "joining" the deceased, whereas in an MDE such thoughts are focused on ending one's own life because of feeling worthless, undeserving of life, or unable to cope with the pain of depression.

Bipolar I Disorder

A. Criteria have been met for at least one manic episode (Criteria A to D under "Manic Episode" earlier).
B. The occurrence of the manic episode and MDE(s) is not better explained by schizoaffective disorder, schizophrenia, schizophreniform disorder, delusional disorder, or other specified or unspecified schizophrenia spectrum and other psychotic disorder.

(Reprinted with permission from the *Diagnostic and Statistical Manual of Mental Disorders*. 5th ed. Arlington, VA: American Psychiatric Publishing; 2013.)

What is your rationale for the diagnosis?

The patient meets *DSM-5* criteria for bipolar disorder, manic with psychotic features because there is a distinct period of abnormally elevated mood lasting at least 1 week requiring hospitalization. During this period there is some grandiosity, flight of ideas, and pressured speech. He has psychotic features (thinking people could read his mind). The episode is not attributable to a substance or another medical condition. The patient's current presentation, the family history as well as the patient's report of his cyclical moods over the past few years support a diagnosis of bipolar disorder.

What tools or tests should be considered to help identify the correct diagnosis?

Blood alcohol level and urine drug screen. If there was evidence of recent alcohol or cannabis use, a diagnosis of substance-induced mood and psychotic disorders would have been considered.

What diagnosis should be considered?

303.90 (F10.20) Alcohol Use Disorder: Moderate

Diagnostic Criteria

A. A problematic pattern of alcohol use leading to clinically significant impairment or distress, as manifested by at least two of the following, occurring within a 12-month period:
   1. Alcohol is often taken in larger amounts or over a longer period than was intended.
   2. There is a persistent desire or unsuccessful efforts to cut down or control alcohol use.
   3. A great deal of time is spent in activities necessary to obtain alcohol, use alcohol, or recover from its effects.
   4. Craving, or a strong desire or urge to use alcohol.
   5. Recurrent alcohol use resulting in a failure to fulfill major role obligations at work, school, or home.
   6. Continued alcohol use despite having persistent or recurrent social or interpersonal problems caused or exacerbated by the effects of alcohol.
   7. Important social, occupational, or recreational activities are given up or reduced because of alcohol use.
   8. Recurrent alcohol use in situations in which it is physically hazardous.
   9. Alcohol use is continued despite knowledge of having a persistent or recurrent physical or psychological problem that is likely to have been caused or exacerbated by alcohol.
   10. Tolerance, as defined by either of the following:
       a. A need for markedly increased amounts of alcohol to achieve intoxication or desired effect.
       b. A markedly diminished effect with continued use of the same amount of alcohol.
   11. Withdrawal, as manifested by either of the following:
       a. The characteristic withdrawal syndrome for alcohol (refer to Criteria A and B of the criteria set for alcohol withdrawal).
       b. Alcohol (or a closely related substance, such as a benzodiazepine) is taken to relieve or avoid withdrawal symptoms.

Specify if:

- **In early remission:** After full criteria for alcohol use disorder were previously met, none of the criteria for alcohol use disorder have been met for at least 3 months but for less than 12 months (with the exception that Criterion A4, "Craving, or a strong desire or urge to use alcohol," may be met).
- **In sustained remission:** After full criteria for alcohol use disorder were previously met, none of the criteria for alcohol use disorder have been met at any time during a period of 12 months or longer (with the exception that Criterion A4, "Craving, or a strong desire or urge to use alcohol," may be met).

Specify if:

- **In a controlled environment:** This additional specifier is used if the individual is in an environment where access to alcohol is restricted.

Code based on current severity: Note for *ICD-10-CM* codes: If an alcohol intoxication, alcohol withdrawal, or another alcohol-induced mental disorder is also present, do not use the codes below for alcohol use disorder. Instead, the comorbid alcohol use disorder is indicated in the 4th character of the alcohol-induced disorder code (see the coding note for alcohol intoxication, alcohol withdrawal, or a specific alcohol-induced mental disorder). For example, if there is comorbid alcohol intoxication and alcohol use disorder, only the alcohol intoxication code is given, with the 4th character indicating whether the comorbid alcohol use disorder is mild, moderate, or severe: F10.129 for mild alcohol use disorder with alcohol intoxication or F10.229 for a moderate or severe alcohol use disorder with alcohol intoxication.

Specify current severity:

- **305.00 (F10.10) Mild:** Presence of two to three symptoms.
- **303.90 (F10.20) Moderate:** Presence of four to five symptoms.
- **303.90 (F10.20) Severe:** Presence of six or more symptoms.

(Reprinted with permission from the *Diagnostic and Statistical Manual of Mental Disorders*. 5th ed. Arlington, VA: American Psychiatric Publishing; 2013.)

What is your rationale for the diagnosis?

The patient meets the criteria of at least four to five symptoms of alcohol use disorder moderate because he has (1) a problematic pattern of alcohol use leading to clinically significant impairment evidenced by consuming larger amounts than was intended ("incessant use"), (2) continued use despite having persistent problems caused by the effects of drinking alcohol, (3) hazardous use ("blackouts"), and (4) his alcohol use is continued regardless of the knowledge of the physical or psychological problems that could occur (describes sporadic episodes of binge drinking since the age of 17).

What differential diagnosis should be considered?

305.20 (F12.10) Cannabis Use Disorders

Although the patient reported a history of cannabis use since the age of 17 in a binge type of pattern, not enough information is available to identify a problematic pattern of use leading to clinically significant impairment or distress. However, the patient or his family may provide additional information that would indicate that he does meet the criteria for cannabis use disorder.

FORMULATING THE TREATMENT STRATEGY

What treatment would you prescribe and what is the rationale?

Psychopharmacology: Valproic acid ER 1,000 mg daily

The first goal of treatment is to control the manic and psychotic symptoms with psychopharmacology. Because the patient understood that he had bipolar disorder and needed treatment, options for medication were reviewed with him (within the constraints of the hospital formulary). He was given a choice between lithium and valproic acid as a mood stabilizer and he chose valproic acid. Current evidence recommends a combination of lithium or valproic acid with an antipsychotic for severe cases of mania.

Risperidone 2 mg BID was started for the psychotic symptoms.

Trazodone 100 mg HS was given for insomnia.

Diagnostic Tests: Laboratory tests to monitor valproic acid levels and to identify hepatotoxicity or pancreatitis are essential. Therapeutic drug levels are 50-100mcg/mL. Initial labs should include liver functions tests, CBC with differential, and coagulation tests. Hereditary mitochondrial disease may predispose a patient to hepatic complications. If the patient is female, a pregnancy test is indicated because valproic acid has potential for teratogenic side effects.

AIMS/evaluation for movement disorders: The patient should be evaluated for medication-induced movement disorders that may be caused by risperidone. Neuroleptic-induced movement disorders include neuroleptic-induced parkinsonism, acute dystonia, acute akathisia, tardive dyskinesia.

Neuroleptic malignant syndrome is another potential complication with neuroleptics. Symptoms include muscular rigidity and dystonia, akinesia, mutism, obtundation and agitation along with fever, sweating, and elevated blood pressure and pulse. It is life threatening and will require intensive care treatment. Laboratory findings include elevated WBC, and CPK, LFTS, plasma myoglobin, and myoglobinuria.

Referrals: Referral options will be limited by his type of insurance. He will be referred to a hospital-affiliated enhanced outpatient program that would provide him with medication monitoring, cognitive behavioral group therapy including groups to address his substance abuse, as well as individual counseling.

His family will be referred to an intensive family support service in order to help them, better understand the patient's illness and need for treatment.

Type of Psychotherapy: See referrals.

Psychoeducation: Depression and Bipolar Support Alliance (DBSA) is a national organization that provides support and education for patients and families affected by bipolar disorder. Local chapters can be accessed at: http://www.dbsalliance.org/site/PageServer?pagename=home

Information about valproic acid can be obtained at:

http://www.nami.org/Learn-More/Treatment/Mental-Health-Medications/Valproate-(Depakote)

Information about risperidone can be obtained at:

http://www.nami.org/Learn-More/Treatment/Mental-Health-Medications/Risperidone-(Risperdal)

What standard guidelines would you use to treat or assess this patient?

The Clinical Management of Bipolar Disorder: A Review of Evidence-Based Guidelines can be retrieved at: https://www.ncbi.nlm.nih.gov/pmc/articles/PMC3219517/?report=classic

CLINICAL NOTE

- If the patient tolerates a starting dose of valproic acid of 1,000 mg daily for at least 3 days and his blood level is within the lower range of 50 to 100, the dose can be increased to 1,500 mg daily. The valproic acid level should be checked after any increases in the medication and particularly before discharge to make sure it is within a safe range. Additionally, his risperidone dose may need to be adjusted depending on the degree of remission of his psychotic thinking or the development of any side effects.
- There is the possibility that the patient may have less binge substance use episodes if his mood is stabilized. However, if his substance use continues to be comorbid, it should be addressed concurrently.
- Among patients taking valproic acid, there is increased risk for hepatotoxicity in the presence of mitochondrial disease.

REFERENCES/RECOMMENDED READINGS

American Psychiatric Association. *Diagnostic and Statistical Manual of Mental Disorders.* 5th ed. Arlington, VA: American Psychiatric Publishing; 2013.

Krähenbühl S, Brandner S, Kleinle S, Liechti S, Straumann D. Mitochondrial diseases represent a risk factor for valproate-induced fulminant liver failure. *Liver* 2000;20(4):346-348.

Sadock BJ, Sadock VA. *Synopsis of Psychiatry*. 10th ed. Philadelphia, PA: Wolters Kluwer Health, Lippincott, Williams & Wilkins; 2007.

Sadock BJ, Sadock VA, Sussman N. *Pocket Handbook of Psychiatric Drug Treatment*. 6th ed. Philadelphia, PA: Wolters Kluwer Health; 2014.

Sajatovic M, Madhusoodanan S, Fuller MA, Aulakh L, Keaton DB. Risperidone for bipolar disorders. *Exp Rev Neurother.* 2005;5(2):177-187.

Sitarz KS, Elliott HR, Karaman BS, Relton C, Chinnery PF, Horvath R. Valproic acid triggers increased mitochondrial biogenesis in POLG-deficient fibroblasts. *Mol Genet Metab.* 2014;112(1):57-63.

Stein DJ, Lerer B, Stahl SM. *Essential Evidence-Based Psychopharmacology*. 2nd ed. Cambridge: Cambridge University Press; 2012.

CASE 33

Depression Post Brain Tumor

IDENTIFICATION: The patient is a 31-year-old single Latino man who lives with his mother. He uses a walker and has left-sided weakness. His speech is impaired due to facial weakness. His mother drove him to this appointment at an outpatient mental health clinic and waited for him in the waiting area.

CHIEF COMPLAINT: "Depression."

HISTORY OF CHIEF COMPLAINT: The patient is seeking treatment for depression. Although he reports a history of depressive symptoms that tend to "wax and wane," he attributes much of his current depressed mood to the postsurgery effect of a brain tumor, which was mostly removed. He feels he is not capable of doing anything. He is unable to enjoy any activity. He has withdrawn from friends and avoids going out. The patient reports that he is anxious in social situations. He was anxious coming to this appointment because of his appearance. He finally came for treatment at his mother's insistence.

PAST PSYCHIATRIC HISTORY: Was depressed with suicidal thoughts at 10 years of age. Treated with sertraline with "no effect." Then attended a partial hospital program. Eventually, he returned to public school full time. No depressive symptoms during high school. At the age of 26, he developed impaired hearing in his left ear, had trouble walking, and his vision became blurry. Eventually, he saw a neurologist. Had three surgeries for a benign brain tumor, a meningioma 7 to 10 cm. Residual effects included left-sided weakness with an unsteady gait and impaired speech. He was treated by a psychiatrist for depression while hospitalized for the brain surgeries and was prescribed sertraline. However, the patient did not think the medication helped and he stopped taking it after several months.

MEDICAL HISTORY: No known allergies. Had three brain surgeries for a benign brain tumor 4 years ago. Currently has left-sided weakness affecting his gait and speech. Takes amlodipine for hypertension. Currently treated by speech therapist.

Reports a good appetite. Able to fall asleep but wakes up throughout the night and has a hard time getting back to sleep.

Denies any pain.

HISTORY OF DRUG OR ALCOHOL ABUSE: Denied any history of drug, alcohol, or nicotine use.

FAMILY HISTORY: The patient's father is Columbian, and his mother is Peruvian. He has one brother, a half brother, and two half sisters. His parents separated when he was 10 years old, after which he became suicidal. The patient lives with his mother. He visits his father occasionally. Said his father has panic attacks. Mother is reported to have hypertension.

PERSONAL HISTORY

Perinatal: No known complications. Met all developmental milestones.

Childhood: Described himself as a "shy" child. Had friends, but was very quiet most of the time. Became depressed and suicidal when his parents separated when he was 10 years old. Was in a partial program briefly and was started on sertraline, but does not think it helped.

Adolescence: Completed high school. Identifies as heterosexual. Described his mood as better during high school.

Adulthood: Attended a community college and has an Associate's Degree in the information technology field. Currently unemployed. Identifies as Latino. Reports he believes in Christianity and Buddhism.

TRAUMA/ABUSE HISTORY: He described the hospital and surgical treatments as being traumatic for him.

MENTAL STATUS EXAMINATION

Appearance: Casually but neatly dressed. Appears his stated age. Limited eye contact. Looks down intermittently avoiding eye contact. Walks very slowly with a walker and exhibits left-sided weakness, including left facial drooping. His skull shows indentation with surgical scars, which he initially covered with a hat. Generally cooperative.

Behavior and psychomotor activity: Left-sided weakness and altered gait. Some psychomotor retardation which does not seem related to his physical limitations.

Consciousness: Alert.

Orientation: Oriented to person, place, and time.

Memory: Recent and remote memory seem intact. Not formally assessed at this visit.

Concentration and attention: Not able to clearly assess as the patient's verbal responses were slow and may have been related to neurologic deficits affecting his speech.

Visuospatial ability: Not assessed.

Abstract thought: Not formally assessed, but his ability to understand concepts seems adequate.

Intellectual functioning: Average.

Speech and language: Normal rate and volume, but he has to focus on articulating due to facial paralysis. Generally the interviewer was able to comprehend his speech. The patient is very agreeable to repeating some of the words and phrases when they are difficult to understand.

Perceptions: No abnormalities elicited.

Thought processes: Logical and coherent.

Thought content: Thinks about wanting to get help and not feeling depressed.

Suicidality or homicidality: Denied.

Mood: Depressed and anxious.

Affect: Congruent with mood, appears very self-conscious.

Impulse control: Good.

Judgment: Good

Insight: Good.

Reliability: Seems like a reliable historian.

FORMULATING THE DIAGNOSIS

Which diagnosis (or diagnoses) should be considered?

296.33 (F33.2) Major Depressive Disorder, Severe, Recurrent

Diagnostic Criteria

A. Five (or more) of the following symptoms have been present during the same 2-week period and represent a change from previous functioning; at least one of the symptoms is either (1) depressed mood or (2) loss of interest or pleasure.
- **Note:** Do not include symptoms that are clearly attributable to another medical condition.
  1. Depressed mood most of the day, nearly every day, as indicated by either subjective report (eg, feels sad, empty, hopeless) or observation made by others (eg, appears tearful). (Note: In children and adolescents, can be irritable mood.)
  2. Markedly diminished interest or pleasure in all, or almost all, activities most of the day, nearly every day (as indicated by either subjective account or observation).
  3. Significant weight loss when not dieting or weight gain (eg, a change of more than 5% of body weight in a month) or decrease or increase in appetite nearly every day. (Note: In children, consider failure to make expected weight gain.)
  4. Insomnia or hypersomnia nearly every day.
  5. Psychomotor agitation or retardation nearly every day (observable by others, not merely subjective feelings of restlessness or being slowed down).
  6. Fatigue or loss of energy nearly every day.
  7. Feelings of worthlessness or excessive or inappropriate guilt (which may be delusional) nearly every day (not merely self-reproach or guilt about being sick).
  8. Diminished ability to think or concentrate, or indecisiveness, nearly every day (either by subjective account or as observed by others).

9. Recurrent thoughts of death (not just fear of dying), recurrent suicidal ideation without a specific plan, or a suicide attempt or a specific plan for committing suicide.

B. The symptoms cause clinically significant distress or impairment in social, occupational, or other important areas of functioning.

C. The episode is not attributable to the physiologic effects of a substance or another medical condition.

Note: Criteria A to C represent a major depressive episode (MDE).

Note: Responses to a significant loss (eg, bereavement, financial ruin, losses from a natural disaster, a serious medical illness or disability) may include the feelings of intense sadness, rumination about the loss, insomnia, poor appetite, and weight loss noted in Criterion A, which may resemble a depressive episode. Although such symptoms may be understandable or considered appropriate to the loss, the presence of an MDE in addition to the normal response to a significant loss should also be carefully considered. This decision inevitably requires the exercise of clinical judgment based on the individual's history and the cultural norms for the expression of distress in the context of loss.

In distinguishing grief from an MDE, it is useful to consider that in grief the predominant affect is feelings of emptiness and loss, while in an MDE it is persistent depressed mood and the inability to anticipate happiness or pleasure. The dysphoria in grief is likely to decrease in intensity over days to weeks and occurs in waves, the so-called pangs of grief. These waves tend to be associated with thoughts or reminders of the deceased. The depressed mood of an MDE is more persistent and not tied to specific thoughts or preoccupations. The pain of grief may be accompanied by positive emotions and humor that are uncharacteristic of the pervasive unhappiness and misery characteristic of an MDE. The thought content associated with grief generally features a preoccupation with thoughts and memories of the deceased, rather than the self-critical or pessimistic ruminations seen in an MDE. In grief, self-esteem is generally preserved, whereas in an MDE feelings of worthlessness and self-loathing are common. If self-derogatory ideation is present in grief, it typically involves perceived failings vis-à-vis the deceased (eg, not visiting frequently enough, not telling the deceased how much he or she was loved). If a bereaved individual thinks about death and dying, such thoughts are generally focused on the deceased and possibly about "joining" the deceased, whereas in an MDE such thoughts are focused on ending one's own life because of feeling worthless, undeserving of life, or unable to cope with the pain of depression.

D. The occurrence of the MDE is not better explained by schizoaffective disorder, schizophrenia, schizophreniform disorder, delusional disorder, or other specified and unspecified schizophrenia spectrum and other psychotic disorders.

E. There has never been a manic episode or a hypomanic episode.

- **Note:** This exclusion does not apply if all of the manic-like or hypomanic-like episodes are substance-induced or are attributable to the physiologic effects of another medical condition.

(Reprinted with permission from the *Diagnostic and Statistical Manual of Mental Disorders*. 5th edition. Arlington, VA: American Psychiatric Publishing; 2013.)

What is the rationale for the diagnosis?

The patient has had a persistent depressed mood. He has not been able to enjoy any previous interests. He has difficulty staying asleep. He seems to have some psychomotor retardation (his slowness, however, may be a neurologic effect). He describes negative thoughts and feels hopeless. Therefore, he meets at least five of the criteria for Major depressive disorder, severe (because the patient is not leaving his house and is totally avoiding social contact), recurrent (because there has been a span of more than 2 years since he was diagnosed with depression as a 10 year old).

What test or tools should be considered to help identify the correct diagnosis?

Beck Depression Inventory (BDI): The BDI is a simple tool which helps identify the severity of the depressive symptoms.

Montreal Cognitive Assessment (MoCA) can help evaluate the patient's cognitive functioning. The patient was very self-conscious and anxious during this assessment, so the MoCA will be completed during the next visit once there is more rapport established with the patient.

What differential diagnosis (or diagnoses) should be considered?

293.83 (F06.31) Depressive Disorder Due to Another Medical Condition

There is a prominent and persistent period of depressed mood, and a temporal association with a medical condition (postmeningioma surgery). However, with a history of depression and the possibility of the diagnosis of an adjustment disorder with depressed features, the diagnosis of Depressive Disorder Due to Another Medical Condition can only be considered as a differential diagnosis because it is not clear that the medical condition is the cause of the depression. However, research has indicated that at least 40% of patients experience depression postmeningoma surgery so there is a distinct possibility that this could be the etiology of depression with this patient.

300.23 (F40.10) Social Anxiety Disorder (Social Phobia)

The patient describes himself as being a very shy child. Currently he reports experiencing anxiety in social situations. However, it is not clear how severe the patient's anxiety was in social situations prior to his appearance being affected by his brain tumor and the surgery. Additional history taking and collateral information may help clarify if the criteria for Social Anxiety Disorder are met. During this initial psychiatric evaluation, the diagnosis will only be considered as a differential diagnosis.

300.4 (F34.1) Persistent Depressive Disorder (Dysthymia)

This diagnosis is considered because the patient reports a history of depressive symptoms "waxing and waning" since he was 10 years old. He has a history of prior treatment for depression and seems to have a long history of low self-esteem. Yet, there is not enough information to determine if he meets the criteria for Persistent Depressive Disorder. He was able to function as evidenced by obtaining a degree in a fairly complex field prior to the meningioma and its treatment.

FORMULATING THE TREATMENT STRATEGY

What treatment would you prescribe and what is the rationale?

Psychopharmacology: Venlafaxine 75 mg daily as an initial dose and titrate as tolerated until symptoms remit. Venlafaxine, a serotonin-norepinephrine reuptake inhibitor (SNRI), was chosen because the patient had failed two previous trials (as a 10 year old and while in the hospital postsurgery) with a selective serotonin reuptake inhibitor (sertraline). Also, he has considerable vegetative symptoms that may be more responsive to an SNRI due to norepinephrine effects.

Diagnostic Tests: Routine diagnostic tests.

Referrals: Individual psychotherapy, see below.

Type of Psychotherapy: Solution-focused therapy was recommended. The patient wanted to increase his level of functioning and was willing to identify specific target goals such as being able to leave his house independently. Because solution-focused therapy utilizes the patient as their own facilitator, this process would allow the patient to gain control in a situation that was predominantly not under his control (physical limitations due to brain tumor). This active involvement in his own treatment could provide a sense of empowerment and be very therapeutic.

Psychoeducation: Advised to contact the American Brain Tumor Association Support Group, which can be accessed online at: http://www.abta.org/brain-tumor-treatment/brain-tumor-support/support-groups/

The patient is very self-conscious about his appearance and is more likely to start engaging socially online rather than in person. Also, some of the other members of this group may be experiencing similar concerns about their appearance.

What standard guidelines would you use to treat or assess this patient?

VA/DoD Clinical Practice Guideline for the Management of Major Depressive Disorder can be accessed at: https://www.healthquality.va.gov/guidelines/MH/mdd/MDDCPGClinicianSummaryFINAL1.pdf

CLINICAL NOTE

- Changes in an individual's appearance can have a profound effect on their self-esteem and their ability to feel comfortable socially. These patients must be offered support and encouragement to maintain social contacts.

REFERENCES/RECOMMENDED READINGS

American Psychiatric Association. *Diagnostic and Statistical Manual of Mental Disorders.* 5th ed. Arlington, VA: American Psychiatric Publishing; 2013.

Boele FW, Rooney AG, Grant R, Klein M. Psychiatric symptoms in glioma patients: from diagnosis to management. *Neuropsychiat Dis Treat* 2015;11:1413-1420. doi:10.2147/NDT.S65874

Van der Vossen S, Schepers VPM, van der Sprenkel JWB, Visser-Meily J, Post MWM. Cognitive and emotional problems in patients after cerebral meningioma surgery. *J Rehabil Med.* 2014;46(5):430-437.

Wheeler K. *Psychotherapy for the Advanced Practice Psychiatric Nurse: A How-to Guide for Evidence-Based Practice.* 2nd ed. New York, NY: Springer Publishing Company; 2013.

CASE 34

Feeling Paranoid

IDENTIFICATION: The patient is a 33-year-old African-American, single man seen in an outpatient clinic.

CHIEF COMPLAINT: "Make sure I get help, so I don't lose my cool."

HISTORY OF CHIEF COMPLAINT: Recently he was riding in a car with his friend when he thought someone was going to kill him so he opened the car door and jumped out while it was moving. After this incident, his friend pleaded with him to get help. So the patient talked to his grandmother, and she made an appointment for him to be evaluated psychiatrically.

The patient is currently hearing voices that are saying, "Why do you need to be alive?" He states that he is always looking over his shoulder and feels afraid around people. He reports having nightmares on most nights. Consequently, he avoids leaving the apartment where he lives alone. He is constantly fearful that he will be harmed.

PAST PSYCHIATRIC HISTORY: The patient has heard voices since the age of 6 telling him, "If you can't do something, take it out on someone else." He was sent to an "alternative" school. He was in physical alterations with other students on a regular basis and he had to be restrained on several occasions. At the age of 13, he was expelled from school and he "went straight to the streets." His family didn't want him to take any medications. He started selling drugs. He reports a "violent period." At one point he was stabbed 17 times. Multiple charges related to drugs contributed to him being incarcerated multiple times as a youth and as an adult. He was prescribed psychiatric medication while he was incarcerated, but does not know what the medication was. Was on probation for 15 years. His brother was in a gang and was shot, but survived. After that, the patient felt like killing people: "I didn't have anything to live for." He said he turned into a "loner" and did not want to be around people. His grandmother took him to see a therapist and then he was referred to a psychiatrist and recalls being prescribed risperidone. He only took it briefly and does not remember if it was helpful.

MEDICAL HISTORY: History of gout. Was hit by a car twice when he was young. He cannot remember if there was any loss of consciousness, but he was taken to a hospital both times.

Currently takes colchicine 0.6 mg daily for his gout.

HISTORY OF DRUG OR ALCOHOL ABUSE: Patient states, "I never got into drugs." Smokes cigarettes, approximately one pack per day.

FAMILY HISTORY: Never knew his father. Was raised by his mother and his grandmother. Has an older brother, age 38, who was in a gang. His mother died from a cardiac condition when he was in his twenties. He is not aware of any psychiatric conditions among family members.

PERSONAL HISTORY

Perinatal: No history available but there is no indication there were any perinatal or birth complications.

Childhood: History of aggression with other children. No history of aggression with animals or any fire setting. He cannot remember if he had nightmares when he was young.

Adolescence: Was expelled from school at age 13 due to violent behavior. Was incarcerated multiple times as a juvenile. Did not complete high school.

Adulthood: No legal employment history. Sold drugs on the street. Lives alone in an apartment in a major city. Supports himself on Social Security Disability. Never married but has a daughter who is 15 years old. He wishes he had more contact with his daughter. Has no current relationship with his daughter's mother.

TRAUMA/ABUSE HISTORY: Was stabbed 17 times in his 20s.

MENTAL STATUS EXAMINATION

Appearance: Well groomed. Clothes neatly pressed. Cooperative. Tattoos on his arm. Muscular build.

Behavior and psychomotor activity: Very polite. No motor abnormalities. Good eye contact.

Consciousness:	Alert.
Orientation:	Oriented to person, place, and time.
Memory:	Not formally assessed but is generally intact.
Concentration and attention:	Not formally assessed but was able to complete a health questionnaire following the directions accurately. Handwriting was neat with a few misspellings.
Visuospatial ability:	Not assessed.
Abstract thought:	Not assessed.
Intellectual functioning:	Average.
Speech and language:	Normal rate and tone.
Perceptions:	When he is alone, he hears voices saying life is over. Has been hearing them for years and usually is able to distract himself with music.
Thought processes:	Thought processes are linear and coherent.
Thought content:	Says he does not feel paranoid during the interview, but when he's walking down the street, he thinks people might be talking about him. He reports "I'm always looking back."
Suicidality or homicidality:	Has had homicidal thoughts in the past but not in the last several years. They were most prominent after his brother was shot. Has suicidal thoughts and hears voices telling him to "end it," but pushes them out of his mind. Thinks about his grandmother and how it would upset her.
Mood:	"Depressed."
Affect:	Congruent with mood. Full range.

Impulse control: Good.

Judgment: Good.

Insight: Fair. Realizes that he needs psychiatric help to treat his symptoms.

Reliability: Seems like a reliable historian.

FORMULATING THE DIAGNOSIS

Which diagnosis (or diagnoses) should be considered?

298.9 (F29) Unspecified Schizophrenia Spectrum and Other Psychotic Disorder

This category applies to presentations in which symptoms characteristic of a schizophrenia spectrum and other psychotic disorders that cause clinically significant distress or impairment in social, occupational, or other important areas of functioning predominate but do not meet the full criteria for any of the disorders in the schizophrenia spectrum and other psychotic disorders diagnostic class. The unspecified schizophrenia spectrum and other psychotic disorder category is used in situations in which the clinician chooses not to specify the reason that the criteria are not met for a specific schizophrenia spectrum and other psychotic disorder, and includes presentations in which there is insufficient information to make a more specific diagnosis (eg, in emergency room settings).

(Reprinted with permission from the *Diagnostic and Statistical Manual of Mental Disorders*. 5th ed. Arlington, VA: American Psychiatric Publishing; 2013.)

What is the rationale for the diagnosis?

This diagnosis is indicated because the patient's symptom presentation includes delusions (paranoid) and hallucinations (mood congruent) for a significant portion of the time since the onset which was at age 6. His level of functioning has been altered and the signs of the disturbance have persisted for at least 6 months continuing until the present. The disturbance is not attributable to a substance, autism spectrum disorder, or a childhood communication disorder. However, it is not clear due to the limited history available if the depressive symptoms are part of a schizoaffective disorder, major depressive disorder with psychotic features, or even posttraumatic distress disorder. Therefore, because there is insufficient information to make a more specific diagnosis, Unspecified Schizophrenia Spectrum and other Psychotic Disorder was chosen.

Which diagnosis (or diagnoses) should be considered?

309.81 (F43.10) Posttraumatic Stress Disorder

Diagnostic Criteria

- **Note:** The following criteria apply to adults, adolescents, and children older than 6 years.

A. Exposure to actual or threatened death, serious injury, or sexual violence in one (or more) of the following ways:
   1. Directly experiencing the traumatic event(s).
   2. Witnessing, in person, the event(s) as it occurred to others.
   3. Learning that the traumatic event(s) occurred to a close family member or close friend. In cases of actual or threatened death of a family member or friend, the event(s) must have been violent or accidental.
   4. Experiencing repeated or extreme exposure to aversive details of the traumatic event(s) (eg, first responders collecting human remains; police officers repeatedly exposed to details of child abuse).
      - **Note:** Criterion A4 does not apply to exposure through electronic media, television, movies, or pictures, unless this exposure is work related.

B. Presence of one (or more) of the following intrusion symptoms associated with the traumatic event(s), beginning after the traumatic event(s) occurred:
   1. Recurrent, involuntary, and intrusive distressing memories of the traumatic event(s).
      - **Note:** In children older than 6 years, repetitive play may occur in which themes or aspects of the traumatic event(s) are expressed.
   2. Recurrent distressing dreams in which the content and/or affect of the dream is related to the traumatic event(s).
      - **Note:** In children, there may be frightening dreams without recognizable content.
   3. Dissociative reactions (eg, flashbacks) in which the individual feels or acts as if the traumatic event(s) were recurring. (Such reactions may occur on a continuum, with the most extreme expression being a complete loss of awareness of present surroundings.)
      - **Note:** In children, trauma-specific reenactment may occur in play.
   4. Intense or prolonged psychological distress at exposure to internal or external cues that symbolize or resemble an aspect of the traumatic event(s).
   5. Marked physiologic reactions to internal or external cues that symbolize or resemble an aspect of the traumatic event(s).

C. Persistent avoidance of stimuli associated with the traumatic event(s), beginning after the traumatic event(s) occurred, as evidenced by one or both of the following:
   1. Avoidance of or efforts to avoid distressing memories, thoughts, or feelings about or closely associated with the traumatic event(s).

2. Avoidance of or efforts to avoid external reminders (people, places, conversations, activities, objects, situations) that arouse distressing memories, thoughts, or feelings about or closely associated with the traumatic event(s).

D. Negative alterations in cognitions and mood associated with the traumatic event(s), beginning or worsening after the traumatic event(s) occurred, as evidenced by two (or more) of the following:
   1. Inability to remember an important aspect of the traumatic event(s) (typically due to dissociative amnesia and not to other factors such as head injury, alcohol, or drugs).
   2. Persistent and exaggerated negative beliefs or expectations about oneself, others, or the world (eg, "I am bad," "No one can be trusted," "The world is completely dangerous," "My whole nervous system is permanently ruined").
   3. Persistent, distorted cognitions about the cause or consequences of the traumatic event(s) that lead the individual to blame himself/herself or others.
   4. Persistent negative emotional state (eg, fear, horror, anger, guilt, or shame).
   5. Markedly diminished interest or participation in significant activities.
   6. Feelings of detachment or estrangement from others.
   7. Persistent inability to experience positive emotions (eg, inability to experience happiness, satisfaction, or loving feelings).

E. Marked alterations in arousal and reactivity associated with the traumatic event(s), beginning or worsening after the traumatic event(s) occurred, as evidenced by two (or more) of the following:
   1. Irritable behavior and angry outbursts (with little or no provocation) typically expressed as verbal or physical aggression toward people or objects.
   2. Reckless or self-destructive behavior.
   3. Hypervigilance.
   4. Exaggerated startle response.
   5. Problems with concentration.
   6. Sleep disturbance (eg, difficulty falling or staying asleep or restless sleep).

F. Duration of the disturbance (Criteria B to E) is more than 1 month.

G. The disturbance causes clinically significant distress or impairment in social, occupational, or other important areas of functioning.

H. The disturbance is not attributable to the physiologic effects of a substance (eg, medication, alcohol) or another medical condition.

Specify whether:

- **With dissociative symptoms:** The individual's symptoms meet the criteria for posttraumatic stress disorder (PTSD), and in addition, in response to the stressor, the individual experiences persistent or recurrent symptoms of either of the following:

1. **Depersonalization:** Persistent or recurrent experiences of feeling detached from, and as if one were an outside observer of, one's mental processes or body (eg, feeling as though one were in a dream; feeling a sense of unreality of self or body or of time moving slowly).
2. **Derealization:** Persistent or recurrent experiences of unreality of surroundings (eg, the world around the individual is experienced as unreal, dreamlike, distant, or distorted).
   - **Note:** To use this subtype, the dissociative symptoms must not be attributable to the physiologic effects of a substance (eg, blackouts, behavior during alcohol intoxication) or another medical condition (eg, complex partial seizures).

Specify if:

- **With delayed expression:** If the full diagnostic criteria are not met until at least 6 months after the event (although the onset and expression of some symptoms may be immediate).

(Reprinted with permission from the *Diagnostic and Statistical Manual of Mental Disorders*. 5th ed. Arlington, VA: American Psychiatric Publishing; 2013.)

What is the rationale for the diagnosis?

The patient was directly exposed to serious injury (stabbed 17 times), experienced nightmares, persistently avoids being in public areas where he can be assaulted, has a diminished interest in activities, has persistent negative emotions such as fear, and is hypervigilant ("I'm always looking back"). The disturbance has lasted for more than 1 month, has caused clinically significant distress, and is not attributable to a substance or medical condition. Therefore, his symptom presentation meets the criteria for PTSD.

What test or tools should be considered to help identify the correct diagnosis?

- Beck's Depression Inventory (BDI) (See list of screening tools in Index.)
- PTSD CheckList—Civilian Version (PCL-C) (http://www.mirecc.va.gov/docs/visn6/3_PTSD_CheckList_and_Scoring.pdf)
- Brief Psychiatric Rating Scale (BRPS), which can indicate the presence of psychotic symptoms (http://www.public-health.uiowa.edu/icmha/outreach/documents/BPRS_expanded.PDF)
- Positive and Negative Syndrome Scale (PANSS) (http://egret.psychol.cam.ac.uk/medicine/scales/PANSS)

What differential diagnosis (or diagnoses) should be considered?

The rationale for Unspecified Schizophrenia Spectrum and other Psychotic Disorder discusses the other diagnoses which should be considered as differentials (see above).

FORMULATING THE TREATMENT STRATEGY

What treatment would you prescribe and what is the rationale?

Psychopharmacology: Lurasidone 20 mg daily with food. Increase as tolerated until symptom remission occurs. The patient is experiencing psychotic symptoms and second-generation antipsychotics (SGAs) have been found efficacious for these symptoms. Lurasidone is well tolerated with a better side-effect profile than some of the older SGAs. Therefore, there will be a better likelihood of medication adherence which is extremely important given the severity of his symptoms.

Prazosin 0.1 mg HS. Prazosin is an alpha-adrenergic agonist and is indicated for the treatment of PTSD symptoms, particularly nightmares. If tolerated, the dose can be increased incrementally up to 0.6 mg HS.

Diagnostic Tests: Routine laboratory tests.

Risk Assessment: Violence risk screening-10 can be accessed at: http://www.forensic-psychiatry.no/violence_risk/v_risk_10_english.pdf. When evaluating the patient for risk using this assessment tool, his risk for violence is determined to be low. Even though he has a history of violence and reports paranoid feelings, he has not exhibited any violent behavior for many years, denies substance use, is insightful about the need for treatment, and has social support (grandmother and friend). He exhibited dangerous behavior when he jumped out of a moving car because of his paranoia, but now recognizes that his paranoia is a symptom that caused impaired judgment and he is seeking treatment for it. He is currently not exhibiting any indication that he would put himself or any one else at risk. However, the patient should be seen frequently because ongoing risk assessment is warranted. The patient is given emergency phone numbers to contact if he feels he is at risk.

Referrals: Individual psychotherapy should be considered after the paranoia decreases.

Type of Psychotherapy: Individual psychotherapy.

Psychoeducation: Advise the patient about the risks and benefits of the prescribed medications, lurasidone and prazosin.

What standard guidelines would you use to treat or assess this patient?

VA/DoD Clinical Practice Guideline for the Management of Posttraumatic Stress Disorder and Acute Stress Disorder can be accessed at: https://www.healthquality.va.gov/guidelines/MH/ptsd/VADoDPTSDCPGClinicianSummaryFinal.pdf

CLINICAL NOTE

- This patient has been exposed to extreme conditions of violence. Providing support and maintaining clear boundaries with this patient are important in developing a therapeutic alliance and promoting compliance with treatment.

REFERENCES/RECOMMENDED READINGS

American Psychiatric Association. *Diagnostic and Statistical Manual of Mental Disorders.* 5th ed. Arlington, VA: American Psychiatric Publishing; 2013.

Buchanan A, Binder R, Norko M, Swartz M. Resource document on psychiatric violence risk assessment. *Focus: Guide AIDS Res.* 2015;13(4):490-498.

Higashi K, Medic G, Littlewood KJ, Diez T, Granström O, De Hert M. Medication adherence in schizophrenia: factors influencing adherence and consequences of nonadherence, a systematic literature review. *Therapeutic Adv Psychopharmacol.* 2013;3(4):200-218.

Stein D, Lerer B, Stahl SM. *Essential evidence-based psychopharmacology.* Cambridge, UK: Cambridge University Press; 2012.

CASE 35

Pregnant and Anxious

IDENTIFICATION: The patient is a 34-year-old white woman who was being treated psychiatrically at an outpatient mental health office. Her psychiatrist recently retired, and she was transferred to this practitioner.

CHIEF COMPLAINT: "I just found out I'm pregnant. My mood is OK since I went back on the Prozac 60 mg."

HISTORY OF CHIEF COMPLAINT: The patient is 12 weeks pregnant. When she first thought she might be pregnant, she tried to reduce her dose of fluoxetine from 60 to 40 mg daily. She became unable to leave the house and was fearful of developing panic symptoms when outside the house. She realized her fear might be irrational but was not able to control it. For the past month, she has not been able to leave the house even to visit her obstetrician. So she resumed her original dose of fluoxetine 60 mg daily. Feeling desperate, she started taking diazepam 10 mg that was leftover from a previous prescription. She was then able to visit her obstetrician. She is feeling nauseous, which triggers anxiety. Patient states, "I'm phobic about nausea." When she tried to stop the diazepam, she "became suicidal."

PAST PSYCHIATRIC HISTORY: Patient was previously in group therapy. She was prescribed alprazolam for anxiety and sertraline for depression 10 years ago. She has a history of periodic preoccupation with suicidal thoughts and occasional bizarre intrusive thoughts such as if she cut off a person's legs, would they still be able to walk. She denies any intent to act on these thoughts and felt very upset by the thoughts. She also described a pattern of meticulousness and scrupulous attention to detail. She has a history of excessive hand washing. Her former psychiatrist diagnosed her with panic disorder with agoraphobia, obsessive-compulsive disorder (OCD), emetophobia, and obsessive compulsive personality disorder. She was prescribed numerous medications over the years, which included diazepam, paroxetine, aripiprazole, pamelor, hydroxyzine, and lorazepam. She has a history of self-injurious behavior by cutting. Most recent episode of self-injury was a year ago. No history of suicidal attempts or psychiatric hospitalizations.

MEDICAL HISTORY: No known allergies. Primigravida 12 weeks. History of asthma, hiatus hernia. Treated for gastroesophageal reflux disease. No history of surgeries. ROS WNL. Appetite fair. Sleep 7 to 8 hours/night. Height 5′6″. Weight 138 lb. BMI 21.0. Denies use of contraceptives.

HISTORY OF DRUG OR ALCOHOL ABUSE: Denied.

FAMILY HISTORY: Has a good relationship with her parents. Is an only child. Her mother takes paroxetine for panic and depression. Her father has been diagnosed with panic disorder with agoraphobia but currently is doing well. No other known family psychiatric history.

PERSONAL HISTORY

Perinatal: Was a full-term vaginal birth. No known developmental delays.

Childhood: No learning disorders.

Adolescence: Graduated from high school.

Adulthood: Started college but dropped out after the first 2 years. Previously employed in a nursery school, but is not currently working. Lives with her fiancé who she describes as very supportive. She and her fiancé are both happy about the pregnancy. Neither she nor her fiancé have any other children. They have a dog.

TRAUMA/ABUSE HISTORY: Denies.

MENTAL STATUS EXAMINATION

Appearance: Neat, casual attire, cooperative. Appears stated age.

Behavior and psychomotor activity: Good eye contact. Psychomotor activity within normal range.

Consciousness: Alert.

Orientation: Oriented to person, place, and time.

Memory:	Recent and remote memory seem intact but not formally assessed.
Concentration and attention:	Not formally assessed but seems satisfactory.
Visuospatial ability:	Not formally assessed.
Abstract thought:	Satisfactory. Not formally assessed.
Intellectual functioning:	Average.
Speech and language:	Normal rate and tone.
Perceptions:	No perceptual disturbances elicited.
Thought processes:	Coherent.
Thought content:	Phobic about nausea. Obsesses about the possibility of vomiting. This has been a long-standing obsession of hers. Otherwise, is very excited about having the baby.
Suicidality or homicidality:	None. Stopped having suicidal thoughts after increasing the fluoxetine dose a month ago. Suicidal thoughts seemed to be obsessive in nature and although the patient had them for years, she has never made any suicide attempts.
Mood:	"I'm not depressed. Just anxious, but not that bad."
Affect:	Congruent with mood.
Impulse control:	Good.
Judgment:	Good.
Insight:	Good.
Reliability:	Good.

FORMULATING THE DIAGNOSIS

Which diagnosis (or diagnoses) should be considered?

300.3 (F42.2) Obsessive Compulsive Disorder, with Fair Insight.

Diagnostic Criteria

A. Presence of obsessions, compulsions, or both:
   - Obsessions are defined by (1) and (2):
     1. Recurrent and persistent thoughts, urges, or images that are experienced, at some time during the disturbance, as intrusive and unwanted, and that in most individuals cause marked anxiety or distress.
     2. The individual attempts to ignore or suppress such thoughts, urges, or images, or to neutralize them with some other thought or action (ie, by performing a compulsion).
   - Compulsions are defined by (1) and (2):
     1. Repetitive behaviors (eg, hand washing, ordering, checking) or mental acts (eg, praying, counting, repeating words silently) that the individual feels driven to perform in response to an obsession or according to rules that must be applied rigidly.
     2. The behaviors or mental acts are aimed at preventing or reducing anxiety or distress, or preventing some dreaded event or situation; however, these behaviors or mental acts are not connected in a realistic way with what they are designed to neutralize or prevent, or are clearly excessive.
        - **Note:** Young children may not be able to articulate the aims of these behaviors or mental acts.

B. The obsessions or compulsions are time-consuming (eg, take more than 1 hour/day) or cause clinically significant distress or impairment in social, occupational, or other important areas of functioning.

C. The obsessive-compulsive symptoms are not attributable to the physiologic effects of a substance (eg, a drug of abuse, a medication) or another medical condition.

D. The disturbance is not better explained by the symptoms of another mental disorder (eg, excessive worries, as in generalized anxiety disorder; preoccupation with appearance, as in body dysmorphic disorder; difficulty discarding or parting with possessions, as in hoarding disorder; hair pulling, as in trichotillomania [hair-pulling disorder]; skin picking, as in excoriation [skin-picking] disorder; stereotypies, as in stereotypic movement disorder; ritualized eating behavior, as in eating disorders; preoccupation with substances or gambling, as in substance-related and addictive disorders; preoccupation with having an illness, as in illness anxiety disorder; sexual urges or fantasies, as in paraphilic disorders; impulses, as in disruptive, impulse-control, and conduct disorders; guilty ruminations, as in major depressive disorder (MDD); thought insertion or delusional preoccupations, as in schizophrenia spectrum and other psychotic disorders; or repetitive patterns of behavior, as in autism spectrum disorder).

Specify if:

- **With good or fair insight:** The individual recognizes that OCD beliefs are definitely or probably not true or that they may or may not be true.
- **With poor insight:** The individual thinks OCD beliefs are probably true.
- **With absent insight/delusional beliefs:** The individual is completely convinced that OCD beliefs are true.

Specify if:

- **Tic-related:** The individual has a current or past history of a tic disorder.

(Reprinted with permission from the *Diagnostic and Statistical Manual of Mental Disorders*. 5th ed. Arlington, VA: American Psychiatric Publishing; 2013.)

What is the rationale for the diagnosis?

The patient's current symptoms meet the diagnostic criteria including the presence of recurrent thoughts that are intrusive and unwanted and cause marked anxiety. She attempts to ignore or suppress these thoughts. The obsessions are time consuming and not attributable to the effects of a substance, or not better explained by another mental disorder. Therefore, the diagnosis of OCD is appropriate.

Which diagnosis (or diagnoses) should be considered?

300.01 (F41.0) Panic Disorder

Diagnostic Criteria

A. Recurrent unexpected panic attacks. A panic attack is an abrupt surge of intense fear or intense discomfort that reaches a peak within minutes, and during which time four (or more) of the following symptoms occur:

Note: The abrupt surge can occur from a calm state or an anxious state.

1. Palpitations, pounding heart, or accelerated heart rate.
2. Sweating.
3. Trembling or shaking.
4. Sensations of shortness of breath or smothering.
5. Feelings of choking.
6. Chest pain or discomfort.
7. Nausea or abdominal distress.
8. Feeling dizzy, unsteady, light-headed, or faint.

9. Chills or heat sensations.
10. Paresthesias (numbness or tingling sensations).
11. Derealization (feelings of unreality) or depersonalization (being detached from oneself).
12. Fear of losing control or "going crazy."
13. Fear of dying.
    - **Note:** Culture-specific symptoms (eg, tinnitus, neck soreness, headache, uncontrollable screaming or crying) may be seen. Such symptoms should not count as one of the four required symptoms.

At least one of the attacks has been followed by 1 month (or more) of one or both of the following:

1. Persistent concern or worry about additional panic attacks or their consequences (eg, losing control, having a heart attack, "going crazy").
2. A significant maladaptive change in behavior related to the attacks (eg, behaviors designed to avoid having panic attacks, such as avoidance of exercise or unfamiliar situations).

B. The disturbance is not attributable to the physiologic effects of a substance (eg, a drug of abuse, a medication) or another medical condition (eg, hyperthyroidism, cardiopulmonary disorders).

C. The disturbance is not better explained by another mental disorder (eg, the panic attacks do not occur only in response to feared social situations, as in social anxiety disorder; in response to circumscribed phobic objects or situations, as in specific phobia; in response to obsessions, as in OCD; in response to reminders of traumatic events, as in posttraumatic stress disorder; or in response to separation from attachment figures, as in separation anxiety disorder).

(Reprinted with permission from the *Diagnostic and Statistical Manual of Mental Disorders*. 5th ed. Arlington, VA: American Psychiatric Publishing; 2013.)

What is the rationale for the diagnosis?

The patient was diagnosed by her psychiatrist with the former *DSM-IV* diagnosis of panic disorder with agoraphobia. In the current *DSM-5*, the diagnoses are separated to either panic disorder or agoraphobia. With her history and her current report of her symptoms, she meets the criteria for panic disorder. Prior to increasing her fluoxetine and taking diazepam in the past month, she reported that she was not able to leave her house due to fear of panic attacks even though she wanted to see her obstetrician. So the diagnosis of panic disorder will be noted even though she is not exhibiting any current panic symptoms.

What test or tools should be considered to help identify the correct diagnosis?

Y-BOCS to monitor the extent of obsessive compulsive symptoms.

What differential diagnosis (or diagnoses) should be considered?

300.22 (F40.00) Agoraphobia

Prior to increasing her medications in the past month, she reported that she was not able to leave her house due to fear of panic attacks. For the *DSM-5* diagnosis of Agoraphobia, there must be at least two out of five situations that are feared and avoided. The patient only avoided one situation (leaving her house) so she did not meet the current criteria for Agoraphobia. In addition, the symptoms have not been present for at least 6 months.

FORMULATING THE TREATMENT STRATEGY

What treatment would you prescribe and what is the rationale?

Consultations:

1. The patent's obstetrician will be contacted to discuss treatment options regarding her pregnancy and the risks and benefits of psychotropic medication.
2. The psychiatrist/Medical Director at the agency was consulted for a second opinion to discuss the risks and benefits of the medication with the pregnancy.

Psychopharmacology: Continue fluoxetine 60 mg daily.

Fluoxetine is a selective serotonin reuptake inhibitor that is FDA approved for MDD, OCD, bulimia nervosa, and panic disorder, with or without agoraphobia. Fluoxetine has been effective in reducing the patient's depressive and panic symptoms so it should be continued. Although she continues to report obsessive thinking, the thoughts are manageable. Because she is pregnant, increasing the dose should be avoided unless her symptoms become more severe.

Diazepam 7.5 mg for 1 week, then diazepam 5 mg daily for 1 week, then 2.5 mg daily for 1 week, then discontinue. Tapering off diazepam should be done as rapidly as possible. Studies have indicated that benzodiazepines can be teratogenic in the first trimester. Also, if used in the third trimester, they can precipitate withdrawal in the newborn. The patient should be able to tolerate the taper since she has resumed a higher dose of fluoxetine that will help control her anxiety. However, a gradual taper is needed because she became suicidal when she abruptly stopped the diazepam before.

Diagnostic Tests: None indicated.

Referrals: Cognitive behavioral therapy (CBT) therapist.

Type of Psychotherapy: CBT is indicated for the treatment of OCD.

Psychoeducation:

1. The patient was advised not to make any medication changes without first discussing them with the provider.
2. The patient was advised to have her fiancé accompany her to the next appointment so the risks and benefits of the medication during pregnancy could be discussed with him too. Literature from womensmentalhealth.org will be provided and reviewed.
3. Relaxation strategies reviewed.

What standard guidelines would you use to treat or assess this patient?

"Antenatal and postnatal mental health: clinical management and service guidance" https://www.nice.org.uk/guidance/cg192/chapter/1-recommendations

CLINICAL NOTE

- Prescribing any medication during pregnancy must be carefully evaluated. Recent research has indicated that there is the potential for teratogenic effects when antidepressants are used, particularly in the first trimester of pregnancy.

REFERENCES/RECOMMENDED READINGS

American Psychiatric Association. *Diagnostic and Statistical Manual of Mental Disorders*. 5th ed. Arlington, VA: American Psychiatric Publishing; 2013.

Behavioral Health Virtual Resource. Prescribing and Tapering Benzodiazepines. http://www.jpshealthnet.org/sites/default/files/prescribing_and_tapering_benzodiapines.pdf. Accessed 2014.

Bérard A, Zhao J-P, Sheehy O. Antidepressant use during pregnancy and the risk of major congenital malformations in a cohort of depressed pregnant women: an updated analysis of the Quebec Pregnancy Cohort. *BMJ Open*. 2017;7(1):e013372.

Ram D, Gandotra S. Antidepressants, anxiolytics, and hypnotics in pregnancy and lactation. *Indian J Psychiatry*. 2015;57(suppl 2):S354-S371. doi:10.4103/0019-5545.161504

Sadock BJ, Sadock V, Sussman N. *Kaplan & Sadock's Pocket Handbook of Psychiatric Drug Treatment*. 6th ed. Philadelphia, PA: Wolters Kluwer; 2013.

Taylor D, Paton C, Kapur S. *The Maudsley Prescribing Guidelines in Psychiatry*. 12th ed. West Sussex, UK: Wiley-Blackwell; 2015. http://www.sssftformulary.nhs.uk/docs/Pregnancy%20 3rd%20Edition.pdf.

CASE 36

Panic Attacks after Traumatic Incident

IDENTIFICATION: The patient is a 35-year-old single Hispanic male in a long-term relationship. He is self-referred.

CHIEF COMPLAINT: "I need medication for my panic attacks."

HISTORY OF CHIEF COMPLAINT: The patient reports intrusive thoughts and nightmares about being thrown off a roof. He describes feelings of impending doom, hypervigilance, and difficulty remembering everyday details. He is fearful of falling asleep due to the occurrence of nightmares. He has lost interest in his children and has to "fake" playing with them. He has lost interest in sex. He avoids leaving his house and sleeps excessively. If he sees the police in person or on TV, he experiences increased anxiety and sometimes has panic attacks. As a result of the panic attacks, he has been unable to work. This has caused him additional anxiety and guilt as he worries about providing for his family.

These symptoms began following an incident with the police that occurred 4 years ago. The patient was detained by the police as he was walking down a street and was accused of criminal activity. He reports being taken inside a building and up to the roof and threatened with being thrown over the roof. Panic attacks started 1 month after the incident. He thought he was having a heart attack and went to the emergency room. He was diagnosed with panic attacks and was prescribed alprazolam. He reported that the alprazolam "calmed him down." He was subsequently prescribed sertraline by his primary care provider, which he did not take. He only took the alprazolam on one or two occasions as it made his face tingle.

PAST PSYCHIATRIC HISTORY: No psychiatric complaints or treatment prior to the incident with the police 4 years ago.

MEDICAL HISTORY: No medical conditions reported. No known allergies. Average height and weight.

HISTORY OF DRUG OR ALCOHOL ABUSE: Drug, alcohol, and cigarette use denied.

FAMILY HISTORY: The patient reports a "normal" family upbringing. He was the oldest son and was raised by both his parents. He lives with his girlfriend and their three children.

PERSONAL HISTORY

Perinatal: Normal vaginal birth. Full term. No developmental delays.

Childhood: Was able to make friends. Described himself as always being a "worrier."

Adolescence: Graduated high school.

Adulthood: The patient had a good work history driving a truck prior to the traumatic incident 4 years ago. Was arrested and charged with "wandering." He had a public defender at that time and was advised to plea bargain. Currently, he is involved in a civil suit related to the same incident. He has not been able to work consistently since then. He is a nonpracticing Catholic. No military history.

TRAUMA/ABUSE HISTORY: None reported prior to the traumatic incident with the police 4 years ago.

MENTAL STATUS EVALUATION:

Appearance: Well groomed. Hip-hop style of clothing. Normal gait and posture.

Behavior and psychomotor activity: Good eye contact. Normal psychomotor activity.

Consciousness: Alert.

Orientation: Oriented to person, place, and time.

Memory: The patient reports gaps in his memory, but when examined, exhibited normal recent and remote memory.

Concentration/attention: Good.

Abstract thought:	Not formally assessed but appears average.
Intellectual functioning:	Average intelligence.
Speech and language:	English speaking. Normal rate and volume.
Perceptions:	No abnormalities.
Thought process/form:	Logical and goal directed.
Thought content:	Preoccupied with concerns about how he will support his family. No hallucinations or delusions. Has flashbacks of the frightening incident with police, particularly when seeing a police car in person or on TV.
Suicidality and homicidality:	Denies any desire to harm himself or others.
Mood:	Anxious and depressed.
Affect:	Congruent with mood.
Impulse control:	Good.
Judgment/insight/reliability:	Good.

FORMULATING THE DIAGNOSIS

Which diagnosis should be considered?

309.81 (F43.10) Posttraumatic Stress Disorder (PTSD)

Diagnostic Criteria

- **Note:** The following criteria apply to adults, adolescents, and children older than 6 years.
- Exposure to actual or threatened death, serious injury, or sexual violence in one (or more) of the following ways:
  - Directly experiencing the traumatic event(s).
  - Witnessing, in person, the event(s) as it occurred to others.

  - Learning that the traumatic event(s) occurred to a close family member or close friend. In cases of actual or threatened death of a family member or friend, the event(s) must have been violent or accidental.
  - Experiencing repeated or extreme exposure to aversive details of the traumatic event(s) (eg, first responders collecting human remains; police officers repeatedly exposed to details of child abuse).
    - **Note:** Criterion A4 does not apply to exposure through electronic media, television, movies, or pictures, unless this exposure is work related.
- Presence of one (or more) of the following intrusion symptoms associated with the traumatic event(s), beginning after the traumatic event(s) occurred:
  - Recurrent, involuntary, and intrusive distressing memories of the traumatic event(s).
    - **Note:** In children older than 6 years, repetitive play may occur in which themes or aspects of the traumatic event(s) are expressed.
  - Recurrent distressing dreams in which the content and/or affect of the dream is related to the traumatic event(s).
    - **Note:** In children, there may be frightening dreams without recognizable content.
  - Dissociative reactions (eg, flashbacks) in which the individual feels or acts as if the traumatic event(s) were recurring. (Such reactions may occur on a continuum, with the most extreme expression being a complete loss of awareness of present surroundings.)
    - **Note:** In children, trauma-specific reenactment may occur in play.
  - Intense or prolonged psychological distress at exposure to internal or external cues that symbolize or resemble an aspect of the traumatic event(s).
  - Marked physiologic reactions to internal or external cues that symbolize or resemble an aspect of the traumatic event(s).
- Persistent avoidance of stimuli associated with the traumatic event(s), beginning after the traumatic event(s) occurred, as evidenced by one or both of the following:
  - Avoidance of or efforts to avoid distressing memories, thoughts, or feelings about or closely associated with the traumatic event(s).
    - Avoidance of or efforts to avoid external reminders (people, places, conversations, activities, objects, situations) that arouse distressing memories, thoughts, or feelings about or closely associated with the traumatic event(s).
- Negative alterations in cognitions and mood associated with the traumatic event(s), beginning or worsening after the traumatic event(s) occurred, as evidenced by two (or more) of the following:
  - Inability to remember an important aspect of the traumatic event(s) (typically due to dissociative amnesia and not to other factors such as head injury, alcohol, or drugs).

  - Persistent and exaggerated negative beliefs or expectations about oneself, others, or the world (eg, "I am bad," "No one can be trusted," "The world is completely dangerous," "My whole nervous system is permanently ruined").
  - Persistent, distorted cognitions about the cause or consequences of the traumatic event(s) that lead the individual to blame himself/herself or others.
  - Persistent negative emotional state (eg, fear, horror, anger, guilt, or shame).
  - Markedly diminished interest or participation in significant activities.
  - Feelings of detachment or estrangement from others.
  - Persistent inability to experience positive emotions (eg, inability to experience happiness, satisfaction, or loving feelings).
- Marked alterations in arousal and reactivity associated with the traumatic event(s), beginning or worsening after the traumatic event(s) occurred, as evidenced by two (or more) of the following:
  - Irritable behavior and angry outbursts (with little or no provocation) typically expressed as verbal or physical aggression toward people or objects.
  - Reckless or self-destructive behavior
  - Hypervigilance
  - Exaggerated startle response
  - Problems with concentration
  - Sleep disturbance (eg, difficulty falling or staying asleep or restless sleep)
- Duration of the disturbance (Criteria B to E) is more than 1 month.
- The disturbance causes clinically significant distress or impairment in social, occupational, or other important areas of functioning.
- The disturbance is not attributable to the physiologic effects of a substance (eg, medication, alcohol) or another medical condition.

Specify whether:

- **With dissociative symptoms:** The individual's symptoms meet the criteria for PTSD, and in addition, in response to the stressor, the individual experiences persistent or recurrent symptoms of either of the following:
  - **Depersonalization:** Persistent or recurrent experiences of feeling detached from, and as if one were an outside observer of, one's mental processes or body (eg, feeling as though one were in a dream; feeling a sense of unreality of self or body or of time moving slowly).
  - **Derealization:** Persistent or recurrent experiences of unreality of surroundings (eg, the world around the individual is experienced as unreal, dreamlike, distant, or distorted).

- **Note:** To use this subtype, the dissociative symptoms must not be attributable to the physiologic effects of a substance (eg, blackouts, behavior during alcohol intoxication) or another medical condition (eg, complex partial seizures).

Specify if:

- **With delayed expression:** If the full diagnostic criteria are not met until at least 6 months after the event (although the onset and expression of some symptoms may be immediate).

(Reprinted with permission from the *Diagnostic and Statistical Manual of Mental Disorders*. 5th ed. Arlington, VA: American Psychiatric Publication; 2013.)

What is your rationale for the diagnosis?

The patient's symptoms meet the criteria for PTSD. He was exposed to a traumatic event. He describes intrusive thoughts and nightmares of the event. He experiences distress when exposed to cues that symbolize or resemble the event (scenes with police on TV). He has a persistent negative emotional state of fear related to the event. He has an inability to experience positive emotions (not able to enjoy playing with his children, not interested in sex). He is hypervigilant and has difficulty falling asleep at night. These disturbances have lasted more than 1 month and have impaired his social and occupation areas of functioning. The disturbances are not due to the effects of a substance or other medical condition.

What tests or tools should be considered to help identify the correct diagnosis?

Clinician-Administered PTSD Scale for *DSM-5* (CAPS-5) which can be accessed at https://www.ptsd.va.gov/PTSD/professional/assessment/adult-int/caps.asp.

What differential diagnosis should be considered?

296.21 (F323.0) Major Depressive Disorder, Single Episode, Mild

The patient reported feelings of depression, loss of interest in activities, and insomnia. These are three of the nine possible symptoms for major depressive disorder; however, five symptoms are required for the diagnosis of major depressive disorder. Therefore, the patient's presentation would not meet the criteria for major depressive disorder.

300.01 (F41.0) Panic Disorder

While the patient has experienced panic symptoms, they have been related to reminders of traumatic events. Therefore, the diagnosis of panic disorder would not be indicated.

FORMULATING THE TREATMENT STRATEGY

What treatment would you prescribe and what is the rationale?

Psychopharmacology

Sertraline 50 mg daily: Selective serotonin reuptake inhibitors are considered first-line treatment for PTSD. However, only sertraline and paroxetine are approved by the Food and Drug Administration for PTSD.

Prazosin 1 mg HS: Recommended for nightmares originating from PTSD. Dose can be increased as tolerated.

Diagnostic Tests: Monitor blood pressure and pulse as prazosin can cause hypotension.

Referral: Individual psychotherapy.

Type of Psychotherapy: Supportive psychotherapy should be initiated. Relaxation techniques can also be taught to help manage anxiety. Exposure and desensitization techniques may help the patient reduce his response to the trauma. Reprocessing therapy (eye movement desensitization and reprocessing, EMDR) has evidence-based data to indicate that it is effective in treating PTSD. Qualified EMDR practitioners can be identified by contacting the EMDR International Association at (866) 451-5200 or at this link http://www.emdria.org/search/custom.asp?id=2337.

Psychoeducation: Provide literature about PTSD from the National Institute of Mental Health.

Provide literature about sertraline and prazosin. Remind the patient that sertraline will take approximately 4 weeks to become effective.

What guidelines would you use to treat or assess this patient?

The Veterans Administration has issued several guidelines that may be valuable in working with individuals with PTSD. VA/DoD Clinical Practice Guidelines: Management of Post-Traumatic Stress Disorder and Acute Stress Reaction. Available at http://www.healthquality.va.gov/guidelines/mh/ptsd/index.asp

CLINICAL NOTE

- An individual's response to trauma will vary depending on their personal history, prior trauma, and other factors influencing their resilience.
- It is recommended that benzodiazepines not be prescribed for PTSD.

REFERENCES/RECOMMENDED READINGS

American Psychiatric Association. *Diagnostic and Statistical Manual of Mental Disorders.* 5th ed. Arlington, VA: American Psychiatric Publishing; 2013.

National Center for PTSD, U.S. Department of Veterans Affairs. (2011). Evidence-Based Treatments for PTSD: What the Research Tells Us About Patient Improvement. http://www.ptsd.va.gov/Public/understanding_TX/CourseList/Course_NCPTSD_Treatment_1435/assets/00015006.PDF

Saddock BJ, Saddock VA. *Synopsis of Psychiatry: Behavioral Sciences/Clinical Psychiatry.* Philadelphia, PA: Lippincott Williams & Wilkins; 2007.

Stahl S. *The Prescriber's Guide: Stahl's Essential Psychopharmacology.* New York, NY: Cambridge University Press; 2011.

Weathers FW, Blake DD, Schnurr PP, Kaloupek DG, Marx BP, Keane TM. The clinician-administered PTSD scale for DSM-5 (CAPS-5). *Interview available from the National Center for PTSD at* www.ptsd.va.gov. Accessed 2013.

CASE 37

Depressed and Worried about Drinking

IDENTIFICATION: The patient is a 35-year-old single white male who lives with his boyfriend.

CHIEF COMPLAINT: "I have phases of depression and am worried about my drinking increasing."

HISTORY OF CHIEF COMPLAINT: Reports drinking two to three bottles of wine a day. Fearful of losing his boyfriend if he keeps drinking. He reports "heavy" drinking since last year.

PAST PSYCHIATRIC HISTORY: Described separation anxiety as a child when starting school, but was never treated. Had depressed mood his "whole life." Started sertraline at 20 years old. Had a suicide attempt while drinking after a breakup with a boyfriend. Was taken to emergency department for an overdose. Stayed in the hospital for 2 weeks and was tried on various medications. Continued drinking while taking the medication after discharge from the hospital. Remembers taking ziprasidone, paroxetine, sertraline, and fluoxetine. Became suicidal while on fluoxetine. Stopped the medications 4 years ago.

MEDICAL HISTORY: No acute or chronic medical conditions.

HISTORY OF DRUG OR ALCOHOL ABUSE: No history of drug use. Reports a history of drinking excessively.

FAMILY HISTORY: Raised by both parents. Mother attends Alcoholics Anonymous (AA) meetings. There are many relatives with alcohol problems. His father passed away 3 years ago from myocardial infarction. He has three brothers but does not have a close relationship with them.

PERSONAL HISTORY

Perinatal: Full-term vaginal birth. No known complications.

Childhood: Was shy but had friends.

Adolescence: Graduated from high school. Was in several school plays.

Adulthood: College graduate and is employed full time. He identifies as gay. In a 6-year monogamous relationship with his boyfriend who complains about his drinking. No military history. Had a DUI at the age of 23.

TRAUMA/ABUSE HISTORY: Denied.

MENTAL STATUS EXAMINATION

Appearance: Casual attire. Appears stated age.

Behavior and psychomotor activity: Cooperative. Good eye contact. No motor abnormalities.

Consciousness:	Alert.
Orientation:	Oriented to person, place, and time.
Memory:	Grossly intact.
Concentration and attention:	Good.
Visuospatial ability:	Not assessed.
Abstract thought:	Satisfactory.
Intellectual functioning:	Average.
Speech and language:	Pressured speech.
Perceptions:	No altered perceptions.
Thought processes:	Tangential and circumstantial.
Thought content:	Relevant to concerns about his drinking. No suicidal or homicidal ideation.
Suicidality or homicidality:	Denied.

Mood: Depressed and anxious.

Affect: Appropriate to content of speech full range. Appeared anxious.

Impulse control: Within normal limits.

Judgment/insight/reliability: Good.

FORMULATING THE DIAGNOSIS

Which diagnosis (or diagnoses) should be considered?

303.90 (F10.20) Alcohol Use Disorder, Severe

Diagnostic Criteria

A. A problematic pattern of alcohol use leading to clinically significant impairment or distress, as manifested by at least two of the following, occurring within a 12-month period:
   1. Alcohol is often taken in larger amounts or over a longer period than was intended.
   2. There is a persistent desire or unsuccessful efforts to cut down or control alcohol use.
   3. A great deal of time is spent in activities necessary to obtain alcohol, use alcohol, or recover from its effects.
   4. Craving, or a strong desire or urge to use alcohol.
   5. Recurrent alcohol use resulting in a failure to fulfill major role obligations at work, school, or home.
   6. Continued alcohol use despite having persistent or recurrent social or interpersonal problems caused or exacerbated by the effects of alcohol.
   7. Important social, occupational, or recreational activities are given up or reduced because of alcohol use.
   8. Recurrent alcohol use in situations in which it is physically hazardous.
   9. Alcohol use is continued despite knowledge of having a persistent or recurrent physical or psychological problem that is likely to have been caused or exacerbated by alcohol.
   10. Tolerance, as defined by either of the following:
       a. A need for markedly increased amounts of alcohol to achieve intoxication or desired effect.
       b. A markedly diminished effect with continued use of the same amount of alcohol.
   11. Withdrawal, as manifested by either of the following:

a. The characteristic withdrawal syndrome for alcohol (refer to Criteria A and B of the criteria set for alcohol withdrawal).
b. Alcohol (or a closely related substance, such as a benzodiazepine) is taken to relieve or avoid withdrawal symptoms.

Specify if:

- **In early remission:** After full criteria for alcohol use disorder were previously met, none of the criteria for alcohol use disorder have been met for at least 3 months but for less than 12 months (with the exception that Criterion A4, "Craving, or a strong desire or urge to use alcohol," may be met).
- **In sustained remission:** After full criteria for alcohol use disorder were previously met, none of the criteria for alcohol use disorder have been met at any time during a period of 12 months or longer (with the exception that Criterion A4, "Craving, or a strong desire or urge to use alcohol," may be met).

Specify if:

- **In a controlled environment:** This additional specifier is used if the individual is in an environment where access to alcohol is restricted.

Code based on current severity: Note for *ICD-10-CM* codes: If an alcohol intoxication, alcohol withdrawal, or another alcohol-induced mental disorder is also present, do not use the codes below for alcohol use disorder. Instead, the comorbid alcohol use disorder is indicated in the fourth character of the alcohol-induced disorder code (see the coding note for alcohol intoxication, alcohol withdrawal, or a specific alcohol-induced mental disorder). For example, if there is comorbid alcohol intoxication and alcohol use disorder, only the alcohol intoxication code is given, with the fourth character indicating whether the comorbid alcohol use disorder is mild, moderate, or severe: F10.129 for mild alcohol use disorder with alcohol intoxication or F10.229 for a moderate or severe alcohol use disorder with alcohol intoxication.

Specify current severity:

- **305.00 (F10.10) Mild:** Presence of two to three symptoms.
- **303.90 (F10.20) Moderate:** Presence of four to five symptoms.
- **303.90 (F10.20) Severe:** Presence of six or more symptoms.

(Reprinted with permission from the *Diagnostic and Statistical Manual of Mental Disorders*. 5th ed. Arlington, VA: American Psychiatric Publishing; 2013.)

What is your rationale for the diagnosis?

The patient self-identifies a problem with excessive drinking. He meets at least six of the diagnostic criteria (1, 2, 4, 6, 8, and 9) for alcohol abuse disorder, severe. Because six or more symptoms were identified, the criterion for a specification of "severe" is met.

Which diagnosis (or diagnoses) should be considered?

311 (F32.9) Unspecified Depressive Disorder

This category applies to presentations in which symptoms characteristic of a depressive disorder that cause clinically significant distress or impairment in social, occupational, or other important areas of functioning predominate but do not meet the full criteria for any of the disorders in the depressive disorders diagnostic class. The unspecified depressive disorder category is used in situations in which the clinician chooses *not* to specify the reason that the criteria are not met for a specific depressive disorder, and includes presentations for which there is insufficient information to make a more specific diagnosis (eg, in emergency room settings).

(Reprinted with permission from the *Diagnostic and Statistical Manual of Mental Disorders*. 5th ed. Arlington, VA: American Psychiatric Publishing; 2013.)

What is your rationale for the diagnosis?

The patient complains of depression. His depressive symptoms may be related to various relationship, employment, or financial issues that have been a consequence of his drinking. His depressive symptoms could be medically related or related to the physiologic effects of the alcohol abuse, or may represent a predisposing tendency for depression. Therefore, a diagnosis of unspecified depressive disorder is used as "the criteria are not met for a specific depressive disorder, and . . . there is insufficient information to make a more specific diagnosis. . ." (American Psychiatric Publishing, 2013).

What tests or tools should be considered to help identify the correct diagnosis?

Alcohol Use Disorder: The patient self-reports excessive drinking so screening for the degree of alcohol use may not be indicated. However, individuals who present with possible alcohol use disorder can be screened using the CAGE questionnaire, which can be accessed at https://pubs.niaaa.nih.gov/publications/inscage.htm. The CAGE questionnaire is a screening tool using four simple questions related to drinking behavior which can indicate potential problems with alcohol.

Unspecified Depressive Disorder: Numerous scales are available to evaluate the severity of depressive symptoms. The Hamilton Rating Scale for Depression, The Montgomery-Åsberg Depression Rating Scale, and The Beck Depression Inventory are commonly used.

A genogram may also help identify family patterns that would indicate a greater familial tendency for major depressive disorder, anxiety, alcohol abuse, or bipolar disorder.

What differential diagnoses should be considered?

300.23 (F40.10) Social Anxiety Disorder (Social Phobia)

The patient describes anxiety as a child but is not reporting anxiety as a current problem. However, anxiety may be a contributing factor to his drinking behavior so it should be thoroughly assessed. Additionally, identification of social anxiety disorder may prompt the patient to address it with self-help manuals or individual therapy to minimize the anxiety response. If diagnosed, there are also pharmacologic treatments (propranolol, selective serotonin reuptake inhibitors) that may be helpful.

296.89 (F31.81) Bipolar II Disorder

Because the patient describes a long history of depression that includes a serious suicidal attempt, it would be prudent to assess for bipolar II disorder. It is known that bipolar depression can take several years to diagnosis. These patients are usually treated for major depressive disorder initially, since hypomanic episodes are either not identified or reported. If hypomanic episodes occurred, they may have been mild. Additional screening with the Mood Disorder Questionnaire and continued observation along with obtaining history from significant others may help rule out this diagnosis.

FORMULATING THE TREATMENT STRATEGY

What treatment would you prescribe and what is the rationale?

Psychopharmacology: Naltrexone 50 mg PO daily. The patient must be opiate free for 7 to 10 days. If there is a risk of withdrawal a naloxone challenge test should be considered. Naltrexone alone or in combination with acamprosate calcium is recommended for the treatment of alcohol use disorder. Naltrexone should be prescribed for patients with moderate to severe alcohol use disorder including those with physical dependence. Individuals with cravings or who have not improved with psychosocial approaches are particularly good candidates for pharmacologic treatments. The patient was advised of improved outcomes with injectable naltrexone long-acting, however at this time he preferred to take the medication orally.

Diagnostic Tests: Routine laboratory tests including liver enzymes should be ordered. Thyroid testing should be included to identify abnormalities that could contribute to anxiety or depression.

Referral: Depending on the results of routine laboratory tests, a referral to the patient's primary care provider (PCP) may be indicated to evaluate and treat any medical conditions that may have occurred with heavy alcohol use. If liver enzymes are elevated, the PCP should be consulted to discuss the risks and benefits of treatment with naltrexone.

Type of Psychotherapy: The patient should be assessed to determine what type of therapy would best help him. AA is one consideration and is helpful for many individuals. However, because this patient reports being "shy," he may not respond well to a group approach to treatment. Individual therapy to help him modify his behavior may be more appropriate. The therapy could include aspects of cognitive behavioral therapy, for instance, identifying triggers and avoiding situations that may expose him to greater risk.

Psychoeducation: The patient was educated about the risks and benefits of naltrexone. The patient should be advised to carry an ID card or wear a medical alert bracelet stating that he is taking naltrexone.

All providers who treat the patient should know he is taking naltrexone.

Web-based therapy can include tools to monitor drinking behavior, exercises to help set goals, and relapse prevention techniques. The Addiction-Comprehensive Health Enhancement Support System (A-CHESS) is a smartphone app that provides patients with other tools and support services.

What guidelines would you use to treat or assess this patient?

Medication for the Treatment of Alcohol Use Disorder: A Brief Guide can be accessed at http://store.samhsa.gov/shin/content/SMA15-4907/SMA15-4907.pdf

CLINICAL NOTE

- There is frequently shame with alcohol use disorders. Therefore, a nonjudgmental attitude is imperative in order to promote a therapeutic alliance.
- Some individuals with a genetic GRIK1 polymorphism may benefit by topiramate 200 mg daily to assist in reducing alcohol intake. If financial resources allow for genetic testing, the patient could be tested for this polymorphism.
- Online AA groups may be beneficial for some individuals with alcohol use disorder. Some options can be accessed at: http://www.aa-intergroup.org/, http://www.aaonline.net/, or http://mobile.intherooms.com/.

REFERENCES/RECOMMENDED READINGS

American Psychiatric Association. *Diagnostic and Statistical Manual of Mental Disorders*. 5th ed. Arlington, VA: American Psychiatric Publishing; 2013.

Bankole AJ. Pharmacotherapy for alcohol use disorder. In: UpToDate, Saitz R (Ed). Waltham, MA: UpToDate; 2014.

Hirschfeld RMA. The Mood Disorder Questionnaire: a simple, patient-rated screening instrument for bipolar disorder. *Primary Care Companion to J Clin Psychiatr.* 2002;4(1):9-11.

Kranzler HR, Covault J, Feinn R, et al. Topiramate treatment of heavy drinkers: moderation by a *GRIK1* polymorphism. *Am J Psychiatr*. 2014;171(4):445-452. doi:10.1176/appi.ajp.2013.13081014

McGoldrick M, Gerson R, Petry S. *Genograms: Assessment and Intervention*. 3rd ed. New York, NY: Norton, W. W. & Co., Inc; 2008.

CASE 38

Telepsychiatry

IDENTIFICATION: The patient is a 35-year-old Caucasian, English speaking, married male on permanent disability who lives with his wife and three children. He is being treated via telepsychiatry.

CHIEF COMPLAINT: "I've been having a lot of trouble with paranoia and anxiety."

HISTORY OF PRESENT ILLNESS: The patient has been in treatment at this community mental health agency continuously for the past several years. His primary complaints are auditory hallucinations, paranoia, and anxiety. The voices tell him he is worthless. They become more intense when he is alone. They bother him almost constantly, to the point that his wife can tell he is "not present." He attempts to participate in the school activities of his children, but admits that he can never stay for a full program because the voices tell him that someone there is going to hurt him. He has terrifying nightmares. The hallucinations and accompanying paranoia cause fears that others are talking about him, that his children may get hurt, etc. These fears precipitate panic attacks with rapid heart rate, difficulty breathing, tingling in hands and feet, upset stomach, and sweating. Due to the panic/fears he isolates himself. He also describes panic symptoms not triggered by any voices. However, he is trying to manage his anxiety by healthy activities such as walking over a mile a day.

PAST PSYCHIATRIC HISTORY: At age 9, the patient was hospitalized for behavior problems. He reports that he had dyslexia, attention deficit problems, and explosiveness. He has been in juvenile treatment centers. He has a history of suicide attempts at age 11 through overdose, at age 12 with shotgun. He had cutting behaviors. First auditory hallucinations occurred when he was around age 17. From age 17 he engaged heavily in drug use which included methamphetamines, heroin, cocaine, marijuana, and alcohol. He stopped using all substances at the age of 25 years when he almost died from an overdose. He was engaged in psychotherapy. He also received pharmacological treatment. Psychotropic medications have included lurasidone, buspirone, asenapine, lithium carbonate, quetiapine, and lorazepam. In the past 2 years, he has had two episodes of mania lasting 2 to 3 days, spaced about 6 months apart.

His current medications are: lithium carbonate ER 300 mg in the AM and 900 mg at HS, quetiapine 300 mg at HS and 50 mg BID, lorazepam 1 mg TID PRN anxiety, and silenor 3 mg one at bedtime.

MEDICAL HISTORY: The patient has no known allergies. He has diabetes mellitus type 1, diabetic neuropathy, elevated liver enzymes, hyperlipidemia, hypertension (systemic), nonorganic sleep apnea, and osteoarthritis. His most recent hemoglobin A1c =8.7 (high). His weight is 304 lb. Body mass index (BMI) is 37.5.

While taking olanzapine and then asenapine, his liver enzymes were elevated. His liver enzymes are currently normal.

He is taking carvedilol 3.125 mg BID; Humalog KwikPen 25 units before meals, Lantus SoloSTAR 68 units at bedtime, atorvastatin 20 mg daily, lisinopril 2.5 mg daily, metformin 1,000 mg BID, ProAir HFA 108 two puffs every 4 hours PRN. Recently started on orlistat 120 mg daily.

His sleep pattern has improved from only 3 to 4 hours nightly to 5 to 7 hours with the use of silenor.

HISTORY OF DRUG OR ALCOHOL ABUSE: The patient is a former cigarette smoker. He reports heavy drug and alcohol use from age 17 to 25. He acknowledges that his use was a form of self-medication for the hallucinations. He states, "I used anything and everything: methamphetamines, heroin, cocaine, pot, and alcohol." He says he almost died at age 25 from overuse, which is what led to his decision to stop. He has not used substances since then. He no longer drinks alcohol due to the impact on his blood sugar. He achieved sobriety through participation in Alcoholics Anonymous meetings and the support of his church.

FAMILY HISTORY: The patient does not know if his biologic heritage includes any mental illness. He says that during his childhood, his father was violent and abusive, angry, yelling, and throwing objects. His father never received any diagnosis or treatment. His parents are alive and still married to each other, but the relationship is characterized by bitterness and fighting. The patient often feels pulled into the conflict and forced to take sides. He has two brothers and one sister. He feels close to his sister.

PERSONAL HISTORY

Perinatal history: No known complications.

Childhood: Was able to make friends and function academically in school. No known learning disabilities.

Adolescence: Completed high school.

Adulthood: After high school he left his family and moved out of state. He was in the Army briefly and was released due to mental health issues. He was married at age 20, and this ended in divorce with one child. He has been with his current spouse now for 10 years. They have two children. His child from his first marriage lives with them. He is on disability. He lives in an area that is underserved by psychiatric providers, so he is being treated via telepsychiatry.

TRAUMA/ABUSE HISTORY: The patient experienced abuse from his father. He does not elaborate on these details other than to say his own anger scares him because he does not want his children to live through what he did.

MENTAL STATUS EXAMINATION

Appearance: Neat, clean, appropriately dressed in casual wear, clean-shaven.

Behavior and psychomotor activity: Cooperative, pleasant, gait normal, posture upright, sits calmly in chair with no fidgeting, does not show or report any involuntary movements or tics.

Consciousness:	Alert and oriented to person, time, and place.
Memory:	Intact. Able to recall distant events of his life, recounts events from yesterday.
Concentration and attention:	Able to do simple arithmetic, spell "world" backward. Stays on topic in conversation during sessions.
Visuospatial ability:	Accurately draws clock-face and puts in stated time.
Abstract thought:	Able to accurately explain proverbs "People who live in glass houses shouldn't throw stones," and "Don't cry over spilled milk."
Intellectual functioning:	Average vocabulary and fund of general knowledge.

Speech and language: Good volume, calm rate of speech, fluid flow.

Perceptions: Auditory hallucinations of voices telling him he is worthless. No visual hallucinations reported.

Thought processes: Clear, linear, logical.

Thought content: Frequent thoughts that others are against him.

Suicidality/homicidality: No thoughts, intentions, or plans to hurt self or others. The patient was evaluated using the Violence Risk Screening-10 tool. See details below.

The Violence Risk Screening-10 tool (can be accessed at http://www.forensic-psychiatry.no/violence_risk/v_risk_10_english.pdf) was used to assess for risk. With his current presentation, he is considered a low risk due to the criteria in this screening tool. Although he does have a major mental illness, there is no previous or current violence, threats, personality disorder, lack of insight, lack of empathy, unrealistic planning, or imminent expectation of unusual stress that might increase the potential for violence. Although there is history of substance abuse, there has not been any for the past 10 years. He does not have access to weapons. He is very insightful and motivated to continue treatment and utilize healthy coping mechanisms.

Mood: Generally somber, serious, sad.

Affect: Pleasant, yet blunted in spontaneity of affect.

Impulse control: Good.

Judgment/Insight/Reliability: The patient is aware that he lives with a chronic mental illness and actively struggles to adjust to it. He works hard to stay active/involved with his children given the limitations due to his mental illness. He seeks out the company/support of his wife, stating at times he just needs to curl up beside her when the voices are intense. He keeps all appointments and reports 100% adherence to medications.

FORMULATING THE DIAGNOSIS

Which diagnosis (or diagnoses) should be considered?

295.70 (F25.0) Schizoaffective Disorder, Bipolar Type, Continuous

Diagnostic Criteria

A. An uninterrupted period of illness during which there is a major mood episode (major depressive or manic) concurrent with Criterion A of schizophrenia.
   - **Note:** The major depressive episode must include Criterion A1: depressed mood.

B. Delusions or hallucinations for 2 or more weeks in the absence of a major mood episode (depressive or manic) during the duration of the illness.

C. Symptoms that meet criteria for a major mood episode are present for the majority of the total duration of the active and residual portions of the illness.

D. The disturbance is not attributable to the effects of a substance (eg, a drug of abuse, a medication) or another medical condition.

Specify whether:

- **295.70 (F25.0) Bipolar type:** This subtype applies if a manic episode is part of the presentation. Major depressive episodes may also occur.
- **295.70 (F25.1) Depressive type:** This subtype applies if only major depressive episodes are part of the presentation.

Specify if:

- **With catatonia** (refer to the criteria for catatonia associated with another mental disorder).
  Coding note: Use additional code 293.89 (F06.1) catatonia associated with schizoaffective disorder to indicate the presence of the comorbid catatonia.

Specify if:
The following course specifiers are only to be used after a 1-year duration of the disorder and if they are not in contradiction to the diagnostic course criteria.

- **First episode, currently in acute episode:** First manifestation of the disorder meeting the defining diagnostic symptom and time criteria. An *acute episode* is a time period in which the symptom criteria are fulfilled.
- **First episode, currently in partial remission:** *Partial remission* is a time period during which an improvement after a previous episode is maintained and in which the defining criteria of the disorder are only partially fulfilled.
- **First episode, currently in full remission:** *Full remission* is a period of time after a previous episode during which no disorder-specific symptoms are present.

- **Multiple episodes, currently in acute episode:** Multiple episodes may be determined after a minimum of two episodes (ie, after a first episode, a remission, and a minimum of one relapse).
- **Multiple episodes, currently in partial remission**
- **Multiple episodes, currently in full remission**
- **Continuous:** Symptoms fulfilling the diagnostic symptom criteria of the disorder are remaining for the majority of the illness course, with subthreshold symptom periods being very brief relative to the overall course.
- **Unspecified**

Specify current severity:

- Severity is rated by a quantitative assessment of the primary symptoms of psychosis, including delusions, hallucinations, disorganized speech, abnormal psychomotor behavior, and negative symptoms. Each of these symptoms may be rated for its current severity (most severe in the last 7 days) on a 5-point scale ranging from 0 (not present) to 4 (present and severe).
- **Note:** Diagnosis of schizoaffective disorder can be made without using this severity specifier.

(Reprinted with permission from the *Diagnostic and Statistical Manual of Mental Disorders*. 5th ed. Arlington, VA: American Psychiatric Publishing; 2013.)

What is the rationale for the diagnosis?

The client fulfills criteria for this diagnosis because he has a continuous experience over more than 15 years of delusions of being in danger from others and of auditory hallucinations. Although he has not exhibited any disorganized speech or grossly abnormal physical behaviors such as catatonia, he does have negative symptoms of reduced facial expressivity and vocal prosody. These have occurred concurrently more times than not in the presence of major depressive symptoms: depressed, sad, loss of interest, feeling guilty/worthless, diminished energy, insomnia. He has also had at least two self-reported episodes of mania (flight of ideas, pressured speech, diminished need for sleep).

Which diagnosis (or diagnoses) should be considered?

300.01 (F41.0) Panic Disorder

Diagnostic Criteria

A. Recurrent unexpected panic attacks. A panic attack is an abrupt surge of intense fear or intense discomfort that reaches a peak within minutes, and during which time four (or more) of the following symptoms occur:

Note: The abrupt surge can occur from a calm state or an anxious state.

1. Palpitations, pounding heart, or accelerated heart rate
2. Sweating
3. Trembling or shaking
4. Sensations of shortness of breath or smothering
5. Feelings of choking
6. Chest pain or discomfort
7. Nausea or abdominal distress
8. Feeling dizzy, unsteady, light-headed, or faint
9. Chills or heat sensations
10. Paresthesias (numbness or tingling sensations)
11. Derealization (feelings of unreality) or depersonalization (being detached from oneself)
12. Fear of losing control or "going crazy"
13. Fear of dying
    - **Note:** Culture-specific symptoms (eg, tinnitus, neck soreness, headache, uncontrollable screaming or crying) may be seen. Such symptoms should not count as one of the four required symptoms.

B. At least one of the attacks has been followed by 1 month (or more) of one or both of the following:
   1. Persistent concern or worry about additional panic attacks or their consequences (eg, losing control, having a heart attack, "going crazy").
   2. A significant maladaptive change in behavior related to the attacks (eg, behaviors designed to avoid having panic attacks, such as avoidance of exercise or unfamiliar situations).

C. The disturbance is not attributable to the physiologic effects of a substance (eg, a drug of abuse, a medication) or another medical condition (eg, hyperthyroidism, cardiopulmonary disorders).

D. The disturbance is not better explained by another mental disorder (eg, the panic attacks do not occur only in response to feared social situations, as in social anxiety disorder; in response to circumscribed phobic objects or situations, as in specific phobia; in response to obsessions, as in obsessive-compulsive disorder; in response to reminders of traumatic events, as in posttraumatic stress disorder; or in response to separation from attachment figures, as in separation anxiety disorder).

(Reprinted with permission from the *Diagnostic and Statistical Manual of Mental Disorders*. 5th ed. Arlington, VA: American Psychiatric Publishing; 2013.)

What is the rationale for the diagnosis?

This diagnosis might be questionable on the basis of Criterion D above. The client's panic often has been precipitated by the fear generated from his delusional beliefs. However, he has also reported episodes of panic where he was in a relatively calm state of mind, in a safe place, and experienced four or more of the symptoms of Criterion A. He does worry about repeated attacks and has resorted to staying home and avoiding being around other people. Therefore, a diagnosis of panic disorder is indicated.

What test or tools should be considered to help identify the correct diagnosis?

The *DSM-5* Cross-cutting symptom measurement to identify patient's symptoms.

World Health Organization Disability Assessment Schedule 2.0

Brief Psychiatric Rating Scale

Positive and Negative Syndrome Scale

Calgary Depression Scale for Schizophrenia (CDSS). The well-known diagnostic screening tools for depression (Hamilton Depression Index, Beck Depression Scale, etc.) were developed for cases without considering psychosis. The CDSS takes the psychosis into account when assessing the level of depression.

What differential diagnoses should be considered?

296.24 (F32.2) Major Depression with Psychotic Features

The depressive symptoms in this client have "waxed and waned" over time, but the psychotic features have been a constant presence, thus major depression has not been the primary diagnosis.

296.44 (F31.2) Bipolar Disorder with Psychotic Features

Although the client did experience two episodes of mania, he has persistent delusions unrelated to the episodes of mania.

300.22 (F40.00) Agoraphobia

Agoraphobia might be considered; however, the client's discomfort around other people seems more due to the hallucinations telling him that the other people are against him or are going to harm him.

FORMULATING THE TREATMENT STRATEGY

What treatment would you prescribe and what is the rationale?

Note: Due to overlapping symptomatology between schizophrenia and schizoaffective disorder, many treatments for schizophrenia will also benefit patients with schizoaffective disorder.

Pharmacology: Continue current medications: Lithium carbonate ER 300 mg in the morning and 900 mg at bedtime for a total of 1,200 mg daily. This medication, the "gold standard" of mood stabilization treatment for mania, was started several years ago when the client experienced a manic episode. The dose has been adjusted several times and the client reports feeling stable, no breakthroughs of mania.

Quetiapine 300 mg at HS and 50 mg BID. Quetiapine is a second-generation antipsychotic medication that is Food and Drug Administration approved for the treatment of schizophrenia and bipolar disorder. Other second-generation medications have been tried and were not effective, not covered by the patient's insurance, or there were significant adverse side effects (elevated liver enzymes with olanzapine and asenapine). He states "although the voices are still present, they are far more manageable than they have been in the past." He has gained weight and that is being monitored carefully. He states that his current combination of medications has allowed him the highest level of functioning he has experienced in many years and he does not want any further changes or adjustments at this time.

Lorazepam 1 mg, up to 3 times a day if needed for anxiety. Lorazepam is indicated for the management of anxiety disorders or for the short-term relief of the symptoms of anxiety. Although antidepressants are typically the first-line treatments for anxiety, they may precipitate a manic episode in someone with bipolar disorder. With benzodiazepines (lorazepam) there is a potential for dependence, particularly with long-term use. This risk needs to be weighed against the benefits for which treatment is being provided. Because the patient's anxiety significantly impairs his functioning, the use of lorazepam is clinically indicated.

Silenor 3 mg one at bedtime for insomnia. Silenor is a recently marketed brand name for the older tricyclic antidepressant doxepin. At this low dose, there is minimal danger of kindling or pushing the client into mania.

Diagnostic Tests: BMI at every visit. Waist circumference at the outset and then annually.

Abnormal Involuntary Movement Scale to detect akathisia and extrapyramidal symptoms (EPS) from antipsychotics.

Fasting plasma glucose at the outset, 12 weeks, and then annually if no abnormal readings.

Fasting lipid profile: baseline, 12 weeks, and then every 5 years if no abnormal readings.

Lithium level, thyroid-stimulating hormone, and creatinine: at 1 week, at 1 to 2 months, then every 12 months if no abnormal readings, or after any dose alteration.

Drug screening at random to monitor use of lorazepam and rule out any illicit drug use.

Referrals: Refer for psychotherapy.

Psychotherapy: Supportive therapy. This therapy focuses on the therapeutic bond between client and provider, responding to whatever the client presents at any given session in ways that are affirming and empowering.

Acceptance and Commitment Therapy (ACT): The use of ACT has been found effective for clients with schizophrenia.

Psychoeducation: Patient should be educated about symptoms of lithium toxicity and instructed to contact the provider or be evaluated promptly. Patient should be educated about the metabolic side effects of second-generation antipsychotic medications.

Provide information on schizophrenia from the following:

National Institutes of Mental Health: www.nimh.nih.gov;

National Alliance for the Mentally Ill in the local community: www.nami.org;

Choices in Recovery: www.choicesinrecovery.com

What standard guidelines would you use to treat or assess this client?

American Psychiatric Association Practice Guidelines for the Treatment of Psychiatric Disorders.

National Institute for Clinical Effectiveness Guidelines for the Treatment of Schizophrenia.

World Federation of Societies of Biological Psychiatry Guidelines for the Treatment of Schizophrenia.

For risk assessment of violence, useful resources can be found at:

https://wwwn.cdc.gov/wpvhc/Course.aspx/Slide/Unit6_8

http://riskassessment.no/

For suicide risk assessment, the Columbia Suicide Severity Rating Scale can be accessed at: https://www.integration.samhsa.gov/clinical-practice/Columbia_Suicide_Severity_Rating_Scale.pdf.

CLINICAL NOTE

- Medications used to treat schizophrenia carry high side effect profiles. Monitor the metabolic side effects of, especially, the second-generation antipsychotics, including hypertension, hyperlipidemia, elevated blood sugars, and increased weight. It is important to address these metabolic issues because studies show that people with serious chronic mental illness have a shortened life expectancy by 25 years.
- Chronic suicidal ideation is also a major concern with individuals with schizophrenia or schizoaffective disorder. Lithium has been shown to be a protective against suicide, even at doses lower than the standard therapeutic recommendation.
- In this case, treating the patient via telepsychiatry is an additional challenge. The establishment of a therapeutic rapport/alliance remains essential to all mental health care treatment settings. Studies have shown that patient satisfaction when treated via telehealth care remains comparable and even greater than in traditional face-to-face treatment. Telehealth increases access to care in underserved areas and has been shown to lower costs of providing care.

- In cases of paranoid-type schizophrenia, the establishment of the therapeutic alliance can be more difficult due to how the disorder can provoke suspicion and distrust. Interacting with the patient across a television monitor in a live video format can raise the levels of distrust in the patient and/or accentuate their ideas of reference such as, "The TV is talking to me." Thus, not all patients with schizophrenia would be candidates for telepsychiatry. However, in this case study, the patient did not have significant impairment in his thought processes, and he responded well to treatment via telepsychiatry.

REFERENCES/RECOMMENDED READINGS

American Psychiatric Association. *Diagnostic and Statistical Manual of Mental Disorders. 5th ed.* Arlington, VA: American Psychiatric Publishing; 2013.

American Psychiatric Association. Telepsychiatry. https://psychiatry.org/psychiatrists/practice/telepsychiatry?_ga=1.178264109.865433774.1485725093. Accessed January 29, 2017.

Bach P, Hayes SC. The use of acceptance and commitment therapy to prevent the rehospitalization of psychotic patients: a randomized controlled study. *J Consult Clin Psychol.* 2002;70(5):1129-1139. doi:10.1037/0022-006X.70.5.1129

Bishop JE, O'Reilly RL, Maddox K, Hutchinson LJ. Client satisfaction in a feasibility study comparing face to face interviews with telepsychiatry. *J Telemed Telecare.* 2002;8(4):217-221.

Carlat D. Telepsychiatry: what you need to know. *Carlat Psychiatr Rep.* 2015;13(10):1-3.

Rogers PG. Telehealth. In Tusaie KR, Fitzpatrick JJ, eds. *Advanced Practice Psychiatric Nursing. Integrating Psychotherapy, Psychopharmacology, and Complementary and Alternative Approaches across the Lifespan* (pp. 225-284). 2nd ed. New York, NY: Springer Publishing; 2017.

Saddock BJ, Saddock VA. *Synopsis of Psychiatry: Behavioral Sciences/Clinical Psychiatry.* 11th ed. Philadelphia, PA: Lippincott Williams & Wilkins; 2015.

Stahl S. *The Prescriber's Guide: Stahl's Essential Psychopharmacology.* 5th ed. New York, NY: Cambridge University Press; 2014.

Tarraza M, Jacobson L. Integrative management of psychotic symptoms. In Tusaie KR, Fitzpatrick JJ, eds. *Advanced Practice Psychiatric Nursing. Integrating Psychotherapy, Psychopharmacology, and Complementary and Alternative Approaches Across the Lifespan* (pp. 699-706). 2nd ed. New York, NY: Springer Publishing; 2017.

Telehealth Resource Centers. HIPAA and Telehealth. Health Resources and Services Administration, Office for the Advancement of Telehealth, Department of Health and Human Resources. http://www.telehealthresourcecenter.org/sites/main/files/fileattachments/hipaa_for_trcs_2014_0.pdf. Accessed 2016.

CASE 38 APPENDIX

Telepsychiatry

To be effective, telepsychiatry must consider these major factors:

1. **Quality and compliance of the technologic platform used to facilitate the telehealth visit.** There are government guidelines that must be followed for the security and privacy of the care. Poor quality equipment and frequent technologic difficulties can impair the communication and negatively impact the treatment experience.
2. **Quality and compliance of the electronic health record system/ electronic prescribing software.** These should be as "user-friendly" as possible so the provider is not unduly distracted navigating forms and efficiently documenting encounters.
3. **The environment of both the locale in which the patient is seen, and the locale from which the provider sees the patient.** Both the ends of the communication need spaces that are clean, comfortable, private, and welcoming.
4. **Presence of support staff where the patient receives treatment to facilitate rooming, monitor behaviors, and coordinate follow-up and laboratory tests.** The support staff must also serve as the "nose" of the provider in situations where the patient's body-odor would indicate a deficit in personal hygiene that might reflect their mental health status.

When these elements are in place, telepsychiatry provides a satisfactory, cost-effective alternative to the traditional face-to-face in-office treatment of mental health disorders, including schizophrenia.

CASE 39

Incarcerated and Substance Use Problems

IDENTIFICATION: Patient is a 37-year-old, single, Caucasian, incarcerated male. Patient was referred by the social worker assigned to his care.

CHIEF COMPLAINT: "I can't handle how I feel; I'm on the verge of exploding at every minute."

HISTORY OF CHIEF COMPLAINT: The patient was sent to jail due to a charge of Driving While Ability Impaired (DWAI), specifically by alcohol, as well as resisting arrest and spitting on an officer. He has been in jail for the past month. This is his first visit with a mental health provider for medication management since coming to jail. He states he started drinking socially at age 16; however, over the past few years he has been drinking excessively to "mask all the rage I have inside." He states that he knew he had a problem with alcohol about a year and a half ago when he received his first charge of driving under the influence of alcohol. His license was suspended; however, he states he drove with a suspended license to get to work as a construction worker. "I needed to get to work to pay my rent so I figured I could get away with it." He states when he received his second DWAI he soon lost his job and began drinking more heavily. He states he needed more and more alcohol to "quiet my mind" and that he began drinking early in the morning to "just feel normal." He states that he went to rehab once, about 8 months ago, then abstained from alcohol for 6 months after he completed the 28-day program. He began drinking again 2 months ago. He states that while he was not drinking, he felt extreme anger and agitation, often getting into fights with his landlord and other neighbors, which he feels led to him back to drinking.

Currently, the patient states that he feels "anger all the time, I feel like I'm going to kill someone or freak out." He has gotten into multiple fights with other inmates and was seen crying or shouting in his cell by numerous correction officers. He was seen by the social worker yesterday who referred him for a psychiatric assessment. He states that he was taking medications in the past, prescribed in jail, but they made him feel worse so he stopped taking them and started drinking again. He does not know the name of the medications and he did not continue them once he left jail.

He reports feeling sad for the past month, angry, difficulty concentrating, poor sleep (about 3 to 4 hours nightly of sleep), and fluctuating appetite. He feels "keyed-up and on edge" constantly. Patient denies a clear history of elevated mood for 2 weeks or more, but does report irritability, anger and rage often, "mood ups and downs," and impulsivity and unpredictable behaviors such as fighting, and intimidation toward his girlfriend. He reports a history of intrusive thoughts recalling his father's death and his father's physical abuse toward his mother. However, he states this has only occurred once or twice in the past 5 years.

PAST PSYCHIATRIC HISTORY: Patient denies any past psychiatric hospitalizations. He denies ever seeing a therapist. He saw a psychiatrist through his rehab facility for the first time this year. He was prescribed fluoxetine, which he states made him feel worse and more irritable. He denies any history of suicide attempts. Patient does not have a current outpatient psychiatric provider.

MEDICAL HISTORY: Patient denies any allergies to medications, foods, or environmental factors. Patient denies any major medical or surgical illnesses. Patient reports multiple concussions from fighting "over the years."

REVIEW OF SYSTEMS

Constitutional:	Negative.
HEENT:	Negative.
Eyes:	Negative.
Respiratory:	Negative.
Cardiovascular:	Negative.
Gastrointestinal:	Negative. Negative for abdominal pain.
Endocrine:	Negative.
Genitourinary:	Negative.
Musculoskeletal:	Negative.

Skin: Negative.

Allergic/immunologic: Negative.

Neurologic: Negative.

Hematologic: Negative.

Psychiatric/behavioral: Positive for sleep disturbance. Positive for anger and irritability. Positive for some symptoms of depression. Negative for anxiety. Negative for psychosis.

HISTORY OF DRUG OR ALCOHOL ABUSE: Patient endorses drinking alcohol socially since age 16. He states he began abusing alcohol at age 27 and currently refers to himself as an alcoholic. He has been to rehab once earlier this year and completed the 28-day program. Patient's last drink was the day he came to jail 1 month ago. Patient reports past cocaine use, over 1 year ago. Patient reports intermittent cannabis use since age 13, "but I don't really like it." Last reported use of cannabis was 6 months ago.

FAMILY HISTORY: The patient's mother is alive with no pertinent health history. She lives nearby with her boyfriend. The patient states that his father died at age 45 due to colon cancer. His father was "alcoholic." The patient has one brother who is 40, and has been incarcerated multiple times and uses "hard drugs." The patient also has a sister who is 35 and lives nearby with her son and husband. She has asthma and a rare blood disorder (unknown type), as well as a history of anxiety.

PERSONAL HISTORY

Perinatal: Patient's mother was 17 when she became pregnant with the patient. She did not use drugs or alcohol during or before pregnancy and received adequate prenatal care. Patient believes he was a full-term vaginal birth. Patient states that his father was an alcoholic and that his mother was once pushed by him during her pregnancy with the patient. Patient states he believes he was bottle fed, but is unsure.

Childhood: Patient states his childhood was "normal" and he dealt with usual childhood experiences. He does endorse a few adverse childhood experiences, but denies that they were symbolic or pertinent to his identity now. He saw his father using alcohol and occasionally drugs in the household. When he was 6, he witnessed his father being arrested for a domestic complaint when his mother called the police after his father held her against the wall by her throat. He states after that his father never physically assaulted his mother again in front of him; however, he states they also did not speak much after that event.

He wet the bed once or twice when 11 years old.

He had some friends growing up but not many. He mainly "hung out" with his brother or stayed to himself. He tried marijuana once or twice when he was 13 years old.

He did poorly in school. He was in normal classes, except for reading. He never enjoyed school and often would try to get out of it by telling his mother that he did not feel well.

Adolescence: His father was verbally abusive toward him and his siblings. His father took his anger out on the patient. He would yell at him, push him, and threaten him. He quit school in the tenth grade after his father died. He began working in construction with his uncle to help support the family. His first time in juvenile detention at the age of 15 was due to stealing from a local department store.

Adulthood: The patient received his GED while in jail when he was 24 during his fifth incarceration. His previous incarcerations were all for fighting or petit larceny. He has had a girlfriend for the past 9 years whom he lives with sometimes. Their relationship is often volatile. She has been to jail a few times, once for not abiding a restraining order that he had against her. The patient denies being religious or having a specific cultural identity. Patient denies history of military duty.

TRAUMA/ABUSE HISTORY: The patient describes an abusive relationship with his father (see Personal History). He states he was also once "touched" by a male family friend who was asked to babysit a few times. The patient states that this babysitter touched his penis and told the patient to touch him back but that his sister was calling so he "got out of it." He states that this only happened once and that, as an adult, he saw the babysitter when they were both incarcerated in jail at the same time and that he "punched him in the stomach." He denies ever receiving therapy or telling anyone about the abuse.

MENTAL STATUS EXAMINATION

Appearance: The patient has facial hair, good grooming and hygiene, is wearing a blue jail jumper.

Behavior and psychomotor activity: Gait is normal, some psychomotor agitation with his leg shaking throughout the interview.

Consciousness:	Alert but distracted at times.
Orientation:	Oriented to person, place, and time.
Memory:	Good memory retention both immediate and 5 minutes later.
Concentration and attention:	Able to spell WORLD forward and backward without issue. Difficulty with counting backward from 100 in serial 3s. Patient refused to continue after two attempts. Patient often looked around at the clock and behind him when there were noises in the clinic.
Visuospatial ability:	Not assessed.
Abstract thought:	Concrete thinking.
Intellectual functioning:	Average.
Speech and language:	Some spontaneous speech, mostly responds to questions, no articulation error noted. Normal rate, rhythm, and volume.
Perceptions:	Patient denies hallucinations and paranoid ideations.
Thought processes:	Linear, goal oriented.
Thought content:	Voices hostility toward others in the jail.
Suicidality or homicidality:	Denies suicidal ideation, denies homicidal ideation but states, "I could kill someone but wouldn't."
Mood:	"Angry and irritable"
Affect:	Constricted but redirectable, congruent.
Impulse control:	Poor per patient.
Judgment/insight/reliability:	Fair/poor/fair.

FORMULATING THE DIAGNOSIS

Which diagnosis (or diagnoses) should be considered?

303.90 (F10.20) Alcohol Use Disorder, Severe

Diagnostic Criteria

A. A problematic pattern of alcohol use leading to clinically significant impairment or distress, as manifested by at least two of the following, occurring within a 12-month period:
   1. Alcohol is often taken in larger amounts or over a longer period than was intended.
   2. There is a persistent desire or unsuccessful efforts to cut down or control alcohol use.
   3. A great deal of time is spent in activities necessary to obtain alcohol, use alcohol, or recover from its effects.
   4. Craving, or a strong desire or urge to use alcohol.
   5. Recurrent alcohol use resulting in a failure to fulfill major role obligations at work, school, or home.
   6. Continued alcohol use despite having persistent or recurrent social or interpersonal problems caused or exacerbated by the effects of alcohol.
   7. Important social, occupational, or recreational activities are given up or reduced because of alcohol use.
   8. Recurrent alcohol use in situations in which it is physically hazardous.
   9. Alcohol use is continued despite knowledge of having a persistent or recurrent physical or psychological problem that is likely to have been caused or exacerbated by alcohol.
   10. Tolerance, as defined by either of the following:
       a. A need for markedly increased amounts of alcohol to achieve intoxication or desired effect.
       b. A markedly diminished effect with continued use of the same amount of alcohol.
   11. Withdrawal, as manifested by either of the following:
       a. The characteristic withdrawal syndrome for alcohol (refer to Criteria A and B of the criteria set for alcohol withdrawal, pp. 499–500).
       b. Alcohol (or a closely related substance, such as a benzodiazepine) is taken to relieve or avoid withdrawal symptoms.

Specify if:

- **In early remission:** After full criteria for alcohol use disorder were previously met, none of the criteria for alcohol use disorder have been met for at least 3 months but for less than 12 months (with the exception that Criterion A4, "Craving, or a strong desire or urge to use alcohol," may be met).

- **In sustained remission:** After full criteria for alcohol use disorder were previously met, none of the criteria for alcohol use disorder have been met at any time during a period of 12 months or longer (with the exception that Criterion A4, "Craving, or a strong desire or urge to use alcohol," may be met).

Specify if:

- **In a controlled environment:** This additional specifier is used if the individual is in an environment where access to alcohol is restricted.

Code based on current severity: Note for *ICD-10-CM* codes: If alcohol intoxication, alcohol withdrawal, or another alcohol-induced mental disorder is also present, do not use the codes below for alcohol use disorder. Instead, the comorbid alcohol use disorder is indicated in the fourth character of the alcohol-induced disorder code (see the coding note for alcohol intoxication, alcohol withdrawal, or a specific alcohol-induced mental disorder). For example, if there is comorbid alcohol intoxication and alcohol use disorder, only the alcohol intoxication code is given, with the fourth character indicating whether the comorbid alcohol use disorder is mild, moderate, or severe: F10.129 for mild alcohol use disorder with alcohol intoxication or F10.229 for a moderate or severe alcohol use disorder with alcohol intoxication.

Specify current severity:

- **305.00 (F10.10) Mild:** Presence of two to three symptoms.
- **303.90 (F10.20) Moderate:** Presence of four to five symptoms.
- **303.90 (F10.20) Severe:** Presence of six or more symptoms.

(Reprinted with permission from the *Diagnostic and Statistical Manual of Mental Disorders*. 5th ed. Arlington, VA: American Psychiatric Publishing; 2013.)

What is the rationale for the diagnosis?

The patient has a problematic pattern of alcohol use that has led to clinically significant impairment as evidenced by taking larger amounts over time, attempting to stop (going to rehab), having a strong urge to use alcohol (relapsing), persistent use despite its use contributing to multiple incarcerations, recurrent use resulting in failure to maintain employment, and use in physically hazardous situations (driving under the influence). Because the use meets at least six of the diagnostic criteria, the diagnosis of alcohol use disorder, severe is applicable. The patient has not been without alcohol for at least 3 months; therefore, the specifier "In early remission," is not used.

Which diagnosis (or diagnoses) should be considered?

296.80 (F31.9) Unspecified Bipolar and Related Disorder

This category applies to presentations in which symptoms characteristic of a bipolar and related disorder that cause clinically significant distress or impairment in social, occupational, or other important areas of functioning predominate but do not meet the full criteria for any of the disorders in the bipolar and related disorders diagnostic class. The unspecified bipolar and related disorder category is used in situations in which the clinician chooses *not* to specify the reason that the criteria are not met for a specific bipolar and related disorder, and includes presentations in which there is insufficient information to make a more specific diagnosis (eg, in emergency room settings).

(Reprinted with permission from the *Diagnostic and Statistical Manual of Mental Disorders*. 5th ed. Arlington, VA: American Psychiatric Publishing; 2013.)

What is the rationale for the diagnosis?

The patient repeatedly describes feeling like he is going to "explode." Said he drinks to "mask all the rage I have inside." He has had extreme anger and agitation, often getting into fights with his landlord and other neighbors. Even after being abstinent from alcohol for 6 months in the past, he continued to experience these feelings. There is limited information to identify a clear pattern of his symptoms. The symptoms he describes do not meet the full criteria for bipolar disorder because he does not describe depressed episodes. Yet there is a strong mood component to his presentation; therefore, the diagnosis of unspecified bipolar and related disorder will be used.

What differential diagnoses should be considered?

309.81 (F43.10) Posttraumatic Stress Disorder

The patient has a long history of trauma including his childhood experiences of seeing his mother abused in the home, his father being taken to jail by the police, sexual abuse by a male babysitter, as well as physical and emotional abuse by his father. Although he denies most symptoms of posttraumatic stress disorder (PTSD) he does report some history of reexperiencing it. PTSD symptoms can surface over time and should be screened for at various time points. At the time of this evaluation, though, the diagnosis of PTSD is not applicable.

301.7 (F60.2) Antisocial Personality Disorder

The patient had been incarcerated repeatedly. He does report being impulsive. He reports persistent irritability and a history of repeated physical fights. He described a long history of not functioning well academically in school, which may have contributed to his truancy. In spite of meeting most of the criteria for antisocial personality disorder, he does not seem to exhibit any deceitfulness or manipulative behavior, which are key features for the diagnosis. Therefore, the diagnosis of antisocial personality disorder will only be considered as a differential.

3114.01 (F90.9) Unspecified Attention-Deficit/Hyperactivity Disorder

The patient described problems academically throughout his education. He currently exhibits some distractibility (he was often looking around at the clock and behind him when there were noises in the clinic). He is not able to subtract serial 3s. There is insufficient information to make a diagnosis of attention-deficit hyperactivity disorder, but, once his mood is more stable, he should be reevaluated.

331.83 (G31.84) Mild Neurocognitive Disorder Due to Traumatic Brain Injury

Although the patient reports a history of multiple concussions from fighting "over the years," it is not known if he experienced a loss of consciousness, posttraumatic amnesia, disorientation and confusion, or neurologic signs. Therefore, the diagnosis of mild neurocognitive disorder due to traumatic brain injury is not applicable without additional information.

312.34 (F63.81) Intermittent Explosive Disorder

This differential diagnosis is included because it describes the impulsivity, rage, irritability, and history of physical fights and arguments that the patient has experienced. However, the patient's rage is constant rather than intermittent with a rapid onset with no prodromal period. Therefore, the diagnosis of intermittent explosive disorder would not be applicable.

What test or tools should be considered to help identify the correct diagnosis?

The Adverse Childhood Experiences (ACE) Questionnaire is a screening tool that was used for the ACE study conducted by Kaiser Permanente in the 1990s. That study assessed the prevalence of adverse childhood events found to correlate with multiple health risks in adulthood leading to potential early demise. (See Appendix.)

Standardized Assessment of Personality: Abbreviated Scale is an eight-item screening interview for personality disorders. The scale aims to produce a dimensional score that, over a certain number, is correlated to having a personality disorder. This scale has utility for the purpose of a valid and reliable way to establish the likelihood of a personality disorder; however, it has multiple limitations including that it does not indicate the specific personality disorder.

There are multiple other diagnostic strategies that may help to understand the brain functioning of the patient, and, therefore, a more thorough understanding of the patient's brain development over time. However, these tests, such as functional magnetic resonance imaging and neurotransmitter genetic testing have little utility in medication management choices and are not accessible in jail settings.

An important part of the diagnostic process that is unfortunately lacking in jail settings is the ability to collect collateral data from family members and friends. Without this information, there is significant missing data that may otherwise be helpful in establishing a more thorough picture of the patient from which to form a diagnosis.

FORMULATING THE TREATMENT STRATEGY

What treatment would you prescribe and what is the rationale?

Psychopharmacology: Valproic acid (VPA) extended release 500 mg liquid nightly and titrate up to 1000 mg PO HS if tolerated. Patient is exhibiting mood instability. He exhibits significant symptoms of agitation, irritability, and aggression. Valproic acid is a mood stabilizer that is Food and Drug Administration approved for mania and mixed mania. Valproic acid is a good choice as it can be dispensed as a liquid and can be monitored through blood testing. This is an important issue in the jail environment where patients may trade, "cheek" (save their medications in their cheeks in order to spit it out later and use it at a later time or give it away), or otherwise misuse the medication. It has not been found to give patients a "high" feeling, such as buspirone, quetiapine, and bupropion; therefore, there is less likelihood of abusing the medication or having it requested by patients in the hopes of getting a high or sedating effect.

Diagnostic Tests: Conduct baseline labs including: review recent liver function tests (LFTs), complete blood count (CBC) w/diff, and electrolytes. After 4 to 6 days of medication continuation or initiation, order VPA level, LFTs, CBC w/diff. After 25 to 35 days of medication continuation or initiation, order LFTs, CBC w/diff, platelets, and VPA level. Repeat every 3 months. Therapeutic range of Depakote is 50 to 100 mcg/mL. Over 100 mcg/mL the patient may have symptoms of toxicity including tachycardia, hypotension, cardiac arrest, coma, confusion, irritability, hallucinations, ataxia, and cerebral edema. Blood pressure, weight, and heart rate are to be monitored at each visit. If necessary, monitor blood glucose levels and A1c.

Referrals: None indicated.

Type of Psychotherapy: Therapy in the jail (and out of the jail once released) including: trauma-informed group therapy, substance abuse treatment groups, and personal therapy such as cognitive behavioral therapy is recommended. Meditation and other stress reduction practices are also recommended.

Psychoeducation: The patient expresses anger toward the correction officers as well as other inmates for "baiting" him into wanting to fight. He reports an inability to relax and usually gets into fights during these times of agitation. Going to his cell during those times to separate from others and practice mindfulness was recommended. Focusing on his breathing, counting backward from 10 with deep breaths, and listening to his inhalations and exhalations are recommended. Education about the effects of childhood trauma and how it is highly correlated to many of the symptoms he is experiencing, such as alcohol abuse and incarceration, was provided. Relaying information in a trauma-informed framework may help the patient gain insight and make connections between past experiences and present dysfunction in behavior.

CLINICAL NOTE

- Adverse childhood experiences may result in consistent stress on the brain that can, over time, alter the brain as well as other important processes in the brain related to development. Jails are an appropriate place to screen patients for childhood trauma because jails are often the first place that patients struggling with mental health and substance abuse are seen by a psychiatric provider. Screening for trauma is important in order to initiate therapy and, if needed, medication management. Many patients in jails consider themselves "black sheep" or victims of the system. To avoid the cycle of recidivism that is so prevalent in this country, mental health screening and treatment are an essential part of the rehabilitation process that is so often missing in jail.
- An ACE score of four or more may indicate a significant risk for medical and psychiatric disorders.

REFERENCES/RECOMMENDED READINGS

American Psychiatric Association. *Diagnostic and Statistical Manual of Mental Disorders.* 5th ed. Arlington, VA: American Psychiatric Publishing; 2013.

American Psychiatric Association. *Psychiatric Services in Correctional Facilities*: Arlington, VA: American Psychiatric Publishing; 2015.

Centers for Disease Control and Prevention. About Adverse Childhood Experiences. https://www.cdc.gov/violenceprevention/acestudy/about_ace.html. Accessed 2016.

Heese M, Moran P. Screening for personality disorder with the standardized assessment of personality: abbreviated scale (SAPAS): further evidence of concurrent validity. *BioMed Central.* 2010;10. doi:10.1186/1471-244X-10-10.

Huband N, Ferriter M, Nathan R, Jones H. Antiepileptics for aggression and associated impulsivity. *Cochrane Database Syst Rev.* 2010;(2):CD003499. doi:10.1002/14651858.CD003499.pub3.

Kamath J, Temporini H, Quarti S, et al. Psychiatric use and utility of divalproex sodium in Connecticut prisons. *Int J Offender Ther Comparat Criminol.* 2008;52:358-370.

Simpson J. Psychopharmacology in Jails: An Introduction. http://thecarlatreport.com/free_articles/psychopharmacology-jails-introduction-free-article. Accessed 2017.

Stankiewicz A, Swiergiel A, Lisowski P. Epigenetics of stress adaptations in the brain. *Brain Res Bull.* 2013;98:76-92.

CASE 39 APPENDIX

Adverse Childhood Experience (ACE) Questionnaire: Finding Your ACE Score

While you were growing up, during your first 18 years of life:

1. Did a parent or other adult in the household **often** . . .

   Swear at you, insult you, put you down, or humiliate you?

   or

   Act in a way that made you afraid that you might be physically hurt?

   Yes No If yes enter 1 ________

2. Did a parent or other adult in the household **often** . . .

   Push, grab, slap, or throw something at you?

   or

   Ever hit you so hard that you had marks or were injured?

   Yes No If yes enter 1 ________

3. Did an adult or person at least 5 years older than you **ever**. . .

   Touch or fondle you or have you touch their body in a sexual way?

   or

   Try to or actually have oral, anal, or vaginal sex with you?

   Yes No If yes enter 1 ________

4. Did you **often** feel that . . .

   No one in your family loved you or thought you were important or special?

   or

   Your family didn't look out for each other, feel close to each other, or support each other?

   Yes No If yes enter 1 ________

5. Did you **often** feel that . . .

   You didn't have enough to eat, had to wear dirty clothes, and had no one to protect you?

   or

   Your parents were too drunk or high to take care of you or take you to the doctor if you needed it?

   Yes No If yes enter 1 ________

6. Were your parents **ever** separated or divorced?

   Yes No If yes enter 1 ________

7. Was your mother or stepmother:

   Often pushed, grabbed, slapped, or had something thrown at her?

   or

   Sometimes or often kicked, bitten, hit with a fist, or hit with something hard?

   or

   Ever repeatedly hit over at least a few minutes or threatened with a gun or knife?

   Yes No If yes enter 1 ________

8. Did you live with anyone who was a problem drinker or alcoholic or who used street drugs?

   Yes No If yes enter 1 ________

9. Was a household member depressed or mentally ill or did a household member attempt suicide?

   Yes No If yes enter 1 ________

10. Did a household member go to prison?

    Yes No If yes enter 1 ________

Now add up your "Yes" answers: _______ This is your ACE Score

CASE 40

Worried about a Brain Tumor

IDENTIFICATION: The patient is a married 40-year-old mother of a 7-year-old daughter. She was referred by her primary care physician (PCP) to the psychiatric nurse practitioner in the primary care practice for evaluation of anxiety symptoms.

CHIEF COMPLAINT: "I think I have a brain tumor."

HISTORY OF CHIEF COMPLAINT: The patient first presented to her primary care provider 2 years ago with symptoms of headache, difficulty sleeping, and light-headedness. She cried during her first office visit when she told her doctor that she was worried that she had a brain tumor. She was evaluated by her PCP and a neurologist. She had magnetic resonance imaging (MRI) of brain with normal result. She takes ibuprofen PRN for headache approximately once per week.

She reports symptoms of apprehension, fear of dying, fear of having a serious medical illness, insomnia, tachycardia, light-headedness, fears of her daughter or husband getting ill or injured, chest tightness, nausea, and loss of appetite. She has had panic attacks. Triggers for her panic attacks include recurrent thoughts that she has a major medical illness, when her daughter or husband is ill, and flying on airplanes. She states, "I have hypochondrias." Her anxiety symptoms are heightened in September when her daughter returns to school and is "around other kids' germs." She reports no anxiety at work and feeling less anxious when she is occupied with activities such as working, spending time with her family, and at yoga class. She has no difficulties at work or in attending to her activities of daily living.

She has been taking clonazepam 0.5 mg one tablet QAM for the past 6 months prescribed by her PCP.

PAST PSYCHIATRIC HISTORY: She saw a therapist while in college for anxiety related to her parents' divorce and her college workload. She reports no history of depression symptoms. No rituals or compulsive behaviors.

She was prescribed paroxetine for anxiety while in college. She stopped taking paroxetine after 3 months due to weight gain and somnolence.

MEDICAL HISTORY: She takes norgestimate/ethinyl estradiol (Ortho Tri-Cyclen Lo) for the past 5 years for birth control, vitamin D 2,000 IU QAM, and loratadine as needed for seasonal allergies.

No history of surgeries. No history of head injury or loss of consciousness.

HISTORY OF DRUG OR ALCOHOL ABUSE: She reports using marijuana "socially," "once or twice per month" during her last year of college. No other drug use and no drug use since age 21. She has a glass of wine with dinner two nights per week. She has one to two cups of black tea per day.

FAMILY HISTORY: Patient was born in a suburban town and raised by her parents. She has one sister, age 38. Her parents divorced amicably when she was age 18. Her father is remarried and her mother resides with her boyfriend. She reports her mother "worries a lot," but is not in mental health treatment. There is no other family history of mental illness.

PERSONAL HISTORY

Perinatal: Full-term vaginal birth. No complications.

Childhood: She reports having "a happy childhood."

Adolescence: She graduated salutatorian of her high school.

Adulthood: She graduated with honors from college. She has a Bachelor's degree in management and works full time for an insurance company. Patient was raised Presbyterian, and currently attends Methodist church with her husband and daughter. She reports being close to her family and her husband's family. She has a social network of friends who she identifies as supportive. No military history. No legal history.

TRAUMA/ABUSE HISTORY: None.

MENTAL STATUS EXAMINATION

Appearance: Well groomed, wearing dress pants and blouse. Normal gait and posture.

Behavior and psychomotor activity: Good eye contact. Normal psychomotor activity. Cooperative.

Consciousness:	Alert.
Orientation:	Oriented to person, place, and time.
Memory:	Normal recent and remote memory recall.
Concentration and attention:	Good.
Abstract thought:	Not assessed but appears intact.
Intellectual functioning:	Above average intelligence.
Speech and language:	English speaking. Normal rate, rhythm, and tone.
Perceptions:	No abnormal perceptions elicited.
Thought process:	Perseverative.
Thought content:	Preoccupied about somatic concerns and thoughts of illness. No hallucinations or delusions.
Suicidality or homicidality:	She denies any thoughts or intent to harm herself or others.
Mood:	Anxious.
Affect:	Congruent with mood.
Impulsivity:	Not observed and none reported.
Judgment/insight/reliability:	Good.

FORMULATING THE DIAGNOSIS

Which diagnosis (or diagnoses) should be considered?

300.7 (F45.21) Illness Anxiety Disorder, Care Seeking Type

Diagnostic Criteria

A. Preoccupation with having or acquiring a serious illness.
B. Somatic symptoms are not present or, if present, are only mild in intensity. If another medical condition is present or there is a high risk for

developing a medical condition (eg, strong family history is present), the preoccupation is clearly excessive or disproportionate.

C. There is a high level of anxiety about health, and the individual is easily alarmed about personal health status.
D. The individual performs excessive health-related behaviors (eg, repeatedly checks his or her body for signs of illness) or exhibits maladaptive avoidance (eg, avoids doctor appointments and hospitals).
E. Illness preoccupation has been present for at least 6 months, but the specific illness that is feared may change over that period of time.
F. The illness-related preoccupation is not better explained by another mental disorder, such as somatic symptom disorder, panic disorder, generalized anxiety disorder, body dysmorphic disorder, obsessive-compulsive disorder, or delusional disorder, somatic type.

Specify whether:

- **Care-seeking type:** Medical care, including physician visits or undergoing tests and procedures, is frequently used.
- **Care-avoidant type:** Medical care is rarely used.

(Reprinted with permission from the *Diagnostic and Statistical Manual of Mental Disorders*. 5th ed. Arlington, VA: American Psychiatric Publishing; 2013.)

What is the rationale for the diagnosis?

The patient is preoccupied with having a serious, undiagnosed medical illness (brain tumor). Her somatic symptoms (headache) are only mild in intensity. A thorough medical and neurologic examination (including an MRI of the brain) has failed to identify a serious medical illness that could account for her concerns. Her distress emanates from the anxiety about the brain tumor. Her preoccupation with thoughts of having a brain tumor is accompanied by substantial anxiety. Her physician's attempts to reassure her have not alleviated her anxiety about having a brain tumor. She has had repeated medical evaluations over the past 2 years and continues to be preoccupied with having a brain tumor. Therefore, she meets the criteria for illness anxiety disorder, care-seeking type.

Which diagnosis (or diagnoses) should be considered?

300.09 (F41.8) Other Specified Anxiety Disorder

This category applies to presentations in which symptoms characteristic of an anxiety disorder that causes clinically significant distress or impairment in social, occupational, or other important areas of functioning predominate but do not meet the full criteria for any of the disorders in the anxiety disorders diagnostic class. The other specified anxiety disorder category is used in situations in which the clinician chooses to communicate the specific reason that the presentation does not meet the criteria for any specific anxiety disorder. This is done by recording "other specified anxiety disorder" followed by the specific reason (eg, "generalized anxiety not occurring more days than not").

Examples of presentations that can be specified using the "other specified" designation include the following:

1. Limited-symptom attacks.
2. Generalized anxiety not occurring more days than not.
3. *Khyâl cap* (wind attacks)
4. *Ataque de nervios* (attack of nerves)

(Reprinted with permission from the *Diagnostic and Statistical Manual of Mental Disorders*. 5th ed.. Arlington, VA: American Psychiatric Association; 2013.)

What is the rationale for the diagnosis?

The patient has a history of anxiety while in college triggered by her parents' divorce and her school workload for which she was treated with psychotherapy and paroxetine. This may have been an adjustment disorder with anxious features. However, there has been a continuation of anxiety triggered when her husband is ill or when her daughter returns to school due to worrying about her being exposed to germs. She also describes a phobia about airplanes. So there seems to be a pattern of excessive anxiety about a number of events or activities. She describes insomnia, tachycardia, light-headedness, chest tightness, nausea, and loss of appetite. She has had panic attacks. This pattern of anxiety resulting in these symptoms would indicate a diagnosis of generalized anxiety disorder. However, her anxiety has not caused impairment in her social, occupational, or other important areas of functioning. In fact, she reports functioning quite well at work. Although some of her anxiety is related to her illness anxiety disorder, there are other situations that cause her considerable worry, which do not fall under that criteria. Therefore, because her symptom presentation meets some but not all of the criteria for general anxiety disorder, a diagnosis of other specified anxiety disorder is applicable.

What test or tools should be considered to help identify the correct diagnosis?

The Health Anxiety Inventory-18 is available for download from the Internet and can be accessed at: serene.me.uk/tests/hai.pdf

What differential diagnosis (or diagnoses) should be considered?

None indicated.

FORMULATING THE TREATMENT STRATEGY

What treatment would you prescribe and what is the rationale?

Psychopharmacology: Sertraline 25 mg daily. A selective serotonin reuptake inhibitor, such as sertraline, may help reduce the patient's anxiety symptoms as there is considerable research for this indication, even if not specifically in the context of illness anxiety disorder. It should be kept in mind that the patient gained weight with paroxetine so her weight should be monitored closely to address any side effects that could contribute to the patient discontinuing the medication.

Clonazepam 0.5 mg in AM. The patient is prescribed clonazepam for anxiety by her PCP. She should continue on clonazepam as prescribed. The use of clonazepam can be reevaluated after the sertraline has had time to provide a therapeutic response.

Consultation: Continue to collaborate with the patient's PCP on management of illness anxiety disorder.

Diagnostic Tests: Patient has had a thorough comprehensive physical exam by her PCP. Medical records from her PCP should be reviewed for any relevant medical issues.

Referrals: Cognitive behavioral therapy (CBT) for anxiety. CBT may be beneficial in treating illness anxiety disorder since it can address the maladaptive thought patterns that support the preoccupation with having a serious medical illness.

Type of Psychotherapy: CBT. Internet-based CBT can be recommended as it may be more accessible and has been demonstrated to be efficacious in treating illness anxiety disorder (see References/Recommended Readings).

Psychoeducation: The Mayo Clinic web site provides information for patients about illness anxiety disorder that can be accessed at: http://www.mayoclinic.org/diseases-conditions/illness-anxiety-disorder/basics/definition/con-20124064

Provide sleep hygiene education, including no caffeine after 4 PM due to insomnia.

Provide education on breathing techniques to reduce anxiety, which patient was instructed to practice twice per day and use as needed.

Encourage to continue weekly yoga class along with additional daily cardio exercise to help reduce her anxiety and improve her sleep.

What standard guidelines would you use to treat or assess this patient?

None.

CLINICAL NOTE

- Individuals with illness anxiety disorder are initially seen in medical settings as are those with somatic symptoms disorder. However, individuals with somatic symptoms disorder present with significant somatic symptoms as opposed to illness anxiety disorder in which the physical symptoms are minimal.
- Illness anxiety disorder was previously called hypochondrias.

REFERENCES/RECOMMENDED READINGS

American Psychiatric Association. *Diagnostic and Statistical Manual of Mental Disorders.* 5th ed. Arlington, VA: American Psychiatric Publishing; 2013.

Barsky AJ, Wyshak G, Klerman GL, Latham KS. The prevalence of hypochondriasis in medical outpatients. *Social Psychiatr Psychiatr Epidemiol.* 1990;25(2):89-94.

Hedman E, Andersson G, Andersson E, et al. Internet-based cognitive–behavioural therapy for severe health anxiety: randomized controlled trial. *Br J Psychiatr.* 2011;198(3):230-236.

Salkovskis PM, Rimes KA, Warwick HMC, Clark DM. The Health Anxiety Inventory: development and validation of scales for the measurement of health anxiety and hypochondriasis. *Psychol Med.* 2002;32(05):843-853.

Warwick HMC. Cognitive therapy in the treatment of hypochondriasis. *Adv Psychiatr Treat.* 1998;4:285-290.

CASE 41

Still Crying about Her Father's Death

IDENTIFICATION: The patient is a 40-year-old white, divorced, professional woman. She is seen for the psychiatric evaluation in an outpatient mental health clinic.

CHIEF COMPLAINT: "Anxiety and panic and depression."

HISTORY OF CHIEF COMPLAINT: The patient became depressed after her father became terminally ill. Went to her primary care provider and was prescribed escitalopram and lorazepam. Was still depressed and gained 15 lb so she stopped the escitalopram. Was only taking lorazepam 0.5 mg PRN for panic. Her panic symptoms included tingling in her arms, crying, and heart palpitations. Her father died 13 months ago. She continued to experience depression and anxiety, so her primary care provider prescribed sertraline, which was increased to 100 mg daily for the past 2 months. The patient thinks it is helping because she has not had any recent panic attacks, but she continues to cry daily at home and work. Her primary care provider advised her to see a psychiatric provider.

PAST PSYCHIATRIC HISTORY: Was prescribed fluoxetine, bupropion, and duloxetine in prior years for depression when she was going through her divorce but she was not sure if any of them helped. No psychiatric hospitalizations, or suicidal attempts, or assaultive behavior.

MEDICAL HISTORY: Tonsillectomy as a toddler (denied any awakening during anesthesia). Denies any history of seizures or head trauma. Regular menses.

Sleep: Denied disturbance.

Appetite: Denied disturbance.

HISTORY OF DRUG OR ALCOHOL ABUSE: Started smoking cigarettes again since her father died.

FAMILY HISTORY: Parents were born in Italy. Has a sister who is 3 years younger. Married at age 28. Moved back to her parents' home following her divorce. Father died 13 months ago. Goes to the cemetery weekly. Crying daily because of his death.

PERSONAL HISTORY

Perinatal: No birth complications, or developmental delays.

Childhood: No social problems. No learning problems.

Adolescence: Denied any self-esteem or body image problems. No history of eating disorders.

Adulthood: She was raised Catholic and attends mass regularly. Went to college and works in the real estate field. Met her husband in college. They have been divorced for 5 years which she described as very stressful. She moved in with her parents following the divorce. Her father, whom she was close to, died 13 months ago. She is still grieving his death.

TRAUMA/ABUSE HISTORY: Denied.

MENTAL STATUS EXAMINATION

Appearance: Well groomed. Good posture. Cooperative.

Behavior and psychomotor activity: Cooperative. Reports continued feeling of sluggishness that became slightly better since starting sertraline.

Consciousness: Alert.

Orientation: Times three.

Memory: Memory intact for recent and remote.

Concentration and attention: Not formally assessed but able to focus when at work.

Visuospatial ability: Not formally assessed.

Abstract thought: Evident.

Intellectual functioning:	Average or above.
Speech and language:	Of normal rate and volume.
Perceptions:	None reported or evident.
Thought processes:	Clear and logical.
Thought content:	Preoccupied with grieving for her father.
Mood:	Depressed, anxious.
Suicidality or homicidality:	None.
Affect:	Appropriate to content of speech. Crying throughout the second half of the interview.
Impulse control:	Good.
Judgment/insight/reliability:	Good/good/good.

FORMULATING THE DIAGNOSIS

What diagnosis should be considered?

309.89 (F43.8) Other Specified Trauma- and Stressor-Related Disorder: Persistent Complex Bereavement Disorder

Diagnostic Criteria

This category applies to presentations in which symptoms characteristic of a trauma- and stressor-related disorder that cause clinically significant distress or impairment in social, occupational, or other important areas of functioning predominate but do not meet the full criteria for any of the disorders in the trauma- and stressor-related disorders diagnostic class. The other specified trauma- and stressor-related disorder category is used in situations in which the clinician chooses to communicate the specific reason that the presentation does not meet the criteria for any specific trauma- and stressor-related disorder. This is done by recording "other specified trauma- and stressor-related disorder" followed by the specific reason (eg, "persistent complex bereavement disorder").

Examples of presentations that can be specified using the "other specified" designation include the following:

1. Adjustment-like disorders with delayed onset of symptoms that occur more than 3 months after the stressor.
2. Adjustment-like disorders with prolonged duration of more than 6 months without prolonged duration of stressor.

3. *Ataque de nervios*
4. Other cultural syndromes
5. Persistent complex bereavement disorder: This disorder is characterized by severe and persistent grief and mourning reactions

(Reprinted with permission from the *Diagnostic and Statistical Manual of Mental Disorders*. 5th ed. Arlington, VA: American Psychiatric Publishing; 2013.)

What is your rationale for the diagnosis?

The patient is experiencing depression and anxiety symptoms related to the death of her father that occurred over a year ago. However, she does not meet the full criteria for any specific trauma or stressor-related disorders.

What test or tools should be considered to help identify the correct diagnosis?

None indicated.

What differential diagnosis should be considered?

296.23 (F32.0) Major Depressive Disorder, Mild

Although the patient has been experiencing a persistent depressed mood related to her father's death, she does not meet the full criteria for a major depressive disorder (MDD). There is no change in her appetite or sleep, feelings of worthlessness or inappropriate guilt, thoughts of death, or suicidal ideation.

"The thought content associated with grief generally features a preoccupation with thoughts and memories of the deceased, rather than the self-critical or pessimistic ruminations seen in major depressive episode. In grief, self-esteem is generally preserved, whereas in major depressive episode feelings of worthlessness and self-loathing are common" (American Psychiatric Association, 2013, p. 161).

Therefore, the diagnosis of MDD would not be appropriate.

FORMULATING THE TREATMENT STRATEGY

What treatment would you prescribe and what is the rationale?

Psychopharmacology: Continue sertraline 100 mg daily. This antidepressant has decreased her symptoms (no more panic attacks, not as lethargic). However, she is anxious about gaining weight, which is a realistic concern with selective serotonin reuptake inhibitors. Weight gain would be an additional stressor and could contribute to more anxiety and depression. Therefore, the dose will be kept at 100 mg daily.

Add bupropion XL 150 mg in AM. This antidepressant can be added to the sertraline as an adjunct. It may reduce her depressive symptoms and sluggishness. Additionally, it may help reduce her smoking. It has not been shown to contribute to weight gain so there may be greater acceptance of this medication. However, bupropion can contribute to increased anxiety and so she will need to be monitored for this possibility. Additionally, patients should be screened for seizure history or current eating disorder before starting bupropion since this medication has the potential to lower the seizure threshold.

Diagnostic Tests: Routine labs.

Referrals: Referral to a local bereavement group.

Type of Psychotherapy: Individual psychotherapy may be indicated to help the patient adjust to the loss of her father and develop additional coping skills.

Psychoeducation: Provide information about the risks and benefits of sertraline and bupropion. Advise the patient to report any increase in anxiety.

What standard guidelines would you use to assess or treat the patient?

None indicated.

CLINICAL NOTE

- Psychiatric practitioners should be aware of cultural attitudes to death in order to provide appropriate care. This patient's Italian heritage must be considered in regard to her response to the loss of her father.
- Any patient who has been under anesthesia for surgery and has a history of anxiety or panic should be evaluated for anesthesia awareness–induced posttraumatic stress disorder. Most cases go undiagnosed and can contribute to anxiety and specific phobias.

REFERENCES/RECOMMENDED READINGS

American Psychiatric Association. *Diagnostic and Statistical Manual of Mental Disorders*. 5th ed. Arlington, VA: American Psychiatric Publishing; 2013.

Kubler-Ross E. *On Death and Dying*. Abingdon: Routledge; 1973.

Prendergast KM, Cullen-Drill M. Anesthesia awareness-induced posttraumatic stress disorder. *J Psychosoc Nurs Mental Health Services*. 2012;50(11):39-44.

CASE 42

Treatment after Rehab for Opiate Addiction

IDENTIFICATION: The patient is a 45-year-old, white, married female with three teenage children.

CHIEF COMPLAINT: "I need my medications reordered."

HISTORY OF CHIEF COMPLAINT: The patient reports arthritic back pain and was prescribed acetaminophen/oxycodone (Percocet) 3 years ago. Saw two different doctors for more prescriptions for this medication. Started buying acetaminophen/oxycodone from friends. Her addiction "skyrocketed." Started stealing money from family members. Lost weight because the food interfered with the effects of the acetaminophen/oxycodone and so she avoided eating. Went to an inpatient rehab hospital for 1 month. Relapsed in 10 days following discharge. Then went to another detox inpatient unit for 4 days. Relapsed again in 1 week. Was admitted to a different rehab inpatient program. Followed up in their partial hospital program and intensive outpatient program, which ended 8 days ago. The patient said she went to some Alcoholics Anonymous meetings but did not think they were helpful. She was not interested in being maintained on methadone or buprenorphine.

PAST PSYCHIATRIC HISTORY: No history of anxiety or shyness. States she "always drank" because "we're Irish." No psychiatric hospitalizations other than in the past year for rehab for opiate addiction. No history of suicidal ideation or attempts. However, the patient reports that she was depressed and crying frequently while in her last rehab program. Also, described being extremely anxious. Currently denies any urge to use opiates.

Current medications include sertraline 100 mg daily, clonidine 0.2 mg QID PRN, gabapentin 400 mg QID, and quetiapine 100 mg HS.

MEDICAL HISTORY: No history of acute or chronic medical conditions. Appetite has increased significantly recently. Reports she gained 25 lb in the past 6 weeks. Height 5′4″ and weight 160 lb.

HISTORY OF DRUG OR ALCOHOL ABUSE: See "History of Chief Complaint." Patient reports a persistent pattern of drinking alcohol, however quantity consumed is not known due to patient's vague description.

FAMILY HISTORY: Parents born in the United States. Raised as the younger of two siblings.

PERSONAL HISTORY

Perinatal: Full-term vaginal birth. No complications.

Childhood: Had many friends. Liked school.

Adolescence: Was a good student. Joined many school clubs.

Adulthood: College graduate. Married her husband after college. Had worked in her parents' family business before having children.

TRAUMA/ABUSE HISTORY: Denied.

MENTAL STATUS EXAMINATION

Appearance: Slightly unkempt. Hair barely combed.

Behavior and psychomotor activity: Cooperative.

Consciousness:	Alert.
Orientation:	Oriented to person, place, and time.
Memory:	Not assessed formally but grossly intact.
Attention and concentration:	Fair attention. Comprehension seems slowed. Information needed to be repeated or clarified.
Visuospatial ability:	Not assessed.
Abstract thought:	Not formally assessed.
Intellectual functioning:	Average or above.

Speech and language:	Normal rate and volume.
Perception:	Not altered.
Thought processes:	Linear.
Thought content:	Described the path of her addiction that led to her hospitalizations. Worried about how it will affect her relationship with her children.
Suicidality and homicidality:	Denied.
Mood:	Anxious.
Affect:	Full range.
Impulse control:	Good during the interview. Patient reports poor impulse control in maintaining abstinence from substances.
Judgment/insight/reliability:	Compromised.

FORMULATING THE DIAGNOSIS

Which diagnosis should be considered?

304.00 (F11.20) Opiate Use Disorder, Severe

Diagnostic Criteria

A. A problematic pattern of opioid use leading to clinically significant impairment or distress, as manifested by at least two of the following, occurring within a 12-month period:
   1. Opioids are often taken in larger amounts or over a longer period than was intended.
   2. There is a persistent desire or unsuccessful efforts to cut down or control opioid use.
   3. A great deal of time is spent in activities necessary to obtain the opioid, use the opioid, or recover from its effects.
   4. Craving, or a strong desire or urge to use opioids.
   5. Recurrent opioid use resulting in a failure to fulfill major role obligations at work, school, or home.
   6. Continued opioid use despite having persistent or recurrent social or interpersonal problems caused or exacerbated by the effects of opioids.
   7. Important social, occupational, or recreational activities are given up or reduced because of opioid use.

8. Recurrent opioid use in situations in which it is physically hazardous.
9. Continued opioid use despite knowledge of having a persistent or recurrent physical or psychological problem that is likely to have been caused or exacerbated by the substance.
10. Tolerance, as defined by either of the following:
    a. A need for markedly increased amounts of opioids to achieve intoxication or desired effect.
    b. A markedly diminished effect with continued use of the same amount of an opioid.
        - **Note:** This criterion is not considered to be met for those taking opioids solely under appropriate medical supervision.

    Withdrawal, as manifested by either of the following:
    a. The characteristic opioid withdrawal syndrome (refer to Criteria A and B of the criteria set for opioid withdrawal).
    b. Opioids (or a closely related substance) are taken to relieve or avoid withdrawal symptoms.
        - **Note:** This criterion is not considered to be met for those individuals taking opioids solely under appropriate medical supervision.

Specify if:

- **In early remission:** After full criteria for opioid use disorder were previously met, none of the criteria for opioid use disorder have been met for at least 3 months but for less than 12 months (with the exception that Criterion A4, "Craving, or a strong desire or urge to use opioids," may be met).
- **In sustained remission:** After full criteria for opioid use disorder were previously met, none of the criteria for opioid use disorder have been met at any time during a period of 12 months or longer (with the exception that Criterion A4, "Craving, or a strong desire or urge to use opioids," may be met).

Specify if:

- **On maintenance therapy:** This additional specifier is used if the individual is taking a prescribed agonist medication such as methadone or buprenorphine and none of the criteria for opioid use disorder have been met for that class of medication (except tolerance to, or withdrawal from, the agonist). This category also applies to those individuals being maintained on a partial agonist, an agonist/antagonist, or a full antagonist such as oral naltrexone or depot naltrexone.
- **In a controlled environment:** This additional specifier is used if the individual is in an environment where access to opioids is restricted.

Coding based on current severity: Note for *ICD-10-CM* codes: If an opioid intoxication, opioid withdrawal, or another opioid-induced mental disorder is also present, do not use the codes below for opioid use disorder. Instead, the comorbid opioid use disorder is indicated in the fourth character of the opioid-induced disorder code (see the coding note for opioid intoxication, opioid withdrawal, or a specific opioid-induced mental disorder). For example, if there is comorbid opioid-induced depressive disorder and opioid use disorder, only the opioid-induced depressive disorder code is given, with the 4th character indicating whether the comorbid opioid use disorder is mild, moderate, or severe: F11.14 for mild opioid use disorder with opioid-induced depressive disorder or F11.24 for a moderate or severe opioid use disorder with opioid-induced depressive disorder.

Specify current severity:

- **305.50 (F11.10) Mild:** Presence of two to three symptoms.
- **304.00 (F11.20) Moderate:** Presence of four to five symptoms.
- **304.00 (F11.20) Severe:** Presence of six or more symptoms.

(Reprinted with permission from the *Diagnostic and Statistical Manual of Mental Disorders*. 5th ed. Arlington, VA: American Psychiatric Publication; 2013.)

What is your rationale for the diagnosis?

The patient describes a pattern of opiate use that includes at least six of the criteria for opioid use disorder: opiates were taken in larger amounts (addiction "skyrocketed"), craving opiates (had difficulty controlling the urges), efforts to cut down or control her use were unsuccessful (went to several rehabs and still relapsed), opioid use contributing to problems fulfilling home responsibilities (is worried how her addiction will affect her children), a great deal of time spent trying to obtain opiates (was stealing money from family to obtain the opiates), and had recurrent opioid use in situations in which it is physically hazardous (avoided eating to increase the effects of the opiates).Therefore, she is diagnosed with opioid use disorder, severe. She has not been opiate free for at least 3 months, so she is not yet considered to be in remission.

What tests or tools should be considered to help identify the correct diagnosis?

Urine drug screens may be used to detect any ongoing drug use.

What diagnosis should be considered?

306 (F10.10) Alcohol Use Disorder, Provisional

Diagnostic Criteria

A. A problematic pattern of alcohol use leading to clinically significant impairment or distress, as manifested by at least two of the following, occurring within a 12-month period:
   1. Alcohol is often taken in larger amounts or over a longer period than was intended.

2. There is a persistent desire or unsuccessful efforts to cut down or control alcohol use.
3. A great deal of time is spent in activities necessary to obtain alcohol, use alcohol, or recover from its effects.
4. Craving, or a strong desire or urge to use alcohol.
5. Recurrent alcohol use resulting in a failure to fulfill major role obligations at work, school, or home.
6. Continued alcohol use despite having persistent or recurrent social or interpersonal problems caused or exacerbated by the effects of alcohol.
7. Important social, occupational, or recreational activities are given up or reduced because of alcohol use.
8. Recurrent alcohol use in situations in which it is physically hazardous.
9. Alcohol use is continued despite knowledge of having a persistent or recurrent physical or psychological problem that is likely to have been caused or exacerbated by alcohol.
10. Tolerance, as defined by either of the following:
    a. A need for markedly increased amounts of alcohol to achieve intoxication or desired effect.
    b. A markedly diminished effect with continued use of the same amount of alcohol.
11. Withdrawal, as manifested by either of the following:
    a. The characteristic withdrawal syndrome for alcohol (refer to Criteria A and B of the criteria set for alcohol withdrawal).
    b. Alcohol (or a closely related substance, such as a benzodiazepine) is taken to relieve or avoid withdrawal symptoms.

Specify if:

- **In early remission:** After full criteria for alcohol use disorder were previously met, none of the criteria for alcohol use disorder have been met for at least 3 months but for less than 12 months (with the exception that Criterion A4, "Craving, or a strong desire or urge to use alcohol," may be met).
- **In sustained remission:** After full criteria for alcohol use disorder were previously met, none of the criteria for alcohol use disorder have been met at any time during a period of 12 months or longer (with the exception that Criterion A4, "Craving, or a strong desire or urge to use alcohol," may be met).

Specify if:

- **In a controlled environment:** This additional specifier is used if the individual is in an environment where access to alcohol is restricted.

Code based on current severity: Note for *ICD-10-CM* codes: If an alcohol intoxication, alcohol withdrawal, or another alcohol-induced mental disorder is also present, do not use the codes below for alcohol use disorder. Instead, the comorbid alcohol use disorder is indicated in the fourth character of the alcohol-induced disorder code (see the coding note for alcohol intoxication, alcohol withdrawal, or a specific alcohol-induced mental disorder). For example, if there is comorbid alcohol intoxication and alcohol use disorder, only the alcohol intoxication code is given, with the fourth character indicating whether the comorbid alcohol use disorder is mild, moderate, or severe: F10.129 for mild alcohol use disorder with alcohol intoxication or F10.229 for a moderate or severe alcohol use disorder with alcohol intoxication.

Specify current severity:

- **305.00 (F10.10) Mild:** Presence of two to three symptoms.
- **303.90 (F10.20) Moderate:** Presence of four to five symptoms.
- **303.90 (F10.20) Severe:** Presence of six or more symptoms.

(Reprinted with permission from the *Diagnostic and Statistical Manual of Mental Disorders*. 5th≈ed. Arlington, VA: American Psychiatric Publishing; 2013.)

What is the rationale for the diagnosis?

The information the patient provided suggests that there may be excessive alcohol use. However, it is unclear if her alcohol use meets the criteria for alcohol use disorder. As a therapeutic alliance is formed, she may provide more information regarding her alcohol use. Also, collateral information from family or her spouse may provide a more accurate history regarding her alcohol use.

What tests or tools should be considered to help identify the correct diagnosis?

The CAGE questionnaire can be used to monitor the patient's alcohol intake and to evaluate the need for treatment.

What differential diagnosis should be considered?

300.00 (F41.9) Unspecified Anxiety Disorder

Although the patient has been prescribed medications that are used to treat anxiety, it is not clear if she had an anxiety disorder prior to her sobriety. Therefore, a differential diagnosis of unspecified anxiety disorder is considered. This diagnosis ". . .includes presentations in which there is not sufficient information to make a more specific diagnosis. . ." (American Psychiatric Publishing, 2013). Collateral information from family members would be helpful in providing more information.

FORMULATING THE TREATMENT STRATEGY

What treatment would you prescribe and what is the rationale?

Psychopharmacology: Continue current medications.

Sertraline 100 mg daily: The patient was treated with sertraline, a selective serotonin reuptake inhibitor, for depression while in the rehab program. Although she does not report any depressed mood at this time she is still very anxious. It would not be prudent to make any changes with the sertraline as it is effective in treating both depression and anxiety. Any change may precipitate additional mood dysregulation, which could contribute to a relapse and impede her recovery.

Gabapentin 400 mg QID: Gabapentin, an anticonvulsant, is used off-label to treat anxiety and neuropathic pain. This will be continued for the time being in order to reduce anxiety. It may also have some benefit in reducing this patient's back pain.

Clonidine 0.2 mg QID PRN: Clonidine is a centrally acting alpha-2 agonist that is commonly used off-label for the treatment of opiate (and alcohol) withdrawal. It is also used to reduce anxiety. Continuation of clonidine is indicated as long as the patient's blood pressure is monitored and complications of hypotension are avoided.

Quetiapine 100 mg HS: Although quetiapine is not Food and Drug Administration approved as a sleep aid, the patient's insomnia was probably quite severe and therefore she was started on this medication as an inpatient. However, attempts should be made to discontinue this medication in the near future as the risks may outweigh the benefits.

Medication-assisted treatment such as buprenorphine or natrexone extended-release injection is strongly recommended to prevent relapse. However, the patient is currently reluctant to proceed with this treatment recommendation.

Diagnostic Tests: Random urine drug screens may be indicated. Monitor blood pressure and if patient is hypotensive, clonidine would need to be adjusted. Due to patient taking quetiapine, monitor for metabolic syndrome.

Referrals: The patient was advised to find alternate means other than medications to manage her back pain, for example, acupuncture or physical therapy.

Psychotherapy: Counseling in combination with medication-assisted treatment has been shown to be more effective in reducing relapse. Treatment of comorbidities should also be addressed. Relapse prevention goals can include learning new coping skills, identifying triggers for relapse, developing a plan to deal with triggers, and promoting healthier life choices in general (adequate sleep, nutrition, exercise, social engagement, etc.).

The family should be involved in treatment in order to address any concerns they may have. Education about addiction, the goals of treatment, and the risk of relapse should be provided.

Psychoeducation: Advise regarding the importance of ongoing therapy to prevent relapse.

Advise to consider medication-assisted treatment such as buprenorphine, naltrexone extended-release injection, or methadone.

Information about opiate addiction and treatment from the NIMH should be provided.

Advise regarding the potential for clonidine abuse and the health risk if stopped abruptly. Advise that a gradual taper should be instituted if discontinuing the clonidine.

Advise of the increased risk of an opiate relapse with the use of alcohol.

What standard guidelines would you use to assess or treat this patient?

"Center for Substance Abuse Treatment: Medication-Assisted Treatment for Opioid Addiction in Opioid Treatment Programs." Rockville, MD: Substance Abuse and Mental Health Services Administration (US); 2005. (Treatment Improvement Protocol (TIP) Series, No. 43.) Chapter 3. Pharmacology of Medications Used to Treat Opioid Addiction. Available at: http://www.ncbi.nlm.nih.gov/books/NBK64158/

CLINICAL NOTE

- Published case studies report clonidine being abused by individuals with addiction disorders. Although clonidine is effective in reducing opiate withdrawal symptoms and can help reduce postwithdrawal anxiety, the potential for abuse must be considered.

REFERENCES/RECOMMENDED READINGS

American Psychiatric Association. *Diagnostic and Statistical Manual of Mental Disorders.* 5th ed. Arlington, VA: American Psychiatric Publishing; 2013.

Seale JP, Dittmer T, Sigman EJ, Clemons H, Johnson JA. Combined abuse of clonidine and amitriptyline in a patient on buprenorphine maintenance treatment. *J Addict Med.* 2014;8(6):476.

Substance Abuse and Mental Health Services Administration. Buprenorphine. http://www.samhsa.gov/medication-assisted-treatment/treatment/buprenorphine. Accessed November 2, 2017.

CASE 43

Depressed and Fatigued

IDENTIFICATION: The patient is a 48-year-old, single, African-American female who was referred by her therapist. She is seen for evaluation in an outpatient mental health clinic.

CHIEF COMPLAINT: "Depressed and anxious."

HISTORY OF CHIEF COMPLAINT: Depressed mood started a year ago when the patient felt overwhelmed by work. She was sleeping excessively, had low energy, and lost interest in previous hobbies. She was extremely depressed, and eventually took an overdose of ibuprofen as a suicide attempt. A friend, whom she was talking to on the phone, called 911 and the patient was taken to the hospital and admitted to the psychiatric unit for 1 week. She followed up in an intensive outpatient program where she was prescribed bupropion extended release 150 mg in the morning, gabapentin 300 mg TID, and amitriptyline 50 mg at bedtime. Prior to these medications she had been tried on numerous antidepressants, however she was unable to remember the names of those medications. She was discharged after several weeks and was referred to the outpatient clinic for medication management and psychotherapy.

PAST PSYCHIATRIC HISTORY: The patient reported a history of severe anxiety and panic had started after a motor vehicle accident over 10 years ago and that caused her to avoid driving. She was treated with amitriptyline and gabapentin which led to symptom remission. She thought the gabapentin helped her anxiety and she was able to drive. She said the amitriptyline helped her sleep. No prior psychiatric hospitalizations or suicidal attempts before the current episode.

MEDICAL HISTORY: History of morbid obesity and gastric sleeve surgery 2 years ago. Patient is currently overweight. However, she reports loss of appetite over the past few months. Takes vitamin D supplements daily since she was previously diagnosed with a vitamin D deficiency. Was diagnosed recently with gout in her right foot and a sprained right ankle. Was prescribed colchicine 0.6 mg daily. By her primary care physician for the gout.

HISTORY OF DRUG OR ALCOHOL ABUSE: Denied.

FAMILY HISTORY: Patient's mother reportedly had a history of schizophrenia and subsequently relinquished custody of the patient when the patient was 3 years old. Patient's father was reported to have alcohol dependence, and a sibling has a history of bipolar disorder. The patient reported a history of abuse and neglect in foster homes until she eventually aged out at 18 years.

PERSONAL HISTORY: Worked for 18 years in tech industry until she took a medical leave due to depression when she was hospitalized one month ago following the overdose. The patient identifies as gay. The patient has been in a relationship with a supportive female partner. She has avoided socializing with friends in the past 2 months.

TRAUMA/ABUSE HISTORY: Physically abused in foster home settings.

MENTAL STATUS EXAMINATION

Appearance: Casual attire, good eye contact.

Behavior and psychomotor activity: Cooperative, no abnormal movements.

Consciousness: Alert.

Orientation: Times three.

Memory: Memory not formally assessed but she reports difficulty remembering appointments and has to write everything down. She had difficulty reporting the history of her recent illness and treatment.

Concentration and attention: Not formally assessed. Reports that her concentration is a struggle when reading or trying to complete a task. Poor concentration and focus observed during the interview.

Visuospatial ability: Not formally assessed.

Abstract thought:	Not formally assessed.
Intellectual functioning:	Average or above.
Speech and language:	Within normal limits.
Perceptions:	No abnormal perceptions.
Thought processes:	Logical.
Thought content:	Reports wanting to feel less depressed and anxious.
Suicidality and homicidality:	Denies suicidal and homicidal thoughts.
Mood:	Depressed.
Affect:	Congruent.
Impulse control:	Not observed or reported.
Judgment/insight/reliability:	Good/good/good.

FORMULATING THE DIAGNOSIS

What diagnosis should be considered?

296.23 (F32.2) Major Depressive Disorder, Severe

Diagnostic Criteria

A. Five (or more) of the following symptoms have been present during the same 2-week period and represent a change from previous functioning; at least one of the symptoms is either (1) depressed mood or (2) loss of interest or pleasure.
   - **Note:** Do not include symptoms that are clearly attributable to another medical condition.
     1. Depressed mood most of the day, nearly every day, as indicated by either subjective report (eg, feels sad, empty, hopeless) or observation made by others (eg, appears tearful). (Note: In children and adolescents, can be irritable mood.)
     2. Markedly diminished interest or pleasure in all, or almost all, activities most of the day, nearly every day (as indicated by either subjective account or observation).

3. Significant weight loss when not dieting or weight gain (eg, a change of more than 5% of body weight in a month), or decrease or increase in appetite nearly every day. (Note: In children, consider failure to make expected weight gain.)
4. Insomnia or hypersomnia nearly every day.
5. Psychomotor agitation or retardation nearly every day (observable by others, not merely subjective feelings of restlessness or being slowed down).
6. Fatigue or loss of energy nearly every day.
7. Feelings of worthlessness or excessive or inappropriate guilt (which may be delusional) nearly every day (not merely self-reproach or guilt about being sick).
8. Diminished ability to think or concentrate, or indecisiveness, nearly every day (either by subjective account or as observed by others).
9. Recurrent thoughts of death (not just fear of dying), recurrent suicidal ideation without a specific plan, or a suicide attempt or a specific plan for committing suicide.

B. The symptoms cause clinically significant distress or impairment in social, occupational, or other important areas of functioning.
C. The episode is not attributable to the physiologic effects of a substance or another medical condition.

Note: Criteria A to C represent a major depressive episode (MDE).

Note: Responses to a significant loss (eg, bereavement, financial ruin, losses from a natural disaster, a serious medical illness or disability) may include the feelings of intense sadness, rumination about the loss, insomnia, poor appetite, and weight loss noted in Criterion A, which may resemble a depressive episode. Although such symptoms may be understandable or considered appropriate to the loss, the presence of an MDE in addition to the normal response to a significant loss should also be carefully considered. This decision inevitably requires the exercise of clinical judgment based on the individual's history and the cultural norms for the expression of distress in the context of loss.

In distinguishing grief from an MDE, it is useful to consider that in grief the predominant affect is feelings of emptiness and loss, whereas in an MDE it is persistent depressed mood and the inability to anticipate happiness or pleasure. The dysphoria in grief is likely to decrease in intensity over days to weeks and occurs in waves, the so-called pangs of grief. These waves tend to be associated with thoughts or reminders of the deceased. The depressed mood of an MDE is more persistent and not tied to specific thoughts or preoccupations. The pain of grief may be accompanied by positive emotions and humor that are uncharacteristic of the pervasive unhappiness and misery characteristic of an MDE. The thought content associated with grief generally features a preoccupation with thoughts and memories of the deceased, rather than the self-critical or pessimistic ruminations seen in an MDE. In grief, self-esteem is generally preserved, whereas in an MDE feelings of worthlessness and self-loathing are common. If self-derogatory ideation is present in grief, it typically involves perceived failings vis-à-vis the deceased (eg, not visiting frequently enough, not telling the deceased how much he or she was loved). If a bereaved individual thinks about death and dying, such thoughts are generally focused on the deceased and possibly about "joining" the deceased, whereas in an MDE such thoughts are focused on ending one's own life because of feeling worthless, undeserving of life, or unable to cope with the pain of depression.

D. The occurrence of the MDE is not better explained by schizoaffective disorder, schizophrenia, schizophreniform disorder, delusional disorder, or other specified and unspecified schizophrenia spectrum and other psychotic disorders.

E. There has never been a manic episode or a hypomanic episode.
   - **Note:** This exclusion does not apply if all of the manic-like or hypomanic-like episodes are substance-induced or are attributable to the physiologic effects of another medical condition.

(Reprinted with permission from the *Diagnostic and Statistical Manual of Mental Disorders*. 5th ed. Arlington, VA: American Psychiatric Publishing; 2013.)

What is your rationale for the diagnosis?

The patient's symptoms of depression, diminished interest, fatigue, feelings of worthlessness, diminished ability to concentrate, and loss of appetite provide at least five of the criteria that are required for a diagnosis of major depressive disorder. The symptoms are considered severe because they are in excess of what is required for a diagnosis of MDD and are distressing and interfere with her social functioning and her ability to work.

What test or tools should be considered to help identify the correct diagnosis?

Beck Depression Inventory would help to assess the severity of the depression.

A Montreal Cognitive Assessment (MoCA) should be administered to assess the patient's current cognitive functioning. A MoCA was scheduled to be completed at the next appointment. http://www.mocatest.org/pdf_files/instructions/MoCA-Instructions-English_2010.pdf and http://echo.unm.edu/wp-content/uploads/2014/07/clinic-dementia-MOCA-English.pdf

What differential diagnosis should be considered?

293.83 (F06.32) Depressive Disorder Due to Another Medical Condition, with Major Depressive-Like Episode

Although the patient has a history of abuse and neglect, which could trigger feelings of abandonment and depression, she had been functioning successfully at a high-level position for 18 years. There is an atypical age of onset with the patient's depression. The only precipitating factor for her depression that she could identify was excessive work hours and stress. It is not known if her cognitive problems with memory and decreased concentration preceded the depressive episode and contributed to her work stress.

She had bariatric surgery 2 years prior, which may have contributed to some vitamin deficiencies, which could affect mood. She has since been treated for vitamin D and vitamin B-12 deficiencies so it is unlikely that they are current contributing factors. General medical tests had been completed by her primary care provider and were all WNL, but additional medical conditions may still need to be investigated.

FORMULATING THE TREATMENT PLAN

What treatment would you prescribe and what is the rationale?

Psychopharmacology: Bupropion extended release (XL) 150 mg in AM
Gabapentin 300 mg TID
Amitriptyline 50 mg HS

Medical conditions need to be ruled out before any medication change. General guidelines recommend avoiding drugs with long stomach absorptive phases and sustained release. Medication absorption alterations should be considered because the patient had gastric sleeve surgery.

Continue current medications until results of lab work are received.

Diagnostic Tests: Lyme disease screen EIA w RFL WB and Sed rate, serum protein, vitamin B-1, vitamin B-3.

Vitamin levels should be evaluated since bariatric surgery may contribute to vitamin deficiencies, particularly pellagra (a lack of vitamin B-3—niacin), beri beri (a lack of vitamin B-1—thiamine), and kwashiorkor (a lack of protein).

Genetic testing: The patient has been tried on several antidepressants and has not experienced symptom relief. It may be beneficial to conduct genetic testing to identify psychotropic medications that could be more effective.

Referrals: Referrals are dependent on results of lab testing. If her memory deficits continue, a referral to a neurologist is indicated.

Type of Psychotherapy: Supportive psychotherapy.

Psychoeducation: Explain reasons for laboratory testing to rule out any contributing medical conditions.

What standard guidelines would you use to assess or treat the patient?

APA Practice Guideline for the Treatment of Patients With Major Depressive Disorder.

CLINICAL NOTE

- General guidelines for individuals who have had bariatric surgery recommend avoiding drugs with long stomach absorptive phases and sustained release. Alternate routes should be considered when possible. For instance, lamotrigine absorption mainly takes place in the stomach and small intestine, so serum blood levels may be helpful in assuring the proper dose. Both quetiapine and olanzapine's absorption takes place in the stomach and duodenum so patients prescribed these medications should be monitored closely in the first few weeks after surgery.
- This patient's history is complicated with significant family mental illness, and foster home placement at an early age. Later events such as bariatric surgery may have contributed to medical conditions that could worsen her mood or reduce her response to medication. There is also the possibility that there may be infective or autoimmune conditions that could contribute to depression and anxiety. In these cases, it is best to take a step-by-step approach to identifying contributing factors and at the same time provide as much psychological support as possible for the patient. Having a strong therapeutic alliance is essential along with careful monitoring for worsening mood and potential suicidal acts.
- If depression is persistent and potential medical conditions have been ruled out, therapies for treatment-resistant depression should be considered. These might include switching to an serotonin norepinephrine reuptake inhibitor medication, adding an adjunctive medication (cytomel, aripiprazole, lithium, ketamine) or electroconvulsive therapy (ECT).

REFERENCES/RECOMMENDED READINGS

American Psychiatric Association. *Diagnostic and Statistical Manual of Mental Disorders.* 5th≈ed. Arlington, VA: American Psychiatric Publishing; 2013.

Chapman DP, Whitfield CL, Felitti VJ, Dube SR, Edwards VJ, Anda RF. Adverse childhood experiences and the risk of depressive disorders in adulthood. *J Affect Disord.* 2004;82(2):217-225.

Cook-Fong SK. *The adult well-being of individuals reared in family foster care placements.* Paper presented at the Child and Youth Care Forum, 2000.

Garakani A, Mitton AG. New-onset panic, depression with suicidal thoughts, and somatic symptoms in a patient with a history of Lyme disease. *Case Rep Psychiatr.* 2015:1-4.

Karmali S. The impact of bariatric surgery on psychological health. *J Obes.* 2013:1-5.

Marian G, Nica EA, Ionescu BE, Carlogea DG, Davila UMFC. Depression as an initial feature of systemic lupus erythematosus? *J Med Life.* 2010;3(2):183-185.

Padwal R, Brocks D, Sharma AM. A systematic review of drug absorption following bariatric surgery and its theoretical implications. *Obes Rev.* 2010;11(1):41-50.

Siddiqui A, Alhajri S, Khalid I, Ahmed A. Lyme disease in a patient who presented with podagra mimicking gout [abstract]. *J Hosp Med.* 2015;10 (suppl 2). http://www.shmabstracts.com/abstract/lyme-disease-in-a-patient-who-presented-with-podagra-mimicking-gout/. Accessed November 29, 2016.

CASE 44

Homeless and Problems with Alcohol

IDENTIFICATION: The patient is a 50-year-old Hispanic, divorced, male with a long history of homelessness. He is currently applying for housing at a facility where a psychiatric evaluation is required.

CHIEF COMPLAINT: "I'm trying to get housing and they told me I have to see you."

HISTORY OF CHIEF COMPLAINT: The patient reported that he had been homeless for the past 3 to 4 years, living in various homeless shelters throughout the city. The patient stated that he became homeless after his wife kicked him out of their home.

When interviewed about his history of homelessness, the patient reported feeling depressed; feeling "useless and worthless." He reported that he is jittery and has trouble staying asleep. He said he usually is "dragging my feet" to do anything. He describes passive suicidal ideation, but no intent, because he said he believed in God and would not do it. He described feeling hopeless and helpless. He reported difficulty concentrating and said he was not able to focus when he was trying to read and would lose his train of thought. He said that his depressive symptoms started when he was in prison for drug related charges, but added that he was not able to remember ever being happy. He said that he would just have a beer when he was angry, and it would take the edge off.

PAST PSYCHIATRIC HISTORY: The patient experienced a traumatic event 20 years ago when he was incarcerated (but did not want to elaborate) and said that for 4 years he experienced nightmares and flashbacks.

He used to have problems with crowds and said that crowds reminded him of prison. He was not able to take a crowded subway, because he felt like he was suffocating. He said those feelings subsided years ago, but they used to be severe.

The patient's first psychiatric hospitalization was 12 years ago for depression. He described feeling useless, "didn't care about himself," and had not been eating or showering. He was isolating and felt like he was "hibernating." His wife called 911, and he was taken to the hospital and admitted for 2 weeks. He was treated with paroxetine and zolpidem.

During other hospitalizations, he was treated with fluoxetine, zolpidem, and valproic acid. He was diagnosed with bipolar disorder during one admission. However, the admission note stated that he denied any symptoms of elevated mood. He only reported a history of mood swings but was unable to endorse any discrete periods of mania separate from substance use. At one point when he was incarcerated, he was prescribed haloperidol and stated that he was "walking around like a zombie."

Patient said that he went to detox at least 4 times and then to three inpatient rehabs. The patient agreed during each detox to go to an inpatient rehab, but then would change his mind after leaving the detox. Consequently, he never received any long-term rehabilitation.

No history of suicidal attempts or assaultive behavior.

MEDICAL HISTORY: ROS negative except for peripheral neuropathy. Patient denied any history of traumatic brain injury. Recent history and physical examination with laboratory tests negative for any medical conditions other than peripheral neuropathy. Patient denied any history of head trauma.

Allergies: NKDA.

HISTORY OF DRUG OR ALCOHOL ABUSE: Alcohol: The patient said that his first drink was when he was around 15 years old. He reports a history of blackouts but denied ever having seizures or delirium tremens. He said that after he stopped using heroin, he started drinking "a little more." Patient denied any drinking for the past 3 or 4 months, but the records from his residence indicate otherwise. They noted that he was under the influence of alcohol almost on a daily basis.

Cannabis: Patient said that he was only using when he was a teenager.

Cocaine: Tried it as a teenager, but said that he did not like it.

Heroin: He started using heroin when he was in his early 20s. At his peak use, he used a minimum of five bags per day. He stopped with the help of a methadone maintenance program, which he attended for 5 years. His last use was 15 years ago. There is no indication that he has used heroin since that time.

Tobacco: Denied.

FAMILY HISTORY: The patient was born in Puerto Rico and moved with his parents to the United States when he was 1 year old. He was raised by both of his parents until he was 16 years. He has two older brothers and one younger sister. His father is reported to have had alcohol use problems.

PERSONAL HISTORY

Perinatal: No known perinatal complications or developmental delays.

Childhood: He described his childhood as "fine."

Adolescence: He dropped out of school when he was 15 years old. Did not get a GED.

Adulthood: The patient was married and lived with his wife until they separated due to his alcohol use when their son was 5 years old. The patient has not had any contact with his son since then. He does not know how old his son is. Patient has had only "off the books" jobs and was mostly self-employed. He reports that he was often fired due to his alcohol and drug use. The patient has a legal history for felony offenses due to drug-related charges. His social support is very limited.

TRAUMA/ABUSE HISTORY: Denied.

MENTAL STATUS EXAMINATION

Appearance: He was wearing casual clothes, appropriate to age and setting. He was well groomed and appeared his chronologic age.

Behavior and psychomotor activity: Cooperative, good eye contact, no abnormal movement, good impulse control during the interview.

Consciousness:	Alert.
Orientation:	Patient was alert and oriented to person, place, date and time, and settings.
Memory:	Immediate recall was 3/3 and short-term memory 2/3.
Concentration and attention:	Not able to complete serial 7s ("100, 97"), good serial 3s (21, 18, 15, 12, 9, 6, 3, 0), good spelling, not able to complete backward spelling.
Visuospatial ability:	Not assessed.
Abstract thought:	Good.
Intellectual functioning:	Average vocabulary. Good fund of knowledge as evidenced by being able to report recent U.S. presidents.

Speech and language:	Normal rate, rhythm, and volume.
Perceptions:	Denied auditory hallucination/visual hallucination.
Thought processes:	Linear and logical, goal oriented.
Thought content:	Denied persecutory delusions.
Suicidality or homicidality:	Denied suicidal/homicidal ideation.
Mood:	"Pretty good," but then said "depressed."
Affect:	Sad.
Impulse control:	Impulse control was good during the interview but may be limited otherwise as evidenced by substance misuse.
Insight:	Poor concerning alcohol use.
Judgment:	Good.
Reliability:	Fair.

FORMULATING THE DIAGNOSIS

Which diagnosis should be considered?

303.90 (F10.20) Alcohol Use Disorder, Severe

Diagnostic Criteria

A. A problematic pattern of alcohol use leading to clinically significant impairment or distress, as manifested by at least two of the following, occurring within a 12-month period:
   1. Alcohol is often taken in larger amounts or over a longer period than was intended.
   2. There is a persistent desire or unsuccessful efforts to cut down or control alcohol use.
   3. A great deal of time is spent in activities necessary to obtain alcohol, use alcohol, or recover from its effects.
   4. Craving, or a strong desire or urge to use alcohol.
   5. Recurrent alcohol use resulting in a failure to fulfill major role obligations at work, school, or home.
   6. Continued alcohol use despite having persistent or recurrent social or interpersonal problems caused or exacerbated by the effects of alcohol.

7. Important social, occupational, or recreational activities are given up or reduced because of alcohol use.
8. Recurrent alcohol use in situations in which it is physically hazardous.
9. Alcohol use is continued despite knowledge of having a persistent or recurrent physical or psychological problem that is likely to have been caused or exacerbated by alcohol.
10. Tolerance, as defined by either of the following:
    a. A need for markedly increased amounts of alcohol to achieve intoxication or desired effect.
    b. A markedly diminished effect with continued use of the same amount of alcohol.
11. Withdrawal, as manifested by either of the following:
    a. The characteristic withdrawal syndrome for alcohol (refer to Criteria A and B of the criteria set for alcohol withdrawal).
    b. Alcohol (or a closely related substance, such as a benzodiazepine) is taken to relieve or avoid withdrawal symptoms.

Specify if:

- **In early remission:** After full criteria for alcohol use disorder were previously met, none of the criteria for alcohol use disorder have been met for at least 3 months but for less than 12 months (with the exception that Criterion A4, "Craving, or a strong desire or urge to use alcohol," may be met).
- **In sustained remission:** After full criteria for alcohol use disorder were previously met, none of the criteria for alcohol use disorder have been met at any time during a period of 12 months or longer (with the exception that Criterion A4, "Craving, or a strong desire or urge to use alcohol," may be met).

Specify if:
- **In a controlled environment:** This additional specifier is used if the individual is in an environment where access to alcohol is restricted.

Code based on current severity: Note for *ICD-10-CM* codes: If an alcohol intoxication, alcohol withdrawal, or another alcohol-induced mental disorder is also present, do not use the codes below for alcohol use disorder. Instead, the comorbid alcohol use disorder is indicated in the fourth character of the alcohol-induced disorder code (see the coding note for alcohol intoxication, alcohol withdrawal, or a specific alcohol-induced mental disorder). For example, if there is comorbid alcohol intoxication and alcohol use disorder, only the alcohol intoxication code is given, with the fourth character indicating whether the comorbid alcohol use disorder is mild, moderate, or severe: F10.129 for mild alcohol use disorder with alcohol intoxication or F10.229 for a moderate or severe alcohol use disorder with alcohol intoxication.

Specify current severity:

- **305.00 (F10.10) Mild:** Presence of two to three symptoms.
- **303.90 (F10.20) Moderate:** Presence of four to five symptoms.
- **303.90 (F10.20) Severe:** Presence of six or more symptoms.

(Reprinted with permission from the *Diagnostic and Statistical Manual of Mental Disorders*. 5th ed. Arlington, VA: American Psychiatric Publishing; 2013.)

What is your rationale for the diagnosis?

The patient uses alcohol and cannot control how much he uses (hospitalized multiple times for alcohol dependency), has continued alcohol use despite have interpersonal problems caused by the effects of alcohol (wife left him), failed many of his social roles (lost contact with his son) due to alcohol use; he has no other recreational activities but alcohol use; he developed tolerance and needs higher quantities (saying that alcohol was not really working for him) and avoids withdrawal symptoms by drinking more. Therefore, because six or more criteria are met, the diagnosis of alcohol use disorder, severe is applicable.

Which diagnosis should be considered?

296.32 (F33.1) Major Depressive Disorder, Recurrent, Moderate

Diagnostic Criteria

A. Five (or more) of the following symptoms have been present during the same 2-week period and represent a change from previous functioning; at least one of the symptoms is either (1) depressed mood or (2) loss of interest or pleasure.
   - **Note:** Do not include symptoms that are clearly attributable to another medical condition.
     1. Depressed mood most of the day, nearly every day, as indicated by either subjective report (eg, feels sad, empty, hopeless) or observation made by others (eg, appears tearful). (Note: In children and adolescents, can be irritable mood.)
     2. Markedly diminished interest or pleasure in all, or almost all, activities most of the day, nearly every day (as indicated by either subjective account or observation).
     3. Significant weight loss when not dieting or weight gain (eg, a change of more than 5% of body weight in a month), or decrease or increase in appetite nearly every day. (Note: In children, consider failure to make expected weight gain.)
     4. Insomnia or hypersomnia nearly every day.
     5. Psychomotor agitation or retardation nearly every day (observable by others, not merely subjective feelings of restlessness or being slowed down).

6. Fatigue or loss of energy nearly every day.
7. Feelings of worthlessness or excessive or inappropriate guilt (which may be delusional) nearly every day (not merely self-reproach or guilt about being sick).
8. Diminished ability to think or concentrate, or indecisiveness, nearly every day (either by subjective account or as observed by others).
9. Recurrent thoughts of death (not just fear of dying), recurrent suicidal ideation without a specific plan, or a suicide attempt or a specific plan for committing suicide.

B. The symptoms cause clinically significant distress or impairment in social, occupational, or other important areas of functioning.
C. The episode is not attributable to the physiologic effects of a substance or another medical condition.

Note: Criteria A to C represent a major depressive episode (MDE).

Note: Responses to a significant loss (eg, bereavement, financial ruin, losses from a natural disaster, a serious medical illness or disability) may include the feelings of intense sadness, rumination about the loss, insomnia, poor appetite, and weight loss noted in Criterion A, which may resemble a depressive episode. Although such symptoms may be understandable or considered appropriate to the loss, the presence of an MDE in addition to the normal response to a significant loss should also be carefully considered. This decision inevitably requires the exercise of clinical judgment based on the individual's history and the cultural norms for the expression of distress in the context of loss.

In distinguishing grief from an MDE, it is useful to consider that in grief the predominant affect is feelings of emptiness and loss, whereas in an MDE it is persistent depressed mood and the inability to anticipate happiness or pleasure. The dysphoria in grief is likely to decrease in intensity over days to weeks and occurs in waves, the so-called pangs of grief. These waves tend to be associated with thoughts or reminders of the deceased. The depressed mood of an MDE is more persistent and not tied to specific thoughts or preoccupations. The pain of grief may be accompanied by positive emotions and humor that are uncharacteristic of the pervasive unhappiness and misery characteristic of an MDE. The thought content associated with grief generally features a preoccupation with thoughts and memories of the deceased, rather than the self-critical or pessimistic ruminations seen in an MDE. In grief, self-esteem is generally preserved, whereas in an MDE feelings of worthlessness and self-loathing are common. If self-derogatory ideation is present in grief, it typically involves perceived failings vis-à-vis the deceased (eg, not visiting frequently enough, not telling the deceased how much he or she was loved). If a bereaved individual thinks about death and dying, such thoughts are generally focused on the deceased and possibly about "joining" the deceased, whereas in an MDE such thoughts are focused on ending one's own life because of feeling worthless, undeserving of life, or unable to cope with the pain of depression.

D. The occurrence of the MDE is not better explained by schizoaffective disorder, schizophrenia, schizophreniform disorder, delusional disorder, or other specified and unspecified schizophrenia spectrum and other psychotic disorders.
E. There has never been a manic episode or a hypomanic episode.
    - **Note:** This exclusion does not apply if all of the manic-like or hypomanic-like episodes are substance-induced or are attributable to the physiologic effects of another medical condition.

(Reprinted with permission from the *Diagnostic and Statistical Manual of Mental Disorders*. 5th ed. Arlington, VA: American Psychiatric Publishing; 2013.)

What is your rationale for the diagnosis?

The patient reports feeling depressed, fatigued ("dragging my feet" to do anything), feeling worthless (feeling "useless and worthless"), diminished ability to think or concentrate (not able to focus when trying to read, losing his train of thoughts), and recurrent suicidal ideation (reported passive suicidal ideation). These symptoms cause distress in important areas of functioning (limited social support). The symptoms are not attributable to the physiologic effects of another medical condition (a recent medical evaluation was negative for any potential contributing medical conditions) or the effects of a substance. Although the patient has an extensive substance abuse history and alcohol dependence, he reports that the depressed mood "started when he was in prison" (a controlled environment). Therefore, the diagnosis of major depressive disorder, recurrent, moderate is appropriate.

Which diagnosis should be considered?

304.00 (F11.20) Opioid Use Disorder, Severe, in Sustained Remission

Diagnostic Criteria

A. A problematic pattern of opioid use leading to clinically significant impairment or distress, as manifested by at least two of the following, occurring within a 12-month period:
    1. Opioids are often taken in larger amounts or over a longer period than was intended.
    2. There is a persistent desire or unsuccessful efforts to cut down or control opioid use.
    3. A great deal of time is spent in activities necessary to obtain the opioid, use the opioid, or recover from its effects.
    4. Craving, or a strong desire or urge to use opioids.
    5. Recurrent opioid use resulting in a failure to fulfill major role obligations at work, school, or home.

6. Continued opioid use despite having persistent or recurrent social or interpersonal problems caused or exacerbated by the effects of opioids.
7. Important social, occupational, or recreational activities are given up or reduced because of opioid use.
8. Recurrent opioid use in situations in which it is physically hazardous.
9. Continued opioid use despite knowledge of having a persistent or recurrent physical or psychological problem that is likely to have been caused or exacerbated by the substance.
10. Tolerance, as defined by either of the following:
    a. A need for markedly increased amounts of opioids to achieve intoxication or desired effect.
    b. A markedly diminished effect with continued use of the same amount of an opioid.
        - **Note**: This criterion is not considered to be met for those taking opioids solely under appropriate medical supervision.

    Withdrawal, as manifested by either of the following:
    c. The characteristic opioid withdrawal syndrome (refer to Criteria A and B of the criteria set for opioid withdrawal).
    d. Opioids (or a closely related substance) are taken to relieve or avoid withdrawal symptoms.
        - **Note**: This criterion is not considered to be met for those individuals taking opioids solely under appropriate medical supervision.

Specify if:

- **In early remission**: After full criteria for opioid use disorder were previously met, none of the criteria for opioid use disorder have been met for at least 3 months but for less than 12 months (with the exception that Criterion A4, "Craving, or a strong desire or urge to use opioids," may be met).
- **In sustained remission**: After full criteria for opioid use disorder were previously met, none of the criteria for opioid use disorder have been met at any time during a period of 12 months or longer (with the exception that Criterion A4, "Craving, or a strong desire or urge to use opioids," may be met).

Specify if:

- **On maintenance therapy**: This additional specifier is used if the individual is taking a prescribed agonist medication such as methadone or buprenorphine and none of the criteria for opioid use disorder have been met for that class of medication (except tolerance to, or withdrawal from, the agonist). This category also applies to those individuals being maintained on a partial agonist, an agonist/antagonist, or a full antagonist such as oral naltrexone or depot naltrexone.

- **In a controlled environment**: This additional specifier is used if the individual is in an environment where access to opioids is restricted.

Coding based on current severity: Note for *ICD-10-CM* codes: If an opioid intoxication, opioid withdrawal, or another opioid-induced mental disorder is also present, do not use the codes below for opioid use disorder. Instead, the comorbid opioid use disorder is indicated in the 4th character of the opioid-induced disorder code (see the coding note for opioid intoxication, opioid withdrawal, or a specific opioid-induced mental disorder). For example, if there is comorbid opioid-induced depressive disorder and opioid use disorder, only the opioid-induced depressive disorder code is given, with the 4th character indicating whether the comorbid opioid use disorder is mild, moderate, or severe: F11.14 for mild opioid use disorder with opioid-induced depressive disorder or F11.24 for a moderate or severe opioid use disorder with opioid-induced depressive disorder.

Specify current severity:

- **305.50 (F11.10) Mild**: Presence of two to three symptoms.
- **304.00 (F11.20) Moderate**: Presence of four to five symptoms.
- **304.00 (F11.20) Severe**: Presence of six or more symptoms.

(Reprinted with permission from the *Diagnostic and Statistical Manual of Mental Disorders*. 5th ed. Arlington, VA: American Psychiatric Publishing; 2013.)

What is your rationale for the diagnosis?

The patient reports heroin use for over a decade culminating in methadone treatment for a period of 5 years. He stopped the methadone maintenance over 15 years and has not relapsed. Because the full criteria for opioid use disorder were previously met and none of the criteria for opioid use disorder have been met for 12 months or longer, a diagnosis of opioid use disorder in sustained remission is appropriate.

What tests or tools should be considered to help identify the correct diagnosis?

The Beck Depression Inventory is a 21-item self-report questionnaire used to assess the severity of depressive symptoms.

The Severity of Alcohol Dependence Questionnaire (SADQ-C) (see Appendix).

What differential diagnoses should be considered?

300.4 (F34.1) Persistent Depressive Disorder (Dysthymia)

There is limited history with which to determine the history of the depressive symptoms. It is known that he currently meets the criteria for major depressive disorder; therefore, persistent depressive disorder is listed as a differential diagnosis until further information obtained.

296.40 (F31.9) Bipolar I Disorder, Unspecified or 296.89 (F31.81) Bipolar II Disorder

Given that the patient was diagnosed with bipolar disorder when hospitalized, he will require a throughout reassessment of manic symptoms. Patient stated that his "manic" symptoms were alcohol related, so until the patient is evaluated following a period of sobriety the diagnosis of bipolar disorder cannot be made.

309.81 (F43.10) Posttraumatic Stress Disorder

The patient reported a history of trauma while incarcerated and endorsed past posttraumatic symptoms (nightmares and flashbacks) that subsided after 4 years. At this time, he is not reporting any specific posttraumatic stress disorder (PTSD) symptoms. Therefore, the diagnosis of PTSD would not be indicated.

FORMULATING THE TREATMENT STRATEGY

What treatment would you prescribe and what is the rationale?

Psychopharmacology: Fluoxetine 20 mg daily. Fluoxetine is Food and Drug Administration approved for the treatment of major depressive disorder and as a selective serotonin reuptake inhibitor is considered a first-line treatment.

Folic acid supplementation of 1 mg daily PO. Folate deficiencies are usually associated with poor diet, common among alcoholics.

Multivitamin, one daily PO with vitamins B-12 and B-6, which promote improved absorption of folate.

Thiamine (vitamin B-1) 100 mg PO daily. Thiamine supplementation prevents the development of Wernicke's encephalopathy. Alcoholism may contribute to thiamine deficiency due to inadequate nutrition, decreased absorption of thiamine from the gastrointestinal system, and reduced uptake by the cells, followed by decreased utilization of thiamine once in the cells. Prolonged thiamine deficiency leads to Wernicke's encephalopathy and eventually to Korsakoff psychosis. Oral thiamine is only minimally absorbed. Thiamine 250 mg IM (plus other B vitamins and ascorbic acid) once daily for 3 to 5 consecutive days is the recommended treatment for at-risk individuals. However, intramuscular or intravenous administration is not usually available in outpatient settings.

Naltrexone 50 mg daily. Naltrexone blocks opioid receptors and works by decreasing the craving for alcohol, which may result in fewer relapses.

Diagnostic Tests: Routine laboratory tests including aspartate aminotransferase, alanine aminotransferase, γ-glutamyltransferase, mean corpuscular volume, and carbohydrate-deficient transferrin, which are the main biomarkers for alcohol use.

Referrals: Refer patient to temporary housing until inpatient rehabilitation placement can be obtained, long term, that is, more than 3 months. Patient may require a treatment program for up to a year, followed by a therapeutic community placement.

Type of Psychotherapy: The patient is being referred for long-term rehabilitation. These types of facilities generally include a 12-step Alcoholics Anonymous model. Other treatment modalities such as dialectical behavior therapy show promise with patients who use substances, in that they teaches coping skills and frustration tolerance, which are usually low in this population.

Psychoeducation: Advise that when taking naltrexone the patient should carry a card stating that he is using it. Educate patient about the importance of taking the vitamin supplements in order to avoid permanent neurologic impairments due to alcohol abuse.

CLINICAL NOTE

- Working with a homeless population poses its own challenges. Often homeless individuals have lost their social network. An additional challenge is treatment nonadherence. Many homeless patients do not follow treatment recommendations, are chronically unreliable in attending appointments, refuse treatment, and may deny having a mental health problem. When working with this vulnerable population, providers must understand that relapse may occur frequently.

REFERENCES/RECOMMENDED READINGS

Agabio R. Thiamine administration in alcohol-dependent patients. *Alcohol Alcoholism.* 2005;40(2):155-156.

American Psychiatric Association. *Diagnostic and Statistical Manual of Mental Disorders.* 5th ed. Arlington, VA: American Psychiatric Publishing; 2013.

Martin PR, Singleton CK, Hiller-Sturmhofel S. The role of thiamine deficiency in alcoholic brain disease. *Alcohol Res Health.* 2003;27(2):134-142.

Substance Abuse and Mental Health Services Administration. Homelessness and Housing. 2016. https://www.samhsa.gov/homelessness-housing.

Stockwell T, Sitharan T, McGrath D, Lang E. The measurement of alcohol dependence and impaired control in community samples. *Addiction.* 1994;89:167-174.

Thomson AD, Guerrini I, Marshall EJ. The evolution and treatment of Korsakoff's syndrome. *Neuropsychol Rev.* 2012;22(2):81-92.

CASE 44 APPENDIX

Severity of Alcohol Dependence Questionnaire (SADQ-C)[1]

*NAME*____*AGE*____________*No.*_______

DATE: ____

Please recall a typical period of heavy drinking in the last 6 months.

When was this? Month:. . .. .
Year. . .. .

Please answer all the following questions about your drinking by circling your most appropriate response.

During that period of heavy drinking

1. The day after drinking alcohol, I woke up feeling sweaty.

   ALMOST NEVER SOMETIMES OFTEN NEARLY ALWAYS

2. The day after drinking alcohol, my hands shook first thing in the morning.

   ALMOST NEVER SOMETIMES OFTEN NEARLY ALWAYS

3. The day after drinking alcohol, my whole body shook violently first thing in the morning if I didn't have a drink.

   ALMOST NEVER SOMETIMES OFTEN NEARLY ALWAYS

4. The day after drinking alcohol, I woke up absolutely drenched in sweat.

   ALMOST NEVER SOMETIMES OFTEN NEARLY ALWAYS

5. The day after drinking alcohol, I dread waking up in the morning.

   ALMOST NEVER SOMETIMES OFTEN NEARLY ALWAYS

[1]Reprinted with permission from Stockwell T, Sitharan T, McGrath D, Lang E. The measurement of alcohol dependence and impaired control in community samples. *Addiction*. 1994;89:167-174.

6. The day after drinking alcohol, I was frightened of meeting people first thing in the morning.

   ALMOST NEVER SOMETIMES OFTEN NEARLY ALWAYS

7. The day after drinking alcohol, I felt at the edge of despair when I awoke.

   ALMOST NEVER SOMETIMES OFTEN NEARLY ALWAYS

8. The day after drinking alcohol, I felt very frightened when I awoke.

   ALMOST NEVER SOMETIMES OFTEN NEARLY ALWAYS

9. The day after drinking alcohol, I liked to have an alcoholic drink in the morning.

   ALMOST NEVER SOMETIMES OFTEN NEARLY ALWAYS

10. The day after drinking alcohol, I always gulped my first few alcoholic drinks down as quickly as possible.

    ALMOST NEVER SOMETIMES OFTEN NEARLY ALWAYS

11. The day after drinking alcohol, I drank more alcohol to get rid of the shakes.

    ALMOST NEVER SOMETIMES OFTEN NEARLY ALWAYS

12. The day after drinking alcohol, I had a very strong craving for a drink when I awoke.

    ALMOST NEVER SOMETIMES OFTEN ALMOST ALWAYS

13. I drank more than a quarter of a bottle of spirits in a day (OR 1 bottle of wine OR 7 beers).

    ALMOST NEVER SOMETIMES OFTEN ALMOST ALWAYS

14. I drank more than half a bottle of spirits per day (OR 2 bottles of wine OR 15 beers).

    ALMOST NEVER SOMETIMES OFTEN ALMOST ALWAYS

15. I drank more than one bottle of spirits per day (OR 4 bottles of wine OR 30 beers).

    ALMOST NEVER SOMETIMES OFTEN ALMOST ALWAYS

16. I drank more than two bottles of spirits per day (OR 8 bottles of wine OR 60 beers).

    ALMOST NEVER SOMETIMES OFTEN ALMOST ALWAYS

Imagine the following situation:

1. You have been **completely off drink for a few weeks**
2. You then drink **very heavily** for **two days**

How would you feel the **morning after** those two days of drinking?

17. I would start to sweat.

    NOT AT ALL SLIGHTLY MODERATELY QUITE A LOT

18. My hands would shake.

    NOT AT ALL SLIGHTLY MODERATELY QUITE A LOT

19. My body would shake.

    NOT AT ALL SLIGHTLY MODERATELY QUITE A LOT

20. I would be craving for a drink.

    NOT AT ALL SLIGHTLY MODERATELY QUITE A LOT

SCORE

CHECKED BY:

ALCOHOL DETOX PRESCRIBED: YES/NO

NOTES ON THE USE OF THE SADQ

The SADQ-C was developed by the Addiction Research Unit at Maudsley Hospital. It is a measure of the severity of dependence. The AUDIT questionnaire, by contrast, is used to assess whether or not there is a problem with dependence.

The SADQ questions cover the following aspects of dependency syndrome:

- Physical withdrawal symptoms
- Affective withdrawal symptoms
- Relief drinking
- Frequency of alcohol consumption
- Speed of onset of withdrawal symptoms

Scoring

Answers to each question are rated on a four-point scale:

Almost never 0
Sometimes 1
Often 2
Nearly always 3

A score of 31 or higher indicates "severe alcohol dependence."
A score of 16 to 30 indicates "moderate dependence."
A score of below 16 usually indicates only a mild physical dependency.
A chlordiazepoxide detoxification regime is usually indicated for someone who scores 16 or over.

It is essential to take account of the amount of alcohol that the patient reports drinking prior to admission as well as the result of the SADQ.

There is no correlation between SADQ and such parameters as the mean corpuscular volume or gamma glutamyltransferase.

CASE 45

Renal Function Decreasing

IDENTIFICATION: The patient is a 52-year old, married, white female accompanied by her husband. She is seen for the evaluation in an outpatient psychiatric clinic.

CHIEF COMPLAINT: "I need a new prescriber because my insurance changed."

HISTORY OF CHIEF COMPLAINT: The patient was hospitalized 10 years ago for symptoms of depression followed by mania. Four years later, she was admitted to the hospital with delusions and paranoia. She was initially started on lithium and then clozapine was added. Two years later, she was prescribed risperidone and developed signs of tardive dyskinesia (TD). The risperidone was stopped, and the TD signs subsided. Later, she was restarted on the Risperdal again with vitamin E. She again developed mild symptoms of TD with involuntary mouth movements. The movements became permanent even after stopping risperidone.

Current medications: clozapine 100 mg BID, lithium ER 450 mg BID, paroxetine 30 mg daily.

PAST PSYCHIATRIC HISTORY: No history prior to her first hospitalization 10 years ago as described earlier. Second psychiatric hospitalization 4 years following the first, as described above.

MEDICAL HISTORY: The patient brought her laboratory results, which were drawn the previous month. Her blood urea nitrogen was elevated at 1.06 mg/dL (0.57 to 1.00). Her glomerular filtration rate was low at 57 mL/min/1.73 m^2 (>59). Her thyroid-stimulating hormone (TSH) was high at 5.480 uIU/mL (0.450 to 4.500).

No history of surgeries. Had two vaginal births without complications. Treated for hyperlipidemia with atorvastatin 20 mg daily. Average height and weight. No disturbance of sleep or appetite. Postmenopausal.

HISTORY OF DRUG OR ALCOHOL ABUSE: Denied.

FAMILY HISTORY: The patient believes her mother may have bipolar disorder but has never been diagnosed.

PERSONAL HISTORY

Perinatal: Information not obtained.

Childhood: Normal milestones and accomplishments.

Adolescence: High school graduate. Active in school organizations.

Adulthood: College educated. The patient is married to a supportive husband and they have two grown children. Stopped working when her first child was born.

TRAUMA/ABUSE HISTORY: Denied.

MENTAL STATUS EXAMINATION

Appearance: Casual, clean attire. Defers to husband to answer questions about her psychiatric history as she says she does not remember all the details. Good eye contact.

Behavior and psychomotor activity: Very cooperative. Abnormal involuntary athetoid movements of the tongue.

Consciousness:	Alert.
Orientation:	Times three.
Memory:	Not formally assessed due to lack of time but will investigate more thoroughly in future visit. Poor recall for some remote events. Relies on her husband to supervise her medications because she thinks she may not remember to take them.
Concentration and attention:	Fair. Her anxiety may be interfering with her attentiveness.
Visuospatial ability:	Not assessed.
Abstract thought:	Needs to be evaluated in more depth when she is less anxious. At present her thinking is fairly concrete.

Intellectual functioning: Average.

Speech and language: Normal rate and volume.

Perceptions: No hallucinations or delusions.

Thought processes: Logical.

Thought content: Worried about getting her medications reordered. Fearful of having a relapse and having to be hospitalized without her medications. Suicidality and homicidality denied.

Mood: Euthymic.

Affect: Full range and congruent to mood.

Impulse control: Good.

Judgment/insight/reliability: Fair.

FORMULATING THE DIAGNOSIS

Which diagnosis should be considered?

295.40 (F31.9) Bipolar Disorder I, Unspecified (Provisional)

Diagnostic Criteria

For a diagnosis of bipolar I disorder, it is necessary to meet the following criteria for a manic episode. The manic episode may have been preceded by and may be followed by hypomanic or major depressive episodes (MDEs).

Manic Episode

A. A distinct period of abnormally and persistently elevated, expansive, or irritable mood and abnormally and persistently increased activity or energy, lasting at least 1 week and present most of the day, nearly every day (or any duration if hospitalization is necessary).

B. During the period of mood disturbance and increased energy or activity, three (or more) of the following symptoms (four if the mood is only irritable) are present to a significant degree and represent a noticeable change from usual behavior:
   1. Inflated self-esteem or grandiosity.
   2. Decreased need for sleep (eg, feels rested after only 3 hours of sleep).
   3. More talkative than usual or pressure to keep talking.
   4. Flight of ideas or subjective experience that thoughts are racing.

5. Distractibility (ie, attention too easily drawn to unimportant or irrelevant external stimuli), as reported or observed.
6. Increase in goal-directed activity (either socially, at work or school, or sexually) or psychomotor agitation (ie, purposeless nongoal-directed activity).
7. Excessive involvement in activities that have a high potential for painful consequences (eg, engaging in unrestrained buying sprees, sexual indiscretions, or foolish business investments).

C. The mood disturbance is sufficiently severe to cause marked impairment in social or occupational functioning or to necessitate hospitalization to prevent harm to self or others, or there are psychotic features.

D. The episode is not attributable to the physiologic effects of a substance (eg, a drug of abuse, a medication, other treatment) or another medical condition.
   - **Note:** A full manic episode that emerges during antidepressant treatment (eg, medication, electroconvulsive therapy) but persists at a fully syndromal level beyond the physiologic effect of that treatment is sufficient evidence for a manic episode and, therefore, a bipolar I diagnosis.

Note: Criteria A to D constitute a manic episode. At least one lifetime manic episode is required for the diagnosis of bipolar I disorder.

Hypomanic Episode

A. A distinct period of abnormally and persistently elevated, expansive, or irritable mood and abnormally and persistently increased activity or energy, lasting at least 4 consecutive days and present most of the day, nearly every day.

B. During the period of mood disturbance and increased energy and activity, three (or more) of the following symptoms (four if the mood is only irritable) have persisted, represent a noticeable change from usual behavior, and have been present to a significant degree:
1. Inflated self-esteem or grandiosity.
2. Decreased need for sleep (eg, feels rested after only 3 hours of sleep).
3. More talkative than usual or pressure to keep talking.
4. Flight of ideas or subjective experience that thoughts are racing.
5. Distractibility (ie, attention too easily drawn to unimportant or irrelevant external stimuli), as reported or observed.
6. Increase in goal-directed activity (either socially, at work or school, or sexually) or psychomotor agitation.
7. Excessive involvement in activities that have a high potential for painful consequences (eg, engaging in unrestrained buying sprees, sexual indiscretions, or foolish business investments).

C. The episode is associated with an unequivocal change in functioning that is uncharacteristic of the individual when not symptomatic.

D. The disturbance in mood and the change in functioning are observable by others.
E. The episode is not severe enough to cause marked impairment in social or occupational functioning or to necessitate hospitalization. If there are psychotic features, the episode is, by definition, manic.
F. The episode is not attributable to the physiologic effects of a substance (eg, a drug of abuse, a medication, other treatment) or another medical condition.
   - **Note:** A full hypomanic episode that emerges during antidepressant treatment (eg, medication, electroconvulsive therapy) but persists at a fully syndromal level beyond the physiologic effect of that treatment is sufficient evidence for a hypomanic episode diagnosis. However, caution is indicated so that one or two symptoms (particularly increased irritability, edginess, or agitation following antidepressant use) are not taken as sufficient for diagnosis of a hypomanic episode, nor necessarily indicative of a bipolar diathesis.

Note: Criteria A to F constitute a hypomanic episode. Hypomanic episodes are common in bipolar I disorder but are not required for the diagnosis of bipolar I disorder.

Major Depressive Episode

A. Five (or more) of the following symptoms have been present during the same 2-week period and represent a change from previous functioning; at least one of the symptoms is either (1) depressed mood or (2) loss of interest or pleasure.
   - **Note:** Do not include symptoms that are clearly attributable to another medical condition.
     1. Depressed mood most of the day, nearly every day, as indicated by either subjective report (eg, feels sad, empty, or hopeless) or observation made by others (eg, appears tearful). (Note: In children and adolescents, can be irritable mood.)
     2. Markedly diminished interest or pleasure in all, or almost all, activities most of the day, nearly every day (as indicated by either subjective account or observation).
     3. Significant weight loss when not dieting or weight gain (eg, a change of more than 5% of body weight in a month), or decrease or increase in appetite nearly every day. (Note: In children, consider failure to make expected weight gain.)
     4. Insomnia or hypersomnia nearly every day.
     5. Psychomotor agitation or retardation nearly every day (observable by others; not merely subjective feelings of restlessness or being slowed down).
     6. Fatigue or loss of energy nearly every day.
     7. Feelings of worthlessness or excessive or inappropriate guilt (which may be delusional) nearly every day (not merely self-reproach or guilt about being sick).

8. Diminished ability to think or concentrate, or indecisiveness, nearly every day (either by subjective account or as observed by others).
9. Recurrent thoughts of death (not just fear of dying), recurrent suicidal ideation without a specific plan, or a suicide attempt or a specific plan for committing suicide.

B. The symptoms cause clinically significant distress or impairment in social, occupational, or other important areas of functioning.
C. The episode is not attributable to the physiologic effects of a substance or another medical condition.

Note: Criteria A to C constitute an MDE. MDEs are common in bipolar I disorder but are not required for the diagnosis of bipolar I disorder.

Note: Responses to a significant loss (eg, bereavement, financial ruin, losses from a natural disaster, a serious medical illness or disability) may include the feelings of intense sadness, rumination about the loss, insomnia, poor appetite, and weight loss noted in Criterion A, which may resemble a depressive episode. Although such symptoms may be understandable or considered appropriate to the loss, the presence of an MDE in addition to the normal response to a significant loss should also be carefully considered. This decision inevitably requires the exercise of clinical judgment based on the individual's history and the cultural norms for the expression of distress in the context of loss.

In distinguishing grief from an MDE, it is useful to consider that in grief the predominant affect is feelings of emptiness and loss, whereas in an MDE it is persistent depressed mood and the inability to anticipate happiness or pleasure. The dysphoria in grief is likely to decrease in intensity over days to weeks and occurs in waves, the so-called pangs of grief. These waves tend to be associated with thoughts or reminders of the deceased. The depressed mood of an MDE is more persistent and not tied to specific thoughts or preoccupations. The pain of grief may be accompanied by positive emotions and humor that are uncharacteristic of the pervasive unhappiness and misery characteristic of an MDE. The thought content associated with grief generally features a preoccupation with thoughts and memories of the deceased, rather than the self-critical or pessimistic ruminations seen in an MDE. In grief, self-esteem is generally preserved, whereas in an MDE, feelings of worthlessness and self-loathing are common. If self-derogatory ideation is present in grief, it typically involves perceived failings vis-à-vis the deceased (eg, not visiting frequently enough, not telling the deceased how much he or she was loved). If a bereaved individual thinks about death and dying, such thoughts are generally focused on the deceased and possibly about "joining" the deceased, whereas in an MDE such thoughts are focused on ending one's own life because of feeling worthless, undeserving of life, or unable to cope with the pain of depression.

Bipolar I Disorder

A. Criteria have been met for at least one manic episode (Criteria A to D under "Manic Episode" above).

B. The occurrence of the manic and MDE(s) is not better explained by schizoaffective disorder, schizophrenia, schizophreniform disorder, delusional disorder, or other specified or unspecified schizophrenia spectrum and other psychotic disorder.

(Reprinted with permission from the *Diagnostic and Statistical Manual of Mental Disorders*, 5th ed. Arlington, VA: American Psychiatric Publishing; 2013.)

What is your rationale for the diagnosis?

The information provided by the patient's husband suggests that the patient was treated for symptoms of bipolar disorder with psychotic symptoms. Until prior psychiatric records are obtained, the diagnosis is considered provisional. However, there is a strong presumption that the full criteria for bipolar disorder will be met. Because it is not known what the most recent episode entailed, the term unspecified was used.

Which diagnosis should be considered?

333.85 (G24.01) Tardive Dyskinesia

Involuntary athetoid or choreiform movements (lasting at least a few weeks) generally of the tongue, lower face and jaw, and extremities (but sometimes involving the pharyngeal, diaphragmatic, or trunk muscles) developing in association with the use of a neuroleptic medication for at least a few months.

Symptoms may develop after a shorter period of medication use in older persons. In some patients, movements of this type may appear after discontinuation, or after change or reduction in dosage, of neuroleptic medications, in which case the condition is called *neuroleptic withdrawal-emergent dyskinesia.* Because withdrawal-emergent dyskinesia is usually time-limited, lasting less than 4 to 8 weeks, dyskinesia that persists beyond this window is considered to be TD.

(Reprinted with permission from the *Diagnostic and Statistical Manual of Mental Disorders*. 5th ed. Arlington, VA: American Psychiatric Publishing; 2013.)

What is your rationale for the diagnosis?

The patient is experiencing involuntary athetoid movements of the tongue that started several years ago in association with the use of a neuroleptic medication (risperidone).

What tests or tools should be considered to help identify the correct diagnosis?

Abnormal Involuntary Movement Scale (AIMS) should be completed on initial examination and at least q 6 months thereafter (see Appendix, http://www.cqaimh.org/pdf/tool_aims.pdf).

What differential diagnosis should be considered?

None indicated.

FORMULATION OF THE TREATMENT STRATEGY

What treatment would you prescribe and what is the rationale?

Psychopharmacology

Lithium ER 450 mg BID
Clozapine 100 mg BID
Paroxetine 30 mg daily

This patient is being seen for the first time by this provider. Her mental status is stable. She is anxious about making sure her medications are reordered and about the possibility of becoming ill again and having to return to the hospital. Although her renal function is abnormal, she is not at risk for immediate complications. Therefore, her current medication will be continued. Plans to increase the clozapine and reduce and discontinue the lithium will be considered after further history is obtained and there is a consultation with a renal specialist. The patient will also need to be followed up for her elevated TSH.

Diagnostic Tests: Besides routine laboratory tests, the following tests are indicated: lithium level, renal function tests, thyroid function tests, electrolytes, calcium, and a urinalysis. Metabolic and renal effects including hypothyroidism, weight gain, and diabetes insipidus can occur with patient's prescribed lithium. A monthly absolute neutrophil count (ANC) is required in order for clozapine to be dispensed from the pharmacy to the patient. When initiating clozapine treatment, ANC is required more frequently as outline by the Risk Evaluation and Mitigation Strategies guidelines (see guidelines section below). An ECG should also be ordered to provide a baseline, as cardiac complications, particularly cardiomyopathy, have been associated with clozapine use.

Referral: Refer to a nephrologist and an endocrinologist. The patient's reduced renal function needs to be addressed as promptly as possible. Chronic lithium use can contribute to nephropathy. End-stage renal disease may occur in a small number of patients. Additionally, she needs to have her thyroid function evaluated and treated.

A referral to a neurologist can be considered in the future depending on the severity of her TD. In the meantime, the risk of TD is less likely with clozapine than with any of the other neuroleptics.

Psychotherapy: Supportive psychotherapy emphasizing stress reduction techniques may be helpful in the patient's anxiety management.

Psychoeducation: The patient should be educated that clozapine is a very effective antimanic drug.

She should also be informed that while she is still taking lithium she should avoid nonsteroidal anti-inflammatory drugs as they increase the risk for renal failure. Instructions regarding maintaining adequate fluid and sodium intake should be provided to the patient to avoid lithium toxicity. The patient should be educated regarding the symptoms of lithium toxicity, which include nausea, constipation, tremors, or swelling of the extremities; these should be reported promptly.

What standard guidelines would you use to treat or assess this patient?

To be qualified to prescribe clozapine, the prescriber must be certified in the clozapine Risk Evaluation and Mitigation Strategies (REMS) program. REMS for clozapine monitoring use can be accessed at:

https://www.clozapinerems.com/CpmgClozapineUI/home.u

CLINICAL NOTE

- Unless there is an urgent need, most patients are more comfortable keeping their current medication regimen until they feel more secure with a new provider.
- Different ethnic groups may have normal low ANCs. Benign ethnic neutropenia is a condition present in some ethnic groups, most commonly in people of African descent and some Middle Eastern ethnic groups. It is also more common in men, for whom average ANCs are lower than the standard range for neutrophil. There is a separate ANC monitoring algorithm for treatment with clozapine. In spite of this condition these individuals are not at higher risk of developing clozapine-induced neutropenia or severe infections.
- It should be kept in mind that fever is often the first sign of a neutropenic infection. In this case clozapine treatment should be interrupted and the patient should be referred to a hematologist.

REFERENCES/RECOMMENDED READINGS

Spivak B, Mester R, Abesgaus J, Wittenberg N, Adlersberg S, Weizman A. Clozapine treatment for neuroleptic-induced tardive dyskinesia, parkinsonism, and chronic akathisia in schizophrenic patients. *J Clin Psychiatr.* 1997;58(7):318-322.

Woods SW, Morgenstern H, Saksa JR, et al. Incidence of tardive dyskinesia with atypical and conventional antipsychotic medications. *J Clin Psychiatr.* 2010;74:463-474.

CASE 45 APPENDIX[1]

Abnormal Involuntary Movement Scale (AIMS)—Overview

- The AIMS records the occurrence of tardive dyskinesia (TD) in patients receiving neuroleptic medications.
- The AIMS test is used to detect TD and to follow the severity of a patient's TD over time.

CLINICAL UTILITY

The AIMS is a 12-item anchored scale that is clinician administered and scored

- Items 1 to 10 are rated on a five-point anchored scale.
  - Items 1 to 4 assess orofacial movements.
  - Items 5 to 7 deal with extremity and truncal dyskinesia.
  - Items 8 to 10 deal with global severity as judged by the examiner, and the patient's awareness of the movements and the distress associated with them.
- Items 11 and 12 are yes–no questions concerning problems with teeth and/or dentures, because such problems can lead to a mistaken diagnosis of dyskinesia.

EXAMINATION PROCEDURE

The indirect observation and the AIMS examination procedure are on the following two pages.

---

[1]Rush JA Jr. *Handbook of Psychiatric Measures*. Washington, DC: American Psychiatric Association;2000: 166-168.

SCORING

- A total score of items 1 to 7 (Categories I, II, III) can be calculated. These represent observed movements.
- Item 8 can be used as an overall severity index.
- Items 9 (incapacitation) and 10 (awareness) provide additional information that may be useful in clinical decision making.
- Items 11 (dental status) and 12 (dentures) provide information that may be useful in determining lip, jaw, and tongue movements.

PSYCHOMETRIC PROPERTIES

The AIMS is a global rating method. The AIMS requires the raters to compare the observed movements to the average movement disturbance seen in persons with TD. Such relative judgments may vary among raters with different backgrounds and experience.

AIMS EXAMINATION PROCEDURE

Either before or after completing the AIMS on the following page, observe the patient unobtrusively at rest (e.g., in the waiting room).

The chair to be used in this examination should be a hard, firm one without arms.

QUESTIONS

1. Ask the patient whether there is anything in his or her mouth (such as gum or candy) and, if so, to remove it.
2. Ask about the *current* condition of the patient's teeth. Ask if he or she wears dentures. Ask whether teeth or dentures bother the patient *now.*
3. Ask whether the patient notices any movements in his or her mouth, face, hands, or feet. If yes, ask the patient to describe them and to indicate to what extent they *currently* bother the patient or interfere with activities.
4. Have the patient sit in chair with hands on knees, legs slightly apart, and feet flat on floor. (Look at the entire body for movements while the patient is in this position.)
5. Ask the patient to sit with hands hanging unsupported—if male, between his legs, if female and wearing a dress, hanging over her knees. (Observe hands and other body areas.)
6. Ask the patient to open his or her mouth. (Observe the tongue at rest within the mouth.) Do this twice.
7. Ask the patient to protrude his or her tongue. (Observe abnormalities of tongue movement.) Do this twice.

8. Ask the patient to tap his or her thumb with each finger as rapidly as possible for 10 to 15 seconds, first with right hand, then with left hand. (Observe facial and leg movements.)
9. Flex and extend the patient's left and right arms, one at a time.
10. Ask the patient to stand up. (Observe the patient in profile. Observe all body areas again, hips included.)
11. Ask the patient to extend both arms out in front, palms down. (Observe trunk, legs, and mouth.)
12. Have the patient walk a few paces, turn, and walk back to the chair. (Observe hands and gait.) Do this twice.

Abnormal Involuntary Movement Scale (AIMS)

Patient Name ______________________ ***Date of Visit*** ______________

Code:

1 = Minimal	*0 = None*
3 = Moderate	*2 = Mild*
	4 = Severe

Movement Ratings: • Rate highest severity observed in category I, II, III • Rate movements that occur upon activation one point less than those observed spontaneously • Circle movements as well as code number that applies		RATER DATE	RATER DATE	RATER DATE	RATER DATE
I FACIAL & ORAL MOVEMENTS	1. **Muscles of Facial Expression,** eg, movements of forehead, eyebrows, periorbital area, cheeks, including frowning, blinking, smiling, grimacing	0 1 2 3 4	0 1 2 3 4	0 1 2 3 4	0 1 2 3 4
	2. **Lips and Perioral Area,** eg, puckering, pouting, smacking	0 1 2 3 4	0 1 2 3 4	0 1 2 3 4	0 1 2 3 4
	3. **Jaw** Biting, clenching, chewing, mouth opening, lateral movement	0 1 2 3 4	0 1 2 3 4	0 1 2 3 4	0 1 2 3 4
	4. **Tongue** Rate only increases in movement both in and out of mouth. NOT inability to sustain movement. Darting in and out of mouth	0 1 2 3 4	0 1 2 3 4	0 1 2 3 4	0 1 2 3 4
II EXTREMITY MOVEMENTS	5. **Upper (arms, wrists, hands, fingers)** Include choreic movements (ie, rapid, objectively purposeless, irregular, spontaneous), athetoid movements. DO NOT INCLUDE TREMOR (ie, repetitive, regular, rhythmic)	0 1 2 3 4	0 1 2 3 4	0 1 2 3 4	0 1 2 3 4
	6. **Lower (legs, knees, ankles, toes)** Lateral knee movement, foot tapping, heel dropping, foot squirming, inversion and eversion of foot	0 1 2 3 4	0 1 2 3 4	0 1 2 3 4	0 1 2 3 4
III TRUNK MOVEMENTS	7. **Neck, shoulders, and hips** Rocking, twisting, squirming, pelvic gyrations	0 1 2 3 4	0 1 2 3 4	0 1 2 3 4	0 1 2 3 4

IV GLOBAL JUDGMENT	**8. Severity of abnormal movements overall**	0 1 2 3 4	0 1 2 3 4	0 1 2 3 4	0 1 2 3 4
	9. Incapacitation due to abnormal movements	0 1 2 3 4	0 1 2 3 4	0 1 2 3 4	0 1 2 3 4
	10. Patient's awareness of abnormal movements. Rate only patients report: No Awareness = 0 Aware, no distress = 1 Aware, mild distress = 2 Aware, moderate distress = 3 Aware, severe distress = 4	0 1 2 3 4	0 1 2 3 4	0 1 2 3 4	0 1 2 3 4
V DENTAL STATUS	**11. Current problems with teeth and/or dentures**	YES NO	YES NO	YES NO	YES NO
	12. Are dentures usually worn	YES NO	YES NO	YES NO	YES NO
	13. Edentia?	YES NO	YES NO	YES NO	YES NO
	14. Do movements disappear with sleep?	YES NO	YES NO	YES NO	YES NO

CASE 46

Very Tired and Cannot Sleep

IDENTIFICATION: The patient is a 58-year-old white, married, male. He is seen in an outpatient mental health clinic.

CHIEF COMPLAINT: "I'm extremely tired. I'm not sleeping. And I've been nauseous."

HISTORY OF CHIEF COMPLAINT: Started having trouble sleeping 5 months ago. At the same time he started taking ledipasvir/sofosbuvir to treat hepatitis C. Patient denies any additional psychosocial stressors that could be contributing to his insomnia. He has no change in medication or medical conditions other than starting ledipasvir/sofosbuvir.

PAST PSYCHIATRIC HISTORY: History of polysubstance abuse. Had court-ordered outpatient treatment after he was in a halfway house 25 years ago. Has been on methadone maintenance since then. No history of suicidal or homicidal symptoms. Has been treated for insomnia with trazodone 50 mg HS for the past 3 years. Insomnia was controlled with the trazodone until 5 months ago.

MEDICAL HISTORY: Has cirrhosis of the liver. Contracted hepatitis C following intravenous (IV) drug abuse. Was started on ledipasvir/sofosbuvir 5 months ago. Has felt nauseous intermittently and has had a poor appetite. Slight weight loss reported.

CURRENT MEDICATIONS: Methadone, ledipasvir/sofosbuvir, trazodone 50 mg HS.

HISTORY OF DRUG OR ALCOHOL ABUSE: Started using alcohol at 16 years old. Drank until he was 32 years old. Smokes two to three cigarettes per day. Used cocaine in the past. Was an IV heroin user, but has been on methadone maintenance for the past 25 years.

FAMILY HISTORY: His father was violent toward his mother and was eventually imprisoned due to the domestic violence.

PERSONAL HISTORY

Perinatal: Information not obtained.

Childhood: Normal developmental achievements.

Adolescence: Started drinking at 16 years old. The patient identifies as heterosexual. He was raised as a Catholic. He obtained his GED.

Adulthood: The patient is married and has one 12-year-old daughter. He currently lives with his wife and daughter. His wife has a history of IV heroin use. He is not currently employed. Several years ago he did light construction work. No military history. Legal history of charge for possession of drugs 25 years ago with subsequent court-ordered treatment.

TRAUMA/ABUSE HISTORY: None reported.

MENTAL STATUS EXAMINATION

Appearance: Well groomed. Distended abdomen. Appears tired.

Behavior and psychomotor activity: Pleasant. Cooperative.

Consciousness:	Alert.
Orientation:	Oriented times three.
Memory:	Grossly intact.
Concentration and attention:	Good.
Mood:	Euthymic.
Visuospatial ability:	Not assessed.
Abstract thought:	Not formally assessed but seems satisfactory.
Intellectual ability:	Average.
Speech and language:	Within normal limits.

Perceptions: No hallucination or delusions.

Thought processes: Organized and logical.

Thought content: Worried about not being able to sleep.

Suicidality and homicidality: Denies.

Mood: Euthymic.

Affect: Congruent to mood. Full range.

Impulse control: Not observed or reported.

Judgment/insight/reliability: Good.

FORMULATING THE DIAGNOSIS

What diagnosis should be considered?

292.85 (F19.282) Substance/Medication-Induced Sleep Disorder

Diagnostic Criteria

A. A prominent and severe disturbance in sleep.
B. There is evidence from the history, physical examination, or laboratory findings of both (1) and (2):
   1. The symptoms in Criterion A developed during or soon after substance intoxication or after withdrawal from or exposure to a medication.
   2. The involved substance/medication is capable of producing the symptoms in Criterion A.
C. The disturbance is not better explained by a sleep disorder that is not substance/medication-induced. Such evidence of an independent sleep disorder could include the following:
   - The symptoms precede the onset of the substance/medication use; the symptoms persist for a substantial period of time (eg, about 1 month) after the cessation of acute withdrawal or severe intoxication; or there is other evidence suggesting the existence of an independent nonsubstance/medication-induced sleep disorder (eg, a history of recurrent nonsubstance/medication-related episodes).
   - The disturbance does not occur exclusively during the course of a delirium.
   - The disturbance causes clinically significant distress or impairment in social, occupational, or other important areas of functioning.

Note: This diagnosis should be made instead of a diagnosis of substance intoxication or substance withdrawal only when the symptoms in Criterion

A predominate in the clinical picture and when they are sufficiently severe to warrant clinical attention.

Coding note: The *ICD-9-CM* and *ICD-10-CM* codes for the [specific substance/medication]-induced sleep disorders are indicated in the table below. Note that the *ICD-10-CM* code depends on whether or not there is a comorbid substance use disorder present for the same class of substance. If a mild substance use disorder is comorbid with the substance-induced sleep disorder, the fourth position character is "1," and the clinician should record "mild [substance] use disorder" before the substance-induced sleep disorder (eg, "mild cocaine use disorder with cocaine-induced sleep disorder"). If a moderate or severe substance use disorder is comorbid with the substance-induced sleep disorder, the fourth position character is "2," and the clinician should record "moderate [substance] use disorder" or "severe [substance] use disorder," depending on the severity of the comorbid substance use disorder. If there is no comorbid substance use disorder (eg, after a one-time heavy use of the substance), then the fourth position character is "9," and the clinician should record only the substance-induced sleep disorder. A moderate or severe tobacco use disorder is required in order to code a tobacco-induced sleep disorder; it is not permissible to code a comorbid mild tobacco use disorder or no tobacco use disorder with a tobacco-induced sleep disorder.

Specify whether:

- **Insomnia type:** Characterized by difficulty falling asleep or maintaining sleep, frequent nocturnal awakenings, or nonrestorative sleep.
- **Daytime sleepiness type:** Characterized by predominant complaint of excessive sleepiness/fatigue during waking hours or, less commonly, a long sleep period.
- **Parasomnia type:** Characterized by abnormal behavioral events during sleep.
- **Mixed type:** Characterized by a substance/medication-induced sleep problem characterized by multiple types of sleep symptoms, but no symptom clearly predominates.

Specify if (see Table in the chapter "Substance-Related and Addictive Disorders" for diagnoses associated with substance class):

- **With onset during intoxication:** This specifier should be used if criteria are met for intoxication with the substance/medication and symptoms developed during the intoxication period.
- **With onset during discontinuation/withdrawal:** This specifier should be used if criteria are met for discontinuation/withdrawal from the substance/medication and symptoms developed during, or shortly after, discontinuation of the substance/medication.

(Reprinted with permission from the *Diagnostic and Statistical Manual of Mental Disorders*. 5th ed. Arlington, VA: American Psychiatric Publishing; 2013.)

What is your rationale for the diagnosis?

The patient started taking ledipasvir/sofosbuvir 5 months ago. Ledipasvir/sofosbuvir is indicated for the treatment of patients with chronic hepatitis C. Common side effects include fatigue and insomnia. It is likely that the insomnia the patient is experiencing is related to this side effect.

What diagnosis should be considered?

292.9 (F18.99) Opioid Use Disorder, in Sustained Remission, on Maintenance Therapy

Diagnostic Criteria

A. A problematic pattern of opioid use leading to clinically significant impairment or distress, as manifested by at least two of the following, occurring within a 12-month period:
   1. Opioids are often taken in larger amounts or over a longer period than was intended.
   2. There is a persistent desire or unsuccessful efforts to cut down or control opioid use.
   3. A great deal of time is spent in activities necessary to obtain the opioid, use the opioid, or recover from its effects.
   4. Craving, or a strong desire or urge to use opioids.
   5. Recurrent opioid use resulting in a failure to fulfill major role obligations at work, school, or home.
   6. Continued opioid use despite having persistent or recurrent social or interpersonal problems caused or exacerbated by the effects of opioids.
   7. Important social, occupational, or recreational activities are given up or reduced because of opioid use.
   8. Recurrent opioid use in situations in which it is physically hazardous.
   9. Continued opioid use despite knowledge of having a persistent or recurrent physical or psychological problem that is likely to have been caused or exacerbated by the substance.
   10. Tolerance, as defined by either of the following:
       a. A need for markedly increased amounts of opioids to achieve intoxication or desired effect.
       b. A markedly diminished effect with continued use of the same amount of an opioid.
          - **Note:** This criterion is not considered to be met for those taking opioids solely under appropriate medical supervision.

       Withdrawal, as manifested by either of the following:
       c. The characteristic opioid withdrawal syndrome (refer to Criteria A and B of the criteria set for opioid withdrawal).

d. Opioids (or a closely related substance) are taken to relieve or avoid withdrawal symptoms.
   - **Note:** This criterion is not considered to be met for those individuals taking opioids solely under appropriate medical supervision.

Specify if:

- **In early remission:** After full criteria for opioid use disorder were previously met, none of the criteria for opioid use disorder have been met for at least 3 months but for less than 12 months (with the exception that Criterion A4, "Craving, or a strong desire or urge to use opioids," may be met).
- **In sustained remission:** After full criteria for opioid use disorder were previously met, none of the criteria for opioid use disorder have been met at any time during a period of 12 months or longer (with the exception that Criterion A4, "Craving, or a strong desire or urge to use opioids," may be met).

Specify if:

- **On maintenance therapy:** This additional specifier is used if the individual is taking a prescribed agonist medication such as methadone or buprenorphine and none of the criteria for opioid use disorder have been met for that class of medication (except tolerance to, or withdrawal from, the agonist). This category also applies to those individuals being maintained on a partial agonist, an agonist/antagonist, or a full antagonist such as oral naltrexone or depot naltrexone.
- **In a controlled environment:** This additional specifier is used if the individual is in an environment where access to opioids is restricted.

Coding based on current severity: Note for *ICD-10-CM* codes: If an opioid intoxication, opioid withdrawal, or another opioid-induced mental disorder is also present, do not use the codes below for opioid use disorder. Instead, the comorbid opioid use disorder is indicated in the fourth character of the opioid-induced disorder code (see the coding note for opioid intoxication, opioid withdrawal, or a specific opioid-induced mental disorder). For example, if there is comorbid opioid-induced depressive disorder and opioid use disorder, only the opioid-induced depressive disorder code is given, with the fourth character indicating whether the comorbid opioid use disorder is mild, moderate, or severe: F11.14 for mild opioid use disorder with opioid-induced depressive disorder or F11.24 for a moderate or severe opioid use disorder with opioid-induced depressive disorder.

Specify current severity:

- **305.50 (F11.10) Mild:** Presence of two to three symptoms.
- **304.00 (F11.20) Moderate:** Presence of four to five symptoms.
- **304.00 (F11.20) Severe:** Presence of six or more symptoms.

(Reprinted with permission from the *Diagnostic and Statistical Manual of Mental Disorders*. 5th ed. Arlington, VA: American Psychiatric Publishing; 2013.)

What is your rationale for the diagnosis?

The patient has been taking a prescribed opiate agonist medication, methadone, for a period of 25 years in order to treat an opioid addiction. He has been on this maintenance treatment for over 12 months and, therefore, meets the criteria for sustained remission. The specifiers indicate that the patient is both in remission and receiving maintenance therapy.

What tests or tools should be considered to help identify the correct diagnosis?

A sleep history calendar can be used to identify the initial occurrence of the insomnia and to track the insomnia once the trial of ledipasvir/sofosbuvir is completed.

What differential diagnosis should be considered?

None indicated.

FORMULATING THE TREATMENT STRATEGY

What treatment would you prescribe and what is the rationale?

Psychopharmacology: None prescribed. Because fatigue and insomnia are known side effects of ledipasvir/sofosbuvir, the patient would be advised to wait until his treatment with ledipasvir/sofosbuvir is completed. If the insomnia persists after that period, medication may be considered.

Diagnostic Tests: None indicated.

Referrals: None indicated.

Type of Psychotherapy: None indicated.

Psychoeducation: The patient should be educated about the side effects of ledipasvir/sofosbuvir and advised to minimize any physical exertion during this period.

Sleep hygiene techniques should be reviewed.

What standard guidelines would you use to treat or assess this patient?

None indicated.

CLINICAL NOTES

- Because this patient is taking multiple medications, it is imperative that a drug interaction assessment be completed. There are several free computerized sites, such as epocrates.com, available to reconcile medications.
- This patient is probably having his urine tested on a regular basis; however, it would be prudent to check pharmacy data systems for any other controlled substances that have been prescribed for this patient. Many states have an online resource for this purpose.
- Methadone is known to have many drug interactions. The most serious interaction can be with benzodiazepines, which can result in respiratory failure.

REFERENCES/RECOMMENDED READINGS

Informed Health Online. Relaxation Techniques and Sleep Hygiene for Insomnia. Cologne, Germany: Institute for Quality and Efficiency in Health Care (IQWiG); 2006 (Updated Sep 24, 2013).

McCance-Katz EF, Sullivan LE, Nallani S. Drug interactions of clinical importance among the opioids, methadone and buprenorphine, and other frequently prescribed medications: a review. *Am J Addict*. 2010;19(1):4-16.

Morin CM, Bootzin RR, Buysse DJ, Edinger JD, Espie CA, Lichstein KL. Psychological and behavioral treatment of insomnia: update of the recent evidence (1998-2004). *Sleep*. 2006;29(11):1398.

SECTION III

Older Adult Case Studies

CASE 47

Withdrawn after Surgery

IDENTIFICATION: The patient is a 65-year-old, African-American, retired, married male who resides with his wife. The patient was referred for psychiatric treatment by his wife. He arrived to the outpatient mental health clinic with his wife but was interviewed alone. Later his wife was invited into the office to discuss the treatment plan.

CHIEF COMPLAINT: "My wife thinks I'm sleeping too much."

HISTORY OF CHIEF COMPLAINT: For the past month, the patient has started going back to bed for several hours in the middle of the day. As the interview proceeded, he confided that everyone "disappeared after I got better" following his hip replacement and stated, "What's the point of getting up?"Patient's wife reports that the patient has been noticeably withdrawn and thinks that he is trying to cover up feeling depressed in the past couple months.

PAST PSYCHIATRIC HISTORY: The patient started seeing a psychiatrist 6 years ago. He was stressed and anxious about work. Was started on sertraline 25 mg daily that he took for a year and that he thought helped. He stopped seeing the psychiatrist and taking the medication because he was feeling better. Reports increased alcohol intake starting approximately 5 years ago. His family had an intervention with him and as a result he went to an alcohol rehab for 2 months. He has been abstinent from alcohol since that time.

MEDICAL HISTORY: History of hip replacement 1 year ago. Had multiple medical complications following the surgery. Diagnosed with septicemia and was in the intensive care unit for 2 months. He went to a rehabilitation center following the hospitalization. He went to outpatient physical therapy for 2 months, which was completed 6 weeks ago.

HISTORY OF DRUG OR ALCOHOL ABUSE: History of alcohol abuse. Went to a rehab 5 years ago. Has abstained since and attends Alcoholics Anonymous (AA) meetings regularly.

FAMILY HISTORY: Mother had dementia. Brother died 10 years ago due to "alcoholism." Son has bipolar II disorder.

PERSONAL HISTORY

Perinatal: No known birth complications or developmental delays.

Childhood: The patient said he does not remember specific details, but that he had a "normal childhood."

Adolescence: Made friends easily. Played on the basketball team throughout high school.

Adulthood: Graduated from college. Married a woman he met in college and had one son. Has worked in a professional capacity with the same company for 45 years. Retired and then shortly after had his hip replacement surgery. Recently competed his physical rehabilitation and now is home without a job ("or purpose") for the first time in his life.

TRAUMA/ABUSE HISTORY: Denies.

MENTAL STATUS EXAMINATION

Appearance: Casual clothing. Good eye contact.

Behavior and psychomotor activity: Cooperative. No motor abnormalities.

Consciousness: Alert.

Orientation: Oriented to person, place, and time.

Memory: Recent memory intact. Had difficulty remembering the past five presidents. Said "Obama, Bush, Bush, Nixon, Johnson." Able to remember three objects after 5 minutes.

Concentration and attention: Fair. Seemed to struggle with naming items that begin with F. Named 12 items but some were duplicates, so he was unable to follow the instructions accurately. Was able to follow a three-stage command.

Visuospatial ability:	Not assessed.
Abstract thought:	Fair.
Intellectual functioning:	Average or above.
Speech and language:	Clear. Normal rate and volume.
Perceptions:	No altered perceptions elicited.
Thought processes:	Slightly tangential.
Thought content:	No obsessions or other preoccupations. Primarily related to numerous specific details about his experiences in his recent hospitalization.
Suicidality or homicidality:	Denied.
Mood:	"I'm fantastic."
Affect:	Full range. The patient seems to be emphasizing how good he feels. Cannot explain why he is going back to bed or has a lack of interest in any activity.
Impulse control:	Good.
Judgment:	Fair.
Insight:	Possibly diminished.
Reliability:	Fair. May not be giving an accurate account of his mood. Appears to not want to be seen as having a problem.

FORMULATING THE DIAGNOSIS

Which diagnosis (or diagnoses) should be considered?

309.0 (F43.21) Adjustment Disorder with Depressed Mood

Diagnostic Criteria

A. The development of emotional or behavioral symptoms in response to an identifiable stressor(s) occurring within 3 months of the onset of the stressor(s).

B. These symptoms or behaviors are clinically significant, as evidenced by one or both of the following:
   1. Marked distress that is out of proportion to the severity or intensity of the stressor, taking into account the external context and the cultural factors that might influence symptom severity and presentation.
   2. Significant impairment in social, occupational, or other important areas of functioning.
C. The stress-related disturbance does not meet the criteria for another mental disorder and is not merely an exacerbation of a preexisting mental disorder.
D. The symptoms do not represent normal bereavement.
E. Once the stressor or its consequences have terminated, the symptoms do not persist for more than an additional 6 months.

Specify whether:

- **309.0 (F43.21) With depressed mood:** Low mood, tearfulness, or feelings of hopelessness are predominant.
- **309.24 (F43.22) With anxiety:** Nervousness, worry, jitteriness, or separation anxiety is predominant.
- **309.28 (F43.23) With mixed anxiety and depressed mood:** A combination of depression and anxiety is predominant.
- **309.3 (F43.24) With disturbance of conduct:** Disturbance of conduct is predominant.
- **309.4 (F43.25) With mixed disturbance of emotions and conduct:** Both emotional symptoms (eg, depression, anxiety) and a disturbance of conduct are predominant.
- **309.9 (F43.20) Unspecified:** For maladaptive reactions that are not classifiable as one of the specific subtypes of adjustment disorder.

Specify if:

- **Acute:** If the disturbance lasts less than 6 months.
- **Persistent (chronic):** If the disturbance lasts for 6 months or longer.

(Reprinted with permission from the *Diagnostic and Statistical Manual of Mental Disorders*. 5th ed. Arlington, VA: American Psychiatric Publishing; 2013.)

What is the rationale for the diagnosis?

The patient experiences behavioral symptom (staying in bed) in response to an identifiable stressor ("lack of purpose" because physical therapy ended), which occurred less than 3 months ago. This behavior is clinically significant because it has contributed to significant impairment in his social functioning (he is isolating himself). The stress-related disturbance does not meet the criteria for another mental disorder and is not an exacerbation of a preexisting mental disorder. Although he has a history of being treated for anxiety associated with work stress 6 years ago, his current symptoms do not seem to be associated with that episode. The symptoms are not associated with bereavement. Therefore, the diagnosis of adjustment disorder with depressed mood is applicable.

Which diagnosis (or diagnoses) should be considered?

303.90 (F10.20) Alcohol Use Disorder, in Sustained Remission

Diagnostic Criteria

A. A problematic pattern of alcohol use leading to clinically significant impairment or distress, as manifested by at least two of the following, occurring within a 12-month period:
  1. Alcohol is often taken in larger amounts or over a longer period than was intended.
  2. There is a persistent desire or unsuccessful efforts to cut down or control alcohol use.
  3. A great deal of time is spent in activities necessary to obtain alcohol, use alcohol, or recover from its effects.
  4. Craving, or a strong desire or urge to use alcohol.
  5. Recurrent alcohol use resulting in a failure to fulfill major role obligations at work, school, or home.
  6. Continued alcohol use despite having persistent or recurrent social or interpersonal problems caused or exacerbated by the effects of alcohol.
  7. Important social, occupational, or recreational activities are given up or reduced because of alcohol use.
  8. Recurrent alcohol use in situations in which it is physically hazardous.
  9. Alcohol use is continued despite knowledge of having a persistent or recurrent physical or psychological problem that is likely to have been caused or exacerbated by alcohol.
  10. Tolerance, as defined by either of the following:
      a. A need for markedly increased amounts of alcohol to achieve intoxication or desired effect.
      b. A markedly diminished effect with continued use of the same amount of alcohol.
  11. Withdrawal, as manifested by either of the following:
      a. The characteristic withdrawal syndrome for alcohol (refer to Criteria A and B of the criteria set for alcohol withdrawal).
      b. Alcohol (or a closely related substance, such as a benzodiazepine) is taken to relieve or avoid withdrawal symptoms.

Specify if:

- **In early remission**: After full criteria for alcohol use disorder were previously met, none of the criteria for alcohol use disorder have been met for at least

3 months but for less than 12 months (with the exception that Criterion A4, "Craving, or a strong desire or urge to use alcohol," may be met).
- **In sustained remission**: After full criteria for alcohol use disorder were previously met, none of the criteria for alcohol use disorder have been met at any time during a period of 12 months or longer (with the exception that Criterion A4, "Craving, or a strong desire or urge to use alcohol," may be met).

Specify if:

- **In a controlled environment**: This additional specifier is used if the individual is in an environment where access to alcohol is restricted.

Code based on current severity: Note for *ICD-10-CM* codes: If an alcohol intoxication, alcohol withdrawal, or another alcohol-induced mental disorder is also present, do not use the codes below for alcohol use disorder. Instead, the comorbid alcohol use disorder is indicated in the fourth character of the alcohol-induced disorder code (see the coding note for alcohol intoxication, alcohol withdrawal, or a specific alcohol-induced mental disorder). For example, if there is comorbid alcohol intoxication and alcohol use disorder, only the alcohol intoxication code is given, with the fourth character indicating whether the comorbid alcohol use disorder is mild, moderate, or severe: F10.129 for mild alcohol use disorder with alcohol intoxication or F10.229 for a moderate or severe alcohol use disorder with alcohol intoxication.

Specify current severity:

- **305.00 (F10.10) Mild**: Presence of two to three symptoms.
- **303.90 (F10.20) Moderate**: Presence of four to five symptoms.
- **303.90 (F10.20) Severe**: Presence of six or more symptoms.

(Reprinted with permission from the *Diagnostic and Statistical Manual of Mental Disorders*. 5th ed. Arlington, VA: American Psychiatric Publishing; 2013.)

What is the rationale for the diagnosis?

The patient has a history of problematic pattern of alcohol use that led to clinically significant distress as evidenced by the need for his family to have an "intervention" with subsequent admission to a detoxification and rehabilitation facility, and then referral and participation in AA. The diagnostic specifier, in sustained remission, is indicated as the patient has not met any of the criteria for alcohol use in the past 12 months.

What test or tools should be considered to help identify the correct diagnosis?

Beck Depression Inventory is a 21-question multiple choice self-report inventory for measuring the severity of depression.

What differential diagnosis (or diagnoses) should be considered?

799.59 (R41.9) Unspecified Neurocognitive Disorder

The patient exhibits minor memory deficits (he was not able to recall the previous five presidents accurately). He struggled to identify words beginning with the letter F. Even though he was able to state 12 words, some were duplicates or proper nouns. This level of functioning does not seem consistent with his education and intelligence level. However, it is not clear if his impaired functioning is related to the concentration and memory impairment, which can be associated with depression or if it is related to a neurocognitive disorder. Additional testing and collateral information would be required to clarify if this diagnosis is indicated.

FORMULATING THE TREATMENT STRATEGY

What treatment would you prescribe and what is the rationale?

Psychopharmacology: Sertraline 50 mg PO daily. Although the patient states he is "OK" the information he provides about his level of activity and motivation indicates otherwise. Additionally, his wife seems to be a reliable historian and is concerned about his mood and thinks he is trying to cover up that he is depressed. He was receptive to starting sertraline. The patient responded well to sertraline in the past so we will restart it and titrate the dose as needed.

Diagnostic Tests: Continue to evaluate his cognitive status with the Montreal Cognitive Assessment, which can be accessed at http://www.mocatest.org/

Referrals: Consider a referral to a neurologist for evaluation if mild neurocognitive deficits do not improve with improvement in his mood.

Type of Psychotherapy: Encouraged to continue attending AA. The patient is not interested in any other therapy currently, but may be receptive to individual psychotherapy in the future.

Psychoeducation: Reminded the patient and his wife that there will be a delayed response to selective serotonin reuptake inhibitor medication. In the meantime, was advised to maintain a steady schedule regarding sleep and wake times, and if possible to avoid isolating himself from family and friends.

What standard guidelines would you use to treat or assess this patient?

Qaseem A, Barry MJ, Kansagara D; for the Clinical Guidelines Committee of the American College of Physicians. Nonpharmacologic versus pharmacologic treatment of adult patients with major depressive disorder: a clinical practice guideline from the American College of Physicians. *Ann Intern Med.* 2016;164:350-359. doi:10.7326/M15-2570.

CLINICAL NOTE

- This patient may be at high risk for a relapse with alcohol due to his depressed mood. This possibility should be discussed with him.

REFERENCES/RECOMMENDED READINGS

Fiske A, Wetherell JL, Gatz M. Depression in older adults. *Annu Rev Clin Psychol.* 2009;5:363-389.

Frank C. Pharmacologic treatment of depression in the elderly. *Canad Fam Physician*. 2014;60(2):121-126.

CASE 48

Lithium and the Older Adult

IDENTIFICATION: The patient is a 72-year-old, widowed white female who resides with her son and daughter-in-law since her husband passed away 3 years ago. She is being followed up for medication management in an outpatient psychiatric office.

CHIEF COMPLAINT: "I feel good."

HISTORY OF CHIEF COMPLAINT: The patient is returning for follow-up medication management of her psychotropic medications. Her mood has been euthymic on her current medications: lithium carbonate 300 mg BID, clonazepam 0.5 mg q 12 hours, duloxetine 60 mg daily, and lamotrigine 200 mg daily.

PAST PSYCHIATRIC HISTORY: The patient has a long history of depression, anxiety, and extreme mood lability. The patient reports her first depressed episode occurring 30 years ago when her mother died. She was subsequently hospitalized for 10 days and was prescribed psychotropic medication, but she cannot remember the names of the medications. She reported ongoing depression and anxiety over the years and was tried on various medications, including fluoxetine, escitalopram, and aripiprazole. She was taking duloxetine 120 mg daily, zolpidem 5 mg at bedtime, lorazepam 2 mg in the AM, and quetiapine 25 mg at bedtime when she was initially evaluated by this writer 6 years ago. Because of her report of feeling like she could not sit still and had to keep moving, and her feet being stiff in the night, the quetiapine was discontinued. These symptoms of akathisia, were probably antipsychotic induced. Over the past 6 years, she has been cross-tapered to the current doses of lamotrigine, lithium, clonazepam along with a reduction of duloxetine to 60 mg daily, which all have helped stabilize her mood. There is no history of suicidal attempts or ideation, or assaultive behavior.

MEDICAL HISTORY: No known allergies. The patient fell on the ice in her 20s and hurt her back. She had spinal surgery with rods and pins inserted. She continues to have intermittent back pain. She has a history of breast cancer with chemotherapy and radiation treatment. She has been diagnosed with hypothyroidism and recently with rheumatoid arthritis. Her current medications include methotrexate, folic acid, levothyroxine, simvastatin, and montelukast PRN. Her gait is slow, and she walks with a cane because of an old foot injury. She fell and hit her head a year ago when she tripped on an area rug. She denies any current unsteadiness or dizziness.

She had blood work drawn prior to the current visit and the following results were abnormal:

Increased creatinine = 1.01 mg/dL (0.57 to 1.00)

Low estimated glomerular filtration rate = 55 mL/min/1.73 (>59)

Lithium level was in the high normal range = 1.1 mmol/L (0.6 to 1.4)

The patient's thyroid-stimulating hormone and free thyroxine were in the normal limits.

HISTORY OF DRUG OR ALCOHOL ABUSE: Denied.

FAMILY HISTORY: Both parents are deceased. Her mother had a history of depression and was treated with electroconvulsive therapy. Her sister has depression and is being treated with antidepressants. The patient has two sons, and she lives with one of the sons and her daughter-in-law. The other son is in the military, and he visits the patient infrequently.

PERSONAL HISTORY

Perinatal: No known complications or developmental delays.

Childhood: No learning disabilities. Was able to make friends without difficulty.

Adolescence: Joined school clubs. Graduated from high school.

Adulthood: Met husband in high school. Married and had two sons. Was mainly a homemaker and raised her sons. No military or legal history. Husband passed away 3 years ago, and the patient moved in with her son. Has numerous friends and goes out to lunch with them regularly. Still drives without any problems.

TRAUMA/ABUSE HISTORY: Denied.

MENTAL STATUS EXAMINATION

Appearance: Well groomed. Cooperative.

Behavior and psychomotor activity: No abnormal movement but walks cautiously to avoid any falls. Walks with a cane.

Consciousness:	Alert.
Orientation:	Oriented times three.
Memory:	Able to state name and date and what she had for breakfast and how she spent the recent holiday. Was able to name the last three presidents. She was able to remember three objects after 5 minutes. She was able to compute serial subtractions of 3 from 100.
Concentration and attention:	Attentive.
Visuospatial ability:	Able to draw a clock face accurately.
Abstract thought:	Her ability for abstraction was limited. She could not understand or interpret any proverbs. She asked, "What is a proverb?"
Intellectual functioning:	Average.
Speech and language:	Normal rate and volume.
Perceptions:	No abnormal perceptions elicited.
Thought processes:	Logical.
Thought content:	No unusual content.
Suicidality or homicidality:	Denied.

Mood: "Good."

Affect: Congruent with mood, euthymic.

Impulse control: Good.

Judgment: Good.

Insight: Fair.

Reliability: Good.

FORMULATING THE DIAGNOSIS

Which diagnosis (or diagnoses) should be considered?

296.26 (F32.5) Major Depressive Disorder, in Full Remission

Diagnostic Criteria

A. Five (or more) of the following symptoms have been present during the same 2-week period and represent a change from previous functioning; at least one of the symptoms is either (1) depressed mood or (2) loss of interest or pleasure.
   - Note: Do not include symptoms that are clearly attributable to another medical condition.
     1. Depressed mood most of the day, nearly every day, as indicated by either subjective report (eg, feels sad, empty, hopeless) or observation made by others (eg, appears tearful). (Note: In children and adolescents, can be irritable mood.)
     2. Markedly diminished interest or pleasure in all, or almost all, activities most of the day, nearly every day (as indicated by either subjective account or observation).
     3. Significant weight loss when not dieting or weight gain (eg, a change of more than 5% of body weight in a month), or decrease or increase in appetite nearly every day. (Note: In children, consider failure to make expected weight gain.)
     4. Insomnia or hypersomnia nearly every day.
     5. Psychomotor agitation or retardation nearly every day (observable by others, not merely subjective feelings of restlessness or being slowed down).
     6. Fatigue or loss of energy nearly every day.
     7. Feelings of worthlessness or excessive or inappropriate guilt (which may be delusional) nearly every day (not merely self-reproach or guilt about being sick).

8. Diminished ability to think or concentrate, or indecisiveness, nearly every day (either by subjective account or as observed by others).
9. Recurrent thoughts of death (not just fear of dying), recurrent suicidal ideation without a specific plan, or a suicide attempt or a specific plan for committing suicide.

B. The symptoms cause clinically significant distress or impairment in social, occupational, or other important areas of functioning.
C. The episode is not attributable to the physiologic effects of a substance or another medical condition.

Note: Criteria A to C represent a major depressive episode (MDE).

Note: Responses to a significant loss (eg, bereavement, financial ruin, losses from a natural disaster, a serious medical illness or disability) may include the feelings of intense sadness, rumination about the loss, insomnia, poor appetite, and weight loss noted in Criterion A, which may resemble a depressive episode. Although such symptoms may be understandable or considered appropriate to the loss, the presence of an MDE in addition to the normal response to a significant loss should also be carefully considered. This decision inevitably requires the exercise of clinical judgment based on the individual's history and the cultural norms for the expression of distress in the context of loss.

In distinguishing grief from an MDE, it is useful to consider that in grief the predominant affect is feelings of emptiness and loss, whereas in an MDE it is persistent depressed mood and the inability to anticipate happiness or pleasure. The dysphoria in grief is likely to decrease in intensity over days to weeks and occurs in waves, the so-called pangs of grief. These waves tend to be associated with thoughts or reminders of the deceased. The depressed mood of an MDE is more persistent and not tied to specific thoughts or preoccupations. The pain of grief may be accompanied by positive emotions and humor that are uncharacteristic of the pervasive unhappiness and misery characteristic of an MDE. The thought content associated with grief generally features a preoccupation with thoughts and memories of the deceased, rather than the self-critical or pessimistic ruminations seen in an MDE. In grief, self-esteem is generally preserved, whereas in an MDE feelings of worthlessness and self-loathing are common. If self-derogatory ideation is present in grief, it typically involves perceived failings vis-à-vis the deceased (eg, not visiting frequently enough, not telling the deceased how much he or she was loved). If a bereaved individual thinks about death and dying, such thoughts are generally focused on the deceased and possibly about "joining" the deceased, whereas in an MDE such thoughts are focused on ending one's own life because of feeling worthless, undeserving of life, or unable to cope with the pain of depression.

D. The occurrence of the MDE is not better explained by schizoaffective disorder, schizophrenia, schizophreniform disorder, delusional disorder, or other specified and unspecified schizophrenia spectrum and other psychotic disorders.

E. There has never been a manic episode or a hypomanic episode.
   - **Note:** This exclusion does not apply if all of the manic-like or hypomanic-like episodes are substance-induced or are attributable to the physiologic effects of another medical condition.

(Reprinted with permission from the *Diagnostic and Statistical Manual of Mental Disorders*. 5th ed. Arlington, VA: American Psychiatric Publishing; 2013.)

What is the rationale for the diagnosis?

The patient previously met the full criteria for major depressive disorder. At the time, she was originally evaluated by this writer, she was extremely depressed, and she cried profusely. She was unable to enjoy activities, she had insomnia, and she expressed feelings of guilt. She ruminated about past events, and she was unable to make decisions without checking with her husband or son. Those depressive symptoms have dissipated. She has been asymptomatic for the past year; therefore, she is considered in full remission.

What test or tools should be considered to help identify the correct diagnosis?

Hamilton Depression Inventory.

What differential diagnosis (or diagnoses) should be considered?

None indicated.

FORMULATING THE TREATMENT STRATEGY

What treatment would you prescribe and what is the rationale?

Psychopharmacology: Reduce the lithium to 450 mg daily. Because the patient is 72 years old, her renal function may be decreasing and she may be more likely to develop toxic levels of lithium. Although the dose has remained the same, her lithium concentration has increased since the last lithium level test 6 months ago. Additional reduction in the dose of lithium should be attempted in collaboration with the patient's primary care provider.

Continue duloxetine 60 mg daily.

Continue clonazepam 0.5 mg q 12 hours.

Continue lamotrigine 200 mg daily.

Diagnostic Tests: Continue monitoring the renal function, thyroid function and lithium level. Evaluate liver function tests since the duloxetine may contribute to hepatotoxicity.

Consultation: Primary care provider contacted regarding abnormal renal function.

Referrals: Referred to her primary care provider for a review of her abnormal renal lab results.

Type of Psychotherapy: None indicated.

Psychoeducation: Provide the patient with information about the risks of renal and thyroid impairment associated with lithium. A fact sheet about lithium can be accessed at:

http://www.namihelps.org/assets/PDFs/fact-sheets/Medications/Lithium.pdf.

Provide the patient with information about the risks versus benefits of clonazepam. Advise that there may be an increased risk for falls. In this case, the patient does not want to change her medication but agreed to pay attention where she walks and to avoid area rugs, etc.

More information about clonazepam can be found at:

https://www.nami.org/Learn-More/Treatment/Mental-Health-Medications/Clonazepam-(Klonopin).

What standard guidelines would you use to treat or assess this patient?

https://www.guideline.gov/summaries/summary/24158/Practice-guideline-for-the-treatment-of-patients-with-major-depressive-disorder-third-edition

CLINICAL NOTE

- Although this patient is diagnosed with a major depressive disorder, she responded to medications that would typically be prescribed for treatment of bipolar disorder (lamotrigine and lithium). However, she never presented with any hypomanic or manic episodes or any mood cycling. Her predominant outstanding symptoms were depressed mood and mood lability, which mainly was evidenced by crying easily and frequently. She never met the criteria for any bipolar spectrum diagnosis. There are considerable data supporting the use of lithium in treatment-resistant depression, which this patient had.
- Risk-benefit analysis requires that the patient be informed accurately in layman's terms about the risks associated with prescribed medications. When prescribing lithium, kidney and thyroid function must be monitored on a regular basis due to the drug's potential for toxicity. Some consumer organizations provide fact sheets to explain the risks involved and may be helpful in this respect (see Appendix).

- Individuals 60 years and older are at greater risk for drug-induced nephrotoxicity. Alternative drugs that are non-nephrotoxic should be substituted whenever possible.
- Methotrexate may increase potential for depression and suicidal ideation. Since this patient's depressive symptoms predate her use of methotrexate it may not be a contributing factor in this case. However, this should be considered in cases when patients taking methotrexate present with depressive symptoms.

REFERENCES/RECOMMENDED READINGS

The Carlat Psychiatry Report. LITHIUM Fact Sheet. 2007. http://www.mainlinefamily.com/wp-content/uploads/2012/08/Lithium_Fact_Sheet.pdf

Connolly MT, Ryan K. Unipolar depression in adults: treatment of resistant depression. *UpToDate*. Philadelphia, PA: Wolters Kluwer; 2016.

PL Detail-Document, Potentially Harmful Drugs in the Elderly: Beers List. Pharmacist's Letter/Prescriber's Letter; June 2012.

Sadock BJ, Sadock V, Sussman N. *Kaplan & Sadock's Pocket Handbook of Psychiatric Drug Treatment*. 6th ed. Philadelphia, PA: Wolters Kluwer; 2013.

Sproule BA, Hardy BG, Shulman KI. Differential pharmacokinetics of lithium in elderly patients. *Drugs Aging*. 2000;16(3):165-177.

CASE 48 APPENDIX

Lithium: AHFS Patient Medication Information

PRONUNCIATION

"lith' ee um"

IMPORTANT WARNING

Keep all appointments with your doctor and the laboratory. Your doctor will order certain lab tests to check your response to lithium.

WHY IS THIS MEDICATION PRESCRIBED?

Lithium is used to treat and prevent episodes of mania (frenzied, abnormally excited mood) in people with bipolar disorder (manic-depressive disorder, a disease that causes episodes of depression, episodes of mania, and other abnormal moods). Lithium is in a class of medications called antimanic agents. It works by decreasing abnormal activity in the brain.

HOW SHOULD THIS MEDICINE BE USED?

Lithium comes as a tablet, capsule, extended-release (long-acting) tablet, and solution (liquid) to take by mouth. The tablets, capsules, and solution are usually taken three to four times a day. The extended-release tablets are usually taken two to three times a day. Take lithium at around the same times every day. Follow the directions on your prescription label carefully, and ask your doctor or pharmacist to explain any part you do not understand. Take lithium exactly as directed. Do not take more or less of it or take it more often than prescribed by your doctor.

Swallow the extended-release tablet whole; do not split, chew, or crush it.

Your doctor may increase or decrease the dose of your medication during your treatment. Follow these directions carefully.

Lithium may help to control your condition but will not cure it. It may take 1 to 3 weeks or longer for you to feel the full benefit of lithium. Continue to take lithium even if you feel well. Do not stop taking lithium without talking to your doctor.

OTHER USES FOR THIS MEDICINE

Lithium is also sometimes used to treat depression, schizophrenia (a mental illness that causes disturbed or unusual thinking, loss of interest in life, and strong or inappropriate emotions), disorders of impulse control (inability to resist the urge to perform a harmful action), and certain mental illnesses in children. Talk to your doctor about the risks of using this medication for your condition.

This medication may be prescribed for other uses; ask your doctor or pharmacist for more information.

WHAT SPECIAL PRECAUTIONS SHOULD I FOLLOW?

Before taking lithium

- Tell your doctor and pharmacist if you are allergic to lithium or any other medications.
- Tell your doctor if you are taking diuretics ("water pills"). Your doctor may tell you not to take lithium if you are taking this medication or will monitor you carefully for side effects.
- Tell your doctor and pharmacist what prescription and nonprescription medications, vitamins, nutritional supplements, and herbal products you are taking or plan to take. Be sure to mention any of the following: acetazolamide (Diamox); aminophylline; angiotensin-converting enzyme inhibitors such as benazepril (Lotensin), captopril (Capoten), enalapril (Vasotec), fosinopril, lisinopril (Prinivil, Zestril), moexipril (Univasc), perindopril (Aceon), quinapril (Accupril), ramipril (Altace), and trandolapril (Mavik); angiotensin II receptor antagonists such as candesartan (Atacand), eprosartan (Teveten), irbesartan (Avapro), losartan (Cozaar), olmesartan (Benicar), telmisartan (Micardis); and valsartan (Diovan); antacids such as sodium bicarbonate; caffeine (found in certain medications to treat drowsiness and headaches); calcium channel blockers such as amlodipine (Norvasc), diltiazem (Cardizem, Dilacor, Tiazac, others), felodipine (Plendil), isradipine (DynaCirc), nicardipine (Cardene), nifedipine (Adalat, Procardia), nimodipine (Nymalize), nisoldipine (Sular), and verapamil (Calan, Covera, Verelan); carbamazepine (Tegretol); medications for mental illness

such as haloperidol (Haldol); methyldopa (Aldomet); metronidazole (Flagyl); nonsteroidal anti-inflammatory drugs such as celecoxib (Celebrex), indomethacin (Indocin), and piroxicam (Feldene); potassium iodide; selective serotonin reuptake inhibitors such as citalopram (Celexa), duloxetine (Cymbalta), escitalopram (Lexapro), fluoxetine (Prozac, Sarafem), fluvoxamine (Luvox), paroxetine (Paxil), and sertraline (Zoloft); and theophylline (Theolair, Theochron). Your doctor may have to change the doses of your medication or monitor you more carefully for side effects.

- Tell your doctor if you have or have ever had heart or kidney disease. Also tell your doctor if you have or develop severe diarrhea, excessive sweating, or fever during your treatment. Your doctor may tell you not to take lithium or may monitor you more carefully for side effects.
- Tell your doctor if you have or have ever had organic brain syndrome (any physical condition that affects the way your brain works) or thyroid disease or if you have ever fainted without an explanation. Also tell your doctor if you or anyone in your family have or have ever had Brugada syndrome (a disorder that can cause a potentially fatal irregular heart rhythm) or if anyone in your family has died suddenly with no explanation before the age of 45 years.
- Tell your doctor if you are pregnant, plan to become pregnant, or are breast-feeding. If you become pregnant while taking lithium, call your doctor. Lithium may harm the fetus.
- If you are having surgery, including dental surgery, tell the doctor or dentist that you are taking lithium.
- You should know that this medication may make you drowsy. Do not drive a car or operate machinery until you know how this medication affects you.

WHAT SPECIAL DIETARY INSTRUCTIONS SHOULD I FOLLOW?

It is important to follow a proper diet, including the right amounts of fluid and salt during your treatment. Your doctor will give you specific directions about the diet that is right for you. Follow these directions carefully.

Talk to your doctor about drinks that contain caffeine, such as tea, coffee, cola, or chocolate milk.

WHAT SHOULD I DO IF I FORGET A DOSE?

Take the missed dose as soon as you remember it. However, if it is almost time for the next dose, skip the missed dose and continue your regular dosing schedule. Do not take a double dose to make up for a missed one.

WHAT SIDE EFFECTS CAN THIS MEDICATION CAUSE?

Lithium may cause side effects. Tell your doctor if any of these symptoms are severe or do not go away:

- restlessness
- fine hand movements that are difficult to control
- mild thirst
- loss of appetite
- stomach pain
- gas
- indigestion
- weight gain or loss
- dry mouth
- excessive saliva in the mouth
- change in the ability to taste food
- swollen lips
- acne
- hair loss
- unusual discomfort in cold temperatures
- constipation
- depression
- joint or muscle pain
- paleness
- thin, brittle fingernails or hair
- itching
- rash

Some side effects may be serious. If you experience any of the following symptoms, call your doctor immediately or get emergency medical help:

- unusual tiredness or weakness
- excessive thirst
- frequent urination
- slow, jerky movements
- movements that are unusual or difficult to control
- blackouts
- seizures
- fainting
- dizziness or light-headedness
- fast, slow, irregular, or pounding heartbeat
- shortness of breath
- chest tightness
- confusion
- hallucinations (seeing things or hearing voices that do not exist)

- crossed eyes
- painful, cold, or discolored fingers and toes
- headache
- pounding noises inside the head
- swelling of the feet, ankles, or lower legs

If you experience any of the following symptoms, stop taking lithium and call your doctor immediately:

- drowsiness
- shaking of a part of your body that you cannot control
- muscle weakness, stiffness, twitching, or tightness
- loss of coordination
- diarrhea
- vomiting
- slurred speech
- giddiness
- ringing in the ears
- blurred vision

Lithium may cause other side effects. Call your doctor if you experience any unusual symptoms while you are taking this medication.

If you experience a serious side effect, you or your doctor may send a report to the Food and Drug Administration's (FDA) MedWatch Adverse Event Reporting program online (http://www.fda.gov/Safety/MedWatch) or by phone (1-800-332-1088).

WHAT SHOULD I KNOW ABOUT STORAGE AND DISPOSAL OF THIS MEDICATION?

Keep this medication in the container it came in, tightly closed, and out of reach of children. Store it at room temperature and away from excess heat and moisture (not in the bathroom).

Unneeded medications should be disposed of in special ways to ensure that pets, children, and other people cannot consume them. However, you should not flush this medication down the toilet. Instead, the best way to dispose of your medication is through a medicine take-back program. Talk to your pharmacist or contact your local garbage/recycling department to learn about take-back programs in your community. See the FDA's Safe Disposal of Medicines website (http://goo.gl/c4Rm4p) for more information if you do not have access to a take-back program.

In case of emergency/overdose

In case of overdose, call your local poison control center at 1-800-222-1222. If the victim has collapsed or is not breathing, call local emergency services at 911.

Symptoms of overdose may include the following:

- diarrhea
- vomiting
- drowsiness
- muscle weakness
- loss of coordination
- giddiness
- blurred vision
- ringing in the ears
- frequent urination

WHAT OTHER INFORMATION SHOULD I KNOW?

Do not let anyone else take your medication. Ask your pharmacist any questions you have about refilling your prescription.

It is important for you to keep a written list of all of the prescription and nonprescription (over-the-counter) medicines you are taking, as well as any products such as vitamins, minerals, or other dietary supplements. You should bring this list with you each time you visit a doctor or if you are admitted to a hospital. It is also important information to carry with you in case of emergencies.

BRAND NAMES

- Eskalith and Eskalith CR brands are no longer on the market; generic alternatives may be available
- Lithobid

CASE 49

Worried about Father Dying

IDENTIFICATION: The patient is a 75-year-old, married, Caucasian female who is the mother of two adult children and grandmother of seven grandchildren, all of whom are very close. The patient is self-referred to a private psychiatric outpatient office and is seeking therapy and medication management.

CHIEF COMPLAINT: "I need help with my medication and managing depression and anxiety, which I've had on and off since high school."

HISTORY OF CHIEF COMPLAINT: The patient reports that her father is dying, and she has been experiencing worsening of depression and anxiety symptoms over the past few months. She is seeking a psychiatric evaluation at her daughter's urging. The patient does not enjoy being with her family, not even her grandchildren. She has difficulty falling asleep, but then spends the day lying on the sofa and reports feeling like she is "moving through molasses." She reports feeling tired all the time. She has also stopped going to her volunteer job at her church. She is not reading as often she used to.

She responded to the practitioner's question of "why depressed now?" by saying that with the imminent death of her beloved father, she is losing her chief ally and support.

In addition to her father's illness, the patient was diagnosed and treated for colon cancer in the past year. She received psychotherapy at that time which focused on her anxiety about the diagnosis, her denial of its severity, her wish to "not know what she knew," and, ultimately, end-of-life issues.

PAST PSYCHIATRIC HISTORY: The patient was never hospitalized for psychiatric reasons. She has no history of suicidal thoughts, gestures, or attempts.

The patient described either a partial or negative response from several medications she had been prescribed from her primary care physician (PCP) over the course of a several years, including duloxetine fluoxetine, paroxetine, venlafaxine, mirtazapine, bupropion, and escitalopram.

She is currently prescribed clonazepam 2 mg TID by her PCP which she has been taking for several years.

MEDICAL HISTORY: Patient has a history of cardiac arrhythmias, irritable bowel syndrome, gastroesophageal reflux disorder, and a recent diagnosis of metastatic colon cancer.

Patient denies being sexually active with her husband.

HISTORY OF DRUG OR ALCOHOL ABUSE: The patient denies history of drug and alcohol abuse. She reports that she had been prescribed clonazepam 2 mg TID by her PCP and has tried repeatedly to decrease the amount unsuccessfully.

FAMILY PSYCHIATRIC HISTORY: Patient reports that her mother had "excessive" cleaning compulsions and expressed many fears about contamination and safety. The patient describes her father as "riddled with anxiety and depression," but neither parent sought treatment for any emotional disturbances. She is an only child and does not recall any emotional difficulties in grandparents or other relatives.

PERSONAL HISTORY

Perinatal: No known perinatal complications.

Childhood: Was a good student. The patient did not develop confidence managing age-appropriate activities, such as picking out her clothing and fixing her own hair because her mother dominated these activities.

Adolescence: The patient's mother dressed her, washed and braided her hair until she was a sophomore in high school, and repeatedly told her that she would never be able to live on her own. Did well academically. Identifies as heterosexual.

Adulthood: The patient's mother discouraged her from taking a job out of state that she was looking forward to. She believes her anxiety and depression began at that time. Besides her mother dissuading her from pursuing her career, she encouraged her to "marry her high school sweetheart and be a stay-at-home mother." Although the patient loved being a mother, the patient reports that her marriage has been a source of anxiety from the very beginning, describing her husband as verbally abusive and a "bully." The patient's mother discouraged her from taking a job out of state that she was looking forward to. She believes her anxiety and depression began at that time. The patient has been married for almost 50 years. She reports that she is very close to her children, her grandchildren, and her five sisters-in-law. The patient has worked in the local rectory and church for the past 25 years and is close to the parish priests as well as to her coworkers at the church.

TRAUMA/ABUSE HISTORY: The patient reports that while she was never physically abused, she felt controlled by her mother's dominance and was verbally and psychologically abused by both her mother and her husband for many years.

MENTAL STATUS EXAMINATION

Appearance: Well-groomed, appropriately dressed, older woman who is slight in stature and of average weight.

Behavior and psychomotor activity: Good eye contact, pleasant, cooperative. Slightly unsteady gait. Patient demonstrated multiple bruises on her arms and legs secondary to ataxia and subsequent falls.

Consciousness:	Alert and able to answer all questions appropriately.
Orientation:	Oriented to person, place, time, and situation.
Memory:	Intact. Good recent and remote memory.
Concentration and attention:	Appears to have good concentration during the interview but reports that she has recently had trouble concentrating while reading.
Visuospatial ability:	Not formally assessed.
Abstract thought:	Within normal limits, appropriate use of metaphors.
Intellectual functioning:	Patient has high school education and some college but demonstrates higher intelligence based on her curiosity, choice of reading material.

Speech and language: Normal rate and rhythm.

Perceptions: No abnormalities present.

Thought processes: Goal directed, but evidence of guilt and rumination consistent with depressive symptomatology.

Thought content: Patient is highly anxious and expresses thoughts of sadness, frustration. She is preoccupied with thoughts about the anticipated loss of her father.

Mood: Depressed and anxious.

Affect: Congruent with mood.

Impulse control: Good.

Judgment/insight/reliability: Good.

FORMULATING THE DIAGNOSIS

Which diagnosis should be considered?

296.32 (F33.1) Major Depressive Disorder, Moderate, with Anxious Distress

Diagnostic Criteria

A. Five (or more) of the following symptoms have been present during the same 2-week period and represent a change from previous functioning; at least one of the symptoms is either (1) depressed mood or (2) loss of interest or pleasure.

Note: Do not include symptoms that are clearly attributable to another medical condition.

1. Depressed mood most of the day, nearly every day, as indicated by either subjective report (eg, feels sad, empty, hopeless) or observation made by others (eg, appears tearful). (Note: in children and adolescents, can be irritable mood.)
2. Markedly diminished interest or pleasure in all, or almost all, activities most of the day, nearly every day (as indicated by either subjective account or observation).

3. Significant weight loss when not dieting or weight gain (eg, a change of more than 5% of body weight in a month), or decrease or increase in appetite nearly every day. (Note: In children, consider failure to make expected weight gain.)
4. Insomnia or hypersomnia nearly every day.
5. Psychomotor agitation or retardation nearly every day (observable by others, not merely subjective feelings of restlessness or being slowed down).
6. Fatigue or loss of energy nearly every day.
7. Feelings of worthlessness or excessive or inappropriate guilt (which may be delusional) nearly every day (not merely self-reproach or guilt about being sick).
8. Diminished ability to think or concentrate, or indecisiveness, nearly every day (either by subjective account or as observed by others).
9. Recurrent thoughts of death (not just fear of dying), recurrent suicidal ideation without a specific plan, or a suicide attempt or a specific plan for committing suicide.

B. The symptoms cause clinically significant distress or impairment in social, occupational, or other important areas of functioning.
C. Episode is not attributable to the physiologic effects of a substance or to another medical condition.

Note: Criteria A to C represent a major depressive episode.

Note: Responses to a significant loss (eg, bereavement, financial ruin, losses from a natural disaster, a serious medical condition, or disability) may include the feelings of intense sadness, rumination about the loss, insomnia, poor appetite, and weight loss noted in Criterion A, which may resemble a depressive episode. Although such symptoms may be understandable or considered appropriate to the loss, the presence of a major depressive episode in addition to the normal response to a significant loss should also be carefully considered. This decision inevitably requires the exercise of clinical judgment based on the individual's history and the cultural norms for the expression of distress in the context of loss.

D. The occurrence of the major depressive episode is not better explained by schizoaffective disorder, schizophrenia, schizophreniform disorder, delusional disorder, or other specified and unspecified schizophrenia spectrum and other psychotic disorders.
E. There has never been a manic episode or a hypomanic episode.

Note: This exclusion does not apply if all of the manic-like or hypomanic-like episodes are substance-induced or are attributable to the physiologic effects of another medical condition.

CODING AND RECORDING PROCEDURES

The diagnostic code for major depressive disorder is based on whether this is a single or recurrent episode, current severity, presence of psychotic features, and remission status. Current severity and psychotic features are only indicated if full criteria are currently met for a major depressive episode. Remission specifiers are only indicated if the full criteria are not currently met for a major depressive episode (Mild, Moderate, Severe, in Partial Remission, in Full Remission, Unspecified).

Specify:

With anxious distress
With mixed features
With melancholic features
With atypical features
With mood-congruent psychotic features
With mood-incongruent psychotic features
With catatonia
With peripartum onset
With seasonal pattern

(Reprinted with permission from the *Diagnostic and Statistical Manual of Mental Disorders*. 5th ed. Arlington, VA: American Psychiatric Publishing; 2013.)

What is your rationale for the diagnosis?

The patient describes a pattern of persistent symptoms of depressed mood, a marked inability to enjoy events (dinners with her family) and people (her grandchildren), insomnia, psychomotor retardation (spending many hours on the couch and reports of feeling like she is "moving through molasses"), fatigue and decreased energy (has stopped going to her volunteer job at her church), and diminished ability to concentrate (inability to read novels, which she had previously been able to do). These symptoms represent at least five of the criteria for the diagnosis of major depressive disorder and they have occurred for most days over a period of several months.

The symptoms cause clinically significant impairment in social, occupational, or other important areas of functioning. (She has stopped going to her volunteer job at her church.)

Her symptoms are not attributable to the effects of a substance or other medical condition, and are not better explained by other disorder, and she has never had a manic or hypomanic episode.

She describes symptoms of anxiety. Therefore, a diagnosis of major depressive disorder, moderate, with anxious distress is indicated.

What tests or tools should be considered to help identify the correct diagnosis?

The Hamilton Depression Rating Scale to determine severity of depression.

What differential diagnosis should be considered?

293.83 (F06.32) Depressive Disorder due to Another Medical Condition, with Major Depressive-Like Episode

The patient has multiple medical comorbidities that could be etiologically associated with her depressive symptoms. However, there is no clear temporal association between the onset, exacerbation of her medical conditions, and her mood disturbance. Therefore, depressive disorder due to another medical condition, with major depressive-like episode should be considered as a differential.

292.82 (F13.24) Substance/Medication-Induced Depressive Disorder

The patient has a prominent and persistent depressed mood. She is currently taking clonazepam, which may contribute to depressive symptoms. However, the disturbance is better explained by psychosocial factors that have become more prominent (father dying). Therefore, the diagnosis of substance/medication-induced depressive disorder would not be applicable.

FORMULATING THE TREATMENT STRATEGY

What treatment would you prescribe and what is the rationale?

Safety: An assessment of the patient's fall risk should be completed. See Appendix for the CDC algorithm. Depending on the severity of the unsteady gait, hospitalization should be considered to fully evaluate the etiology and treat accordingly. If a benzodiazepine taper is indicated, inpatient detox treatment may be required.

Psychopharmacology: Start sertraline 50 mg QD. Sertraline is FDA approved for the treatment of major depressive disorder. Start with divided doses to improve tolerability and increase gradually until symptom remission.

Reduce clonazepam by 0.5 mg every 2 weeks until 1 mg per day is reached. Then decrease by 0.25 mg per week. Clonazepam has the potential to contribute to the patient's ataxia and recent history of falls. When tapering benzodiazepines, it is generally recommended to use a benzodiazepine which has a longer half-life, such as clonazepam with a half-life of 20-50 hours.

If there is no satisfactory response to the sertraline in 4 to 6 weeks, the dose should be increased to the maximum level as long as there are no adverse effects. If symptom remission is not achieved with an adequate trial of sertraline, other options for treatment-resistant depression exist. In general, options for treatment-resistant depression include augmentation with a second generation antipsychotic, lithium, or liothyronine. Another option is to switch treatment to a different antidepressant, transcranial electromagnetic stimulation, electroconvulsive therapy, or ketamine therapy. Treatment with an off-label option could also include lamotrigine.

Diagnostic Tests: Test B/P sitting and standing to evaluate for possible orthostatic hypotension that may be contributing to her falls.

Urine for drug screening.

Obtain results from her other treating providers and review with the patient.

Consultations: Contact patient's medical providers to collaborate regarding treatment.

Referrals: Refer to a medical provider for a history and physical to evaluate the etiology of the falls. May require a neurologic referral.

Psychotherapy: Treatment recommendation included weekly psychodynamic psychotherapy, which has been shown to be as effective as cognitive behavior therapy for the treatment of major depressive disorder.

Psychoeducation: The patient should be educated that it may take several weeks for sertraline to improve her mood. Fall prevention strategies should be reviewed with the patient. The "Stay Independent" brochure from the CDC can be accessed at: https://www.cdc.gov/steadi/pdf/stay_independent_brochure-a.pdf

What standard guidelines would you use to treat or assess this patient?

"Practice Guideline for the Treatment of Major Depressive Disorder," which is available through: American Psychiatric Association (2010) Practice Guidelines and retrievable on-line at

https://psychiatryonline.org/pb/assets/raw/sitewide/practice_guidelines/guidelines/mdd.pdf.

CLINICAL NOTE

- Depression should not be considered a normal part of the aging process. Depression in the older adult may be underdiagnosed and undertreated.

If depression is evident, a thorough evaluation should be conducted. Neurocognitive functioning should be evaluated to identify dementia-related depressive symptoms.

REFERENCES AND RECOMMENDED READINGS

American Psychiatric Association. *Diagnostic and Statistical Manual for Mental Disorder, DSM 5*. 5th ed. Arlington, VA: American Psychiatric Publishing; 2013.

American Psychiatric Association. *APA Practice Guidelines for the Psychiatric Evaluation of Adults*. 3rd ed. Arlington, VA: American Psychiatric Publishing; 2016.

Calabrese JR, Shelton MD, Rapport DJ, et al. Long-term treatment of bipolar disorder with lamotrigine. *J Clin Psychiatr*. 2002;63(Supp 10):18-22.

Gwande A. *Being Mortal: Medicine and What Matters in the End*. New York, NY: Metropolitan Books, Henry Holt and Company; 2014.

Kalinithi P. *When Breath Becomes Air*. New York, NY: Random House; 2016.

Lydiard RB. Irritable bowel syndrome, anxiety, and depression: what are the links? *J Clin Psychiatr*. 2001;62(suppl 8):38-45.

Parker GB, Graham RK. Determinants of treatment-resistant depression: the salience of benzodiazepines. *J Nervous Mental Dis*. 2015;203(9):659-663.

Sadock BJ, Sadock VA, Ruiz P. *Kaplan & Sadock's Synopsis of Psychiatry: Behavioral Sciences/ Clinical Psychiatry*. 11th ed. In Chapter 34.2 *Palliative Care*. Philadelphia, PA: Lippincott, Williams & Wilkins; 2014:1359–1369

Shah D, Borresen D. Benzodiazepines: a guide to safe prescribing. *The Carlat Report Psychiatry*. 2017. http://thecarlatreport.com/free_articles/benzodiazepines-guide-safe-prescribing

Shedler J. The efficacy of psychodynamic psychotherapy. *Am Psychol*. 2010;February-March:98-109.

Solmi M, Veronese N, Zaninotto L, et al. Lamotrigine compared to placebo and other agents with antidepressant activity in patients with unipolar and bipolar depression: a comprehensive meta-analysis of efficacy and safety outcomes in short-term trials. *CNS Spectrums*. 2016;21(5):403-418.

Voshaar RCO, Couvée JE, Van Balkom AJLM, Mulder PGH, Zitman FG. Strategies for discontinuing long-term benzodiazepine use. *Meta-analysis*. 2006;189(3):213-220. doi:10.1192/bjp.189.3.213.

CASE 49 APPENDIX

Fall Risk Assessment and Interventions

Algorithm for Fall Risk Assessment and Interventions

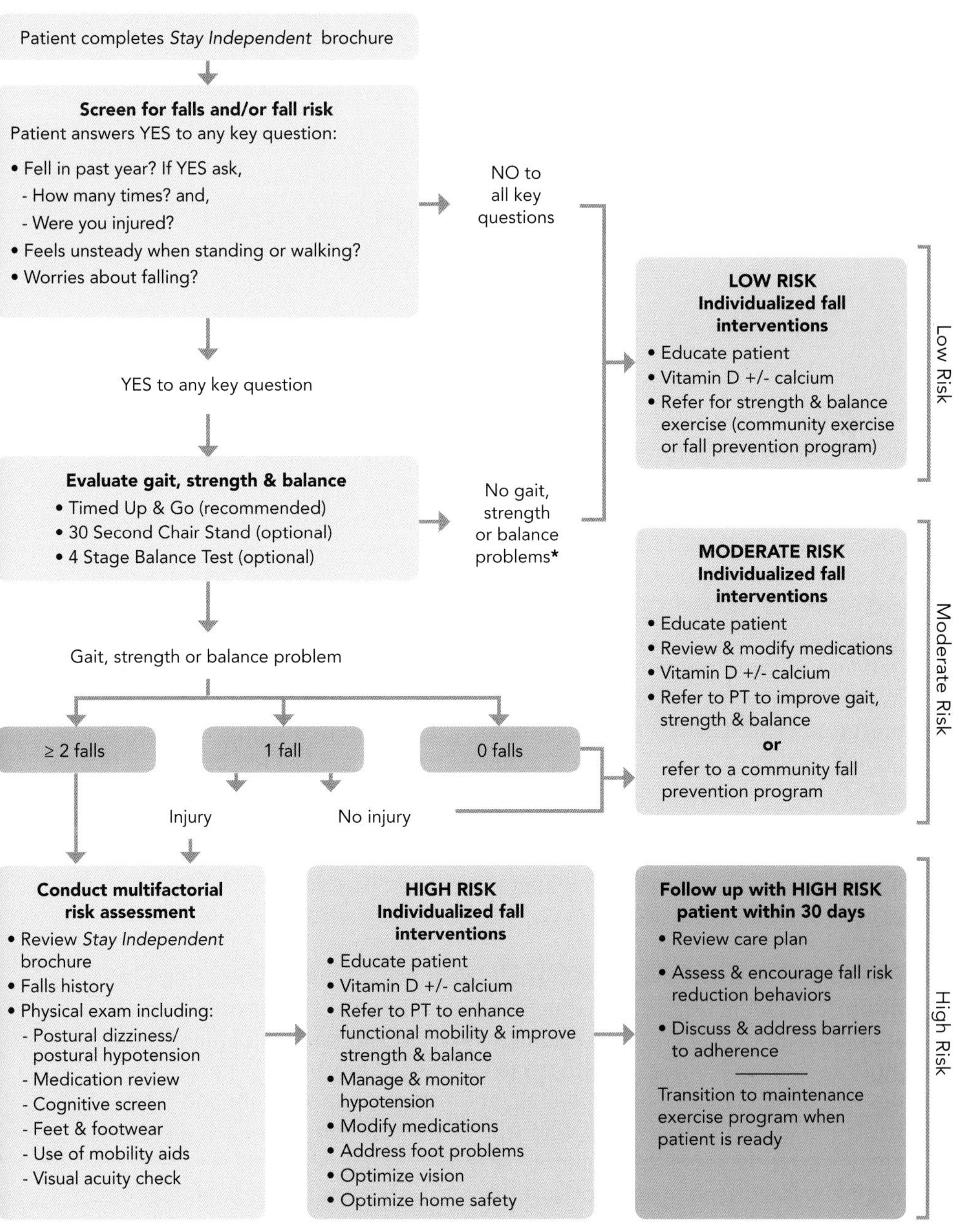

Patient completes *Stay Independent* brochure
Screen for falls and/or fall risk
Patient answers YES to any key question:
• Fell in past year? If YES ask,
- How many times? and,
- Were you injured?
• Feels unsteady when standing or walking?
• Worries about falling?
NO to all key questions
YES to any key question
Evaluate gait, strength & balance
• Timed Up & Go (recommended)
• 30 Second Chair Stand (optional)
• 4 Stage Balance Test (optional)
No gait, strength or balance problems*
Gait, strength or balance problem
≥ 2 falls
1 fall
0 falls
Injury
No injury
LOW RISK Individualized fall interventions
• Educate patient
• Vitamin D +/- calcium
• Refer for strength & balance exercise (community exercise or fall prevention program)
Low Risk
MODERATE RISK Individualized fall interventions
• Educate patient
• Review & modify medications
• Vitamin D +/- calcium
• Refer to PT to improve gait, strength & balance
or
refer to a community fall prevention program
Moderate Risk
Conduct multifactorial risk assessment
• Review *Stay Independent* brochure
• Falls history
• Physical exam including:
- Postural dizziness/ postural hypotension
- Medication review
- Cognitive screen
- Feet & footwear
- Use of mobility aids
- Visual acuity check
HIGH RISK Individualized fall interventions
• Educate patient
• Vitamin D +/- calcium
• Refer to PT to enhance functional mobility & improve strength & balance
• Manage & monitor hypotension
• Modify medications
• Address foot problems
• Optimize vision
• Optimize home safety
Follow up with HIGH RISK patient within 30 days
• Review care plan
• Assess & encourage fall risk reduction behaviors
• Discuss & address barriers to adherence
Transition to maintenance exercise program when patient is ready
High Risk

*For these patients, consider additional risk assessment (eg, medication review, cognitive screen, syncope)

eprinted from the Centers for Disease Control, National Center for Injury Prevention and Control, with permission.

CASE 50

Older and Depressed

IDENTIFICATION: The patient is a 76-year-old single white female accompanied to the interview by her caseworker. The patient is seen for evaluation at an outpatient mental health clinic.

CHIEF COMPLAINT: "I miss my sister."

HISTORY OF CHIEF COMPLAINT: The patient's twin sister moved into a residential facility from the apartment they used to share 2 months ago. The patient has had limited opportunity to visit her. The patient plans to move to the same facility and is waiting for the arrangements to be made. In the meantime, she has not been sleeping well, is crying frequently, and her appetite has decreased. She cannot remember when she last ate or drank. Her sister used to do the shopping and the cooking. Although the patient wears adult diapers, the diaper is dry. She reports that she typically has urinary incontinence and has to change the diaper 2 to 3 times a day; however, she has not needed to change the diaper yet today. She complains of abdominal pain.

PAST PSYCHIATRIC HISTORY: The patient has a long history of bipolar disorder since her teens. She was first hospitalized at the age of 55 due to symptoms of depression. She had three subsequent hospitalizations mainly attributed to nonadherence to her medications. After her last hospitalization, she attended a partial hospitalization outpatient program and then was treated in an outpatient clinic. She was diagnosed with bipolar II disorder and is currently prescribed valproic acid ER 250 mg daily and sertraline 100 mg daily. Her psychiatric records show a Mini-Mental Status Examination completed 3 years ago with a score of 30/30. She reported that until her sister moved to the residential facility recently, her mood had been stable and she had not been depressed.

MEDICAL HISTORY: No known allergies. History of uterine cancer with subsequent hysterectomy and radiation treatment 15 years prior. Has chronic urinary incontinence and irritable bowel syndrome. Has had surgical treatment for the urinary incontinence but it persists.

The patient has considerable kyphosis. History of osteoporosis and vitamin D deficiency.

HISTORY OF DRUG OR ALCOHOL ABUSE: Denied.

FAMILY HISTORY: The patient's mother had a history of depression and was treated with electroconvulsive therapy. The mother also had a history of Alzheimer's disease. Her mother passed away 10 years ago. The patient has one sibling, her twin sister, who has a history of depression.

PERSONAL HISTORY

Perinatal: No known birth complications.

Childhood: No history of separation anxiety, problems with friendships, intellectual or learning disabilities, nightmares, phobias, fire setting, or cruelty to animals.

Adolescence: No problems with body image or eating disorders. She developed depression initially as a teen. No self-injurious behaviors.

Adulthood: Never completed high school. Worked at a family business as a receptionist. Later worked as a waitress off and on. Has not worked for the past 20 years. She identified as an atheist even though she was raised as a Catholic. The patient was married and divorced twice. Has one adult daughter who lives in California. Does not have much contact with her. She has limited leisure activities other than reading. Her only current friend is her sister who recently moved to a senior residential care facility. They were previously living in the same apartment.

TRAUMA/ABUSE HISTORY: Denied.

MENTAL STATUS EXAMINATION

Appearance: Casual clothing. Wears a wig. Appears older than stated age. Good eye contact. Cooperative. Lips appear dry and skin turgor is poor.

Behavior and psychomotor activity: Psychomotor activity slow. Has significant altered posture due to kyphosis. Trembling.

Consciousness:	Alert.
Orientation:	Oriented times three.
Memory:	Grossly intact. Not formally evaluated.
Concentration and attention:	Attentive.
Visuospatial ability:	Not assessed.
Abstract thought:	Not formally assessed but seems to comprehend concepts without difficulty.
Intellectual functioning:	Average.
Speech and language:	Normal rate and tone.
Perceptions:	No perceptual disturbances elicited.
Thought processes:	Logical and coherent.
Thought content:	Preoccupied with no longer living with her sister.
Suicidality or homicidality:	Denies.
Mood:	Depressed.
Affect:	Depressed. Crying. Tearful.
Impulse control:	Good.
Judgment:	Fair.
Insight:	Able to identify that she is missing her sister, which is contributing to her depressed mood.
Reliability:	Seems like a reliable historian.

FORMULATING THE DIAGNOSIS

Which diagnosis (or diagnoses) should be considered?

309.0 (F43.21) Adjustment Disorder, with Depressed Mood

Diagnostic Criteria

A. The development of emotional or behavioral symptoms in response to an identifiable stressor(s) occurring within 3 months of the onset of the stressor(s).
B. These symptoms or behaviors are clinically significant, as evidenced by one or both of the following:
    1. Marked distress that is out of proportion to the severity or intensity of the stressor, taking into account the external context and the cultural factors that might influence symptom severity and presentation.
    2. Significant impairment in social, occupational, or other important areas of functioning.
C. The stress-related disturbance does not meet the criteria for another mental disorder and is not merely an exacerbation of a preexisting mental disorder.
D. The symptoms do not represent normal bereavement.
E. Once the stressor or its consequences have terminated, the symptoms do not persist for more than an additional 6 months.

Specify whether:

- **309.0 (F43.21) With depressed mood:** Low mood, tearfulness, or feelings of hopelessness are predominant.
- **309.24 (F43.22) With anxiety:** Nervousness, worry, jitteriness, or separation anxiety is predominant.
- **309.28 (F43.23) With mixed anxiety and depressed mood:** A combination of depression and anxiety is predominant.
- **309.3 (F43.24) With disturbance of conduct:** Disturbance of conduct is predominant.
- **309.4 (F43.25) With mixed disturbance of emotions and conduct:** Both emotional symptoms (eg, depression, anxiety) and a disturbance of conduct are predominant.
- **309.9 (F43.20) Unspecified:** For maladaptive reactions that are not classifiable as one of the specific subtypes of adjustment disorder.

Specify if:

- **Acute:** If the disturbance lasts less than 6 months.
- **Persistent (chronic):** If the disturbance lasts for 6 months or longer.

What is the rationale for the diagnosis?

The patient developed emotional and behavioral symptoms in response to the absence of her sister that began 2 months ago. She is crying frequently and having difficulty sleeping. The patient is significantly impaired regarding maintaining adequate nutrition since her sister moved. This stress-related disturbance does not meet the criteria for another mental disorder and is not an exacerbation of a preexisting mental disorder. Although the patient has a history of depression, her mood had been stable prior to the absence of her sister. The symptoms do not represent bereavement. It is not expected that the symptoms will persist once the patient is reunited with her sister. Therefore, this single event has triggered this response and the symptoms and their course meet the criteria for adjustment disorder, with depressed mood.

Which diagnosis (or diagnoses) should be considered?

296.89 (F31.81) Bipolar II Disorder

Diagnostic Criteria

For a diagnosis of bipolar II disorder, it is necessary to meet the following criteria for a current or past hypomanic episode *and* the following criteria for a current or past major depressive episode (MDE).

Hypomanic Episode

A. A distinct period of abnormally and persistently elevated, expansive, or irritable mood and abnormally and persistently increased activity or energy, lasting at least 4 consecutive days and present most of the day, nearly every day.
B. During the period of mood disturbance and increased energy and activity, three (or more) of the following symptoms have persisted (four if the mood is only irritable), represent a noticeable change from usual behavior, and have been present to a significant degree:
   1. Inflated self-esteem or grandiosity.
   2. Decreased need for sleep (eg, feels rested after only 3 hours of sleep).
   3. More talkative than usual or pressure to keep talking.
   4. Flight of ideas or subjective experience that thoughts are racing.
   5. Distractibility (ie, attention too easily drawn to unimportant or irrelevant external stimuli), as reported or observed.
   6. Increase in goal-directed activity (socially, at work or school, or sexually) or psychomotor agitation.
   7. Excessive involvement in activities that have a high potential for painful consequences (eg, engaging in unrestrained buying sprees, sexual indiscretions, or foolish business investments).
C. The episode is associated with an unequivocal change in functioning that is uncharacteristic of the individual when not symptomatic.

D. The disturbance in mood and the change in functioning are observable by others.
E. The episode is not severe enough to cause marked impairment in social or occupational functioning or to necessitate hospitalization. If there are psychotic features, the episode is, by definition, manic.
F. The episode is not attributable to the physiologic effects of a substance (eg, a drug of abuse, a medication, other treatment) or another medical condition.
   - **Note:** A full hypomanic episode that emerges during antidepressant treatment (eg, medication, electroconvulsive therapy) but persists at a fully syndromal level beyond the physiologic effect of that treatment is sufficient evidence for a hypomanic episode diagnosis. However, caution is indicated so that one or two symptoms (particularly increased irritability, edginess, or agitation following antidepressant use) are not taken as sufficient for diagnosis of a hypomanic episode, nor necessarily indicative of a bipolar diathesis.

Major Depressive Episode

A. Five (or more) of the following symptoms have been present during the same 2-week period and represent a change from previous functioning; at least one of the symptoms is either (1) depressed mood or (2) loss of interest or pleasure.
   - **Note:** Do not include symptoms that are clearly attributable to a medical condition.
     1. Depressed mood most of the day, nearly every day, as indicated by either subjective report (eg, feels sad, empty, or hopeless) or observation made by others (eg, appears tearful). (Note: In children and adolescents, can be irritable mood.)
     2. Markedly diminished interest or pleasure in all, or almost all, activities most of the day, nearly every day (as indicated by either subjective account or observation).
     3. Significant weight loss when not dieting or weight gain (eg, a change of more than 5% of body weight in a month), or decrease or increase in appetite nearly every day. (Note: In children, consider failure to make expected weight gain.)
     4. Insomnia or hypersomnia nearly every day.
     5. Psychomotor agitation or retardation nearly every day (observable by others; not merely subjective feelings of restlessness or being slowed down).
     6. Fatigue or loss of energy nearly every day.
     7. Feelings of worthlessness or excessive or inappropriate guilt (which may be delusional) nearly every day (not merely self-reproach or guilt about being sick).
     8. Diminished ability to think or concentrate, or indecisiveness, nearly every day (either by subjective account or as observed by others).

9. Recurrent thoughts of death (not just fear of dying), recurrent suicidal ideation without a specific plan, a suicide attempt, or a specific plan for committing suicide.

B. The symptoms cause clinically significant distress or impairment in social, occupational, or other important areas of functioning.
C. The episode is not attributable to the physiologic effects of a substance or another medical condition.

Note: Criteria A to C constitute an MDE.

Note: Responses to a significant loss (eg, bereavement, financial ruin, losses from a natural disaster, a serious medical illness, or disability) may include the feelings of intense sadness, rumination about the loss, insomnia, poor appetite, and weight loss noted in Criterion A, which may resemble a depressive episode. Although such symptoms may be understandable or considered appropriate to the loss, the presence of an MDE in addition to the normal response to a significant loss should be carefully considered. This decision inevitably requires the exercise of clinical judgment based on the individual's history and the cultural norms for the expression of distress in the context of loss.

In distinguishing grief from an MDE, it is useful to consider that in grief the predominant affect is feelings of emptiness and loss, whereas in an MDE it is persistent depressed mood and the inability to anticipate happiness or pleasure. The dysphoria in grief is likely to decrease in intensity over days to weeks and occurs in waves, the so-called pangs of grief. These waves tend to be associated with thoughts or reminders of the deceased. The depressed mood of an MDE is more persistent and not tied to specific thoughts or preoccupations. The pain of grief may be accompanied by positive emotions and humor that are uncharacteristic of the pervasive unhappiness and misery characteristic of an MDE. The thought content associated with grief generally features a preoccupation with thoughts and memories of the deceased, rather than the self-critical or pessimistic ruminations seen in an MDE. In grief, self-esteem is generally preserved, whereas in an MDE feelings of worthlessness and self-loathing are common. If self-derogatory ideation is present in grief, it typically involves perceived failings vis-à-vis the deceased (eg, not visiting frequently enough, not telling the deceased how much he or she was loved). If a bereaved individual thinks about death and dying, such thoughts are generally focused on the deceased and possibly about "joining" the deceased, whereas in an MDE such thoughts are focused on ending one's own life because of feeling worthless, undeserving of life, or unable to cope with the pain of depression.

Bipolar II Disorder

A. Criteria have been met for at least one hypomanic episode (Criteria A to F under "Hypomanic Episode") and at least one MDE (Criteria A to C under "Major Depressive Episode").
B. There has never been a manic episode.

C. The occurrence of the hypomanic episode(s) and MDE(s) is not better explained by schizoaffective disorder, schizophrenia, schizophreniform disorder, delusional disorder, or other specified or unspecified schizophrenia spectrum and other psychotic disorder.
D. The symptoms of depression or the unpredictability caused by frequent alternation between periods of depression and hypomania causes clinically significant distress or impairment in social, occupational, or other important areas of functioning.

(Reprinted with permission from the *Diagnostic and Statistical Manual of Mental Disorders*. 5th ed. Arlington, VA: American Psychiatric Publishing; 2013.)

What is the rationale for the diagnosis?

Although this provider has not witnessed any hypomanic/manic episodes, the patient was previously diagnosed with bipolar II disorder and has a long history of being treated with medications to stabilize her mood, which have been effective. Therefore, this diagnosis will be considered to be accurate unless additional information is received to suggest otherwise.

Which diagnosis (or diagnoses) should be considered?

E86.0 Dehydration.

This is the clinical information listed for this diagnosis with the ICD-10. Clinical Information

- A condition caused by the loss of too much water from the body. Severe diarrhea or vomiting can cause dehydration.
- A condition resulting from the excessive loss of water from the body. It is usually caused by severe diarrhea, vomiting, or diaphoresis.
- A disorder characterized by excessive loss of water from the body. It is usually caused by severe diarrhea, vomiting, or diaphoresis.
- Decreased intravascular, interstitial, and/or intracellular fluid. This refers to dehydration, water loss alone without change in sodium.
- State of excessively reduced body water or water deficit.
- The condition that results from excessive loss of water from a living organism.
- When you are dehydrated, your body does not have enough fluid to work properly. An average person on an average day needs about 3 quarts of water. But if you are out in the hot sun, you will need a lot more than that. Most healthy bodies are very good at regulating water. Elderly people, young children, and some special cases—like people taking certain medications—need to be a little more careful. Signs of dehydration in adults include
    - being thirsty
    - urinating less often than usual
    - dark-colored urine

- dry skin
- feeling tired
- dizziness and fainting

Signs of dehydration in babies and young children include a dry mouth and tongue, crying without tears, no wet diapers for 3 hours or more, a high fever, and being unusually sleepy or drowsy. If you think you are dehydrated, drink small amounts of water over a period of time. Taking too much all at once can overload your stomach and make you throw up. For people exercising in the heat and losing a lot of minerals in sweat, sports drinks can be helpful. Avoid any drinks that have caffeine.

(Reprinted with permission from World Health Organization. *The ICD-10 Classification of Mental and Behavioural Disorders: Clinical Descriptions and Diagnostic Guidelines*. Geneva: World Health Organization; 1992.)

What is the rationale for the diagnosis?

The patient's skin and lips are dry. She reports that she has had a decreased appetite and cannot remember when she last ate or drank. Her skin turgor is poor. Her adult diaper is dry.

What test or tools should be considered to help identify the correct diagnosis?

None indicated in this facility. Should be referred for immediate medical evaluation and treatment via the emergency department.

What differential diagnosis (or diagnoses) should be considered?

None.

FORMULATING THE TREATMENT STRATEGY

What treatment would you prescribe and what is the rationale?

The patient was referred directly to the emergency department at the closest hospital. She was informed that she appeared to be dehydrated and was experiencing abdominal pain and these symptoms indicated that she needed immediate medical evaluation. The patient was agreeable with this plan.

Psychopharmacology: The patient's current medications should be continued: valproic acid ER 250 mg daily and sertraline 100 mg daily. There was no indication that her medications should be changed because her mood had been stable and euthymic on them and her depressive symptoms seemed related to an identifiable stressor, the absence of her sister.

Diagnostic Tests: It was not possible to obtain an accurate blood pressure as the patient could not hold her arm still. Valproic acid level should be obtained.

Referrals: Referred to the emergency department to be evaluated for dehydration.

Type of Psychotherapy: Supportive.

Psychoeducation: Advised of the importance of adequate fluid intake.

What standard guidelines would you use to treat or assess this patient?

None.

CLINICAL NOTE

- Prompt treatment of the early stages of dehydration is indicated in order to reduce the morbidity and mortality resulting from this condition.
- It was expected that this patient's mood would improve and her depressive symptoms would subside once she was reunited with her sister, which was expected to occur shortly.

REFERENCES/RECOMMENDED READINGS

American Psychiatric Association. *Diagnostic and Statistical Manual for Mental Disorder, DSM 5*. 5th ed. Washington, DC: American Psychiatric Publishing; 2013.

Bryant H. Dehydration in older people: assessment and management: Hannah Bryant relates the importance of assessing and managing dehydration in older people. *Emergency Nurse*. 2007;15(4):22-26.

Frank C. Pharmacologic treatment of depression in the elderly. *Canad Fam Physician*. 2014; 60(2):121-126.

World Health Organization. *The ICD-10 Classification of Mental and Behavioural Disorders: Clinical Descriptions and Diagnostic Guidelines*. Geneva: World Health Organization; 1992.

CASE 51

Seeing Dead People

IDENTIFICATION: The patient is a 78-year-old female in general good health living in an assisted living facility. She is a retired executive secretary.

CHIEF COMPLAINT: "Every once in awhile, I see my dead mother laying on the bed, I get scared and run out of the room and get a staff member to come in here. I'm so embarrassed because nothing is in the bed when I return. This happens a lot and sometimes I see people I never met before standing in my kitchen. I get scared, and they disappear."

HISTORY OF CHIEF COMPLAINT: The patient was referred for a psychiatric evaluation following the incidents described in the Chief Complaint, which began 3 months ago with abrupt onset. These incidents did not occur while sleeping or waking up from sleep.

PAST PSYCHIATRIC HISTORY: No history of mental illness. Denied any symptoms of mental illness other than the information described earlier.

MEDICAL HISTORY: Her vital signs were normal following the hallucinatory events, that is, pulse 90, BP 130/88. A medical consultation was ordered. The primary care provider ordered an electroencephalogram (EEG)/MRI of the brain to r/o seizures, brain tumors, or encephalopathy, and the results were within normal limits (WNLs) other than periventricular white matter changes associated with age. Comprehensive metabolic panel (CMP), urinalysis (UA), thyroid-stimulating hormone (TSH), triiodothyronine (T_3), thyroxine (T_4), B_{12}, RBC folate, RPR, and complete blood count (CBC) were all normal. A 48-hour Holter monitor was also ordered. Immediately before her hallucinatory events, distinct episodes of bradycardia of 30 beats/minutes were identified. This cardiac insufficiency would likely contribute to hypoxia. Due to the bradycardia identified with the 48-hour monitor, a pacemaker was inserted. Taking cholesterol medication atorvastatin once a day for several years with normal cholesterol for past 2 years. Taking aspirin 81 mg daily.

HISTORY OF DRUG OR ALCOHOL ABUSE: Denied.

FAMILY HISTORY: Enjoyed living in the assisted living for the past 3 years, had many friends, family visited often, she went to church every Sunday and was well liked.

PERSONAL HISTORY

Perinatal: No known complications.

Childhood: Developmental milestones achieved WNL.

Adolescence: She was on the honor roll in high school and attended 2 years of college for secretarial training with an all A average.

Adulthood: She worked as an executive secretary for an auto company for 30 years until her retirement 10 years ago. After the death of her husband of 50 years, she moved to the assisted living facility about 5 years ago. She said that taking care of the house had become too much of a responsibility for her. She has three children and five grandchildren and is “close” with all of them. They visit often. Her apartment at the assisted living facility is neat and clean and well furnished.

TRAUMA/ABUSE HISTORY: Denied.

MENTAL STATUS EXAMINATION

Appearance: Well dressed, attractive, with weight in proportion to height. She smiles easily.

Behavior and psychomotor activity: Cooperative. Good eye contact. No abnormal movements.

Consciousness	No rmal. Alert.
Orientation	Oriented to person, place and time.
Memory	No indications of dementia, mini-mental state examination normal, up-to-date on current events with rapid response time to questions asked. No indication of even mild neurocognitive decline.

Concentration and attention	Normal. No distractibility.
Abstract thought	Normal.
Speech and language	Normal rate and volume. Clear. Full vocabulary.
Perceptions	No abnormal perceptions during the interview but describes visual hallucinations that occur at intervals when she is wide awake in the morning, evening or midday. They frighten her and she seeks staff help.
Thought processes	Organized and logical.
Thought content	No unusual content other than fear of hallucinations recurring.
Suicidality or homicidality	None.
Mood	Euthymic.
Affect	Full range and congruent to mood.
Impulse control	Good.
Judgment	Good.
Insight	Good, aware that hallucinations cannot be real.
Reliability	Seems like a reliable historian.

FORMULATING THE DIAGNOSIS

Which diagnosis (or diagnoses) should be considered?

780.09 (R41.0) Other Specified Delirium, Attenuated Delirium Syndrome

This category applies to presentations in which symptoms characteristic of delirium that cause clinically significant distress or impairment in social, occupational, or other important areas of functioning predominate but do not meet the full criteria for delirium or any of the disorders in the neurocognitive disorders diagnostic class. The other specified delirium category is used in situations in which the clinician chooses to communicate the specific reason that the presentation does not meet the criteria for delirium or any specific neurocognitive disorder. This is done by recording "other specified delirium" followed by the specific reason (eg, "attenuated delirium syndrome").

An example of a presentation that can be specified using the "other specified" designation is the following:

- **Attenuated delirium syndrome:** This syndrome applies in cases of delirium in which the severity of cognitive impairment falls short of that required for the diagnosis, or in which some, but not all, diagnostic criteria for delirium are met.

(Reprinted with permission from the *Diagnostic and Statistical Manual of Mental Disorders*, 5th ed. Arlington, VA: American Psychiatric Publishing; 2013.)

What is the rationale for the diagnosis?

The patient does not meet the full criteria for dementia, because there is no disturbance in the patient's attention and awareness, and the disturbance has been occurring for the past 3 months intermittently rather than over a few hours or days. However, she does report a disturbance in perception (with the visual hallucinations of her mother and others occurring intermittently). The disturbances are not better explained by another preexisting neurocognitive disorder (she does not exhibit any decline in cognition that would suggest Lewy body disease, a diagnosis that can include hallucinations as a symptom). The disturbance does not occur in the context of a reduced level of arousal or during sleep (in fact she is frightened and runs out of the room to tell the nursing staff), which would rule out narcolepsy. A brief neurologic examination does not indicate any gross abnormalities. At the time of the initial evaluation, there is inconclusive evidence from laboratory findings that the disturbance is a direct physiologic result of a medical condition.

What test or tools should be considered to help identify the correct diagnosis?

A timeline was made to examine the relationship of hallucinatory events with episodes of bradycardia. UA with culture and sensitivity to rule out any urinary tract infection that could be contributing to a delirium. However, there are many medical conditions that cause psychosis, such as systemic lupus erythematosus, Cushing syndrome, HIV, neurosyphilis, thyroiditis seizures, and brain cancer or tumor to name a few.

For further information about differential diagnosis of psychotic symptoms see: http://www.psychiatrictimes.com/forensic-psychiatry/differential-diagnosis-psychotic-symptoms-medical-%E2%80%9Cmimics%E2%80%9D

A neurological examination form can be accessed at: http://www.cliniciansbrief.com/sites/default/files/neuro_form_4.pdf

Diagnosis of delirium can be aided by using the Confusion Assessment Method diagnostic algorithm (see Appendix), which can be accessed at: http://www.dementiamanagementstrategy.com/File.axd?id=bf5c8939-fbe1-4c57-9e64-2ba7c3bd5022.

The Montreal Cognitive Assessment (MoCA) is a rapid screening instrument for mild cognitive dysfunction which assesses multiple domains (see Appendix).

What differential diagnosis (or diagnoses) should be considered?

294.11 (F02.81) Major or Mild Neurocognitive Disorder with Lewy Bodies

Although the patient has visual hallucinations that occur on an intermittent basis, which would indicate the possibility of major or mild neurocognitive disorder with Lewy bodies, she does not exhibit any neurocognitive decline and has not had any impairment in her capacity for independence in everyday activities. However, the patient should continue to be evaluated for this diagnosis.

347.00 (G47.419) Narcolepsy without Cataplexy

The hallucinations did not occur during times of "dozing off" or "just waking up from sleep," which can occur in narcolepsy with hypnogogic and hypnopompic hallucinations. Therefore, a diagnosis of narcolepsy would not be applicable.

FORMULATING THE TREATMENT STRATEGY

What treatment would you prescribe and what is the rationale?

Psychopharmacology: None indicated.

Diagnostic Tests: The patient had already completed extensive diagnostic testing, so no further testing indicated at this time.

Referrals: Continue to follow up with medical/cardiac providers

Type of Psychotherapy: None indicated.

Psychoeducation: Advise the patient that the hallucinatory episodes may be related to her medical condition.

What standard guidelines would you use to treat or assess this patient?

American Psychiatric Association. Practice guideline for the treatment of patients with delirium. *Am J Psychiatr*. 1999;156(5)(suppl):1-20.

CLINICAL NOTE

- Differentiating between delirium and dementia requires attention to the patient's history. Delirium is usually an abrupt process occurring within hours or days, whereas dementia is a slower process with a gradual onset of symptoms. Delirium is usually reversible if treated promptly, whereas symptoms of dementia are not. Most importantly delirium requires immediate medical attention as it may be life threatening.
- In this specific case, the hallucinatory events subsided following placement of the pacemaker. This supports a delirium diagnosis since hypoxia (related to the bradycardia) can contribute to hallucinations.

REFERENCES/RECOMMENDED READINGS

American Psychiatric Association. *Diagnostic and Statistical Manual for Mental Disorder, DSM 5.* 5th ed. Arlington, VA: American Psychiatric Publishing; 2013.

Fong TG, Tulebaev SR, Inouye SK. Delirium in elderly adults: diagnosis, prevention and treatment. *Nat Rev Neurol.* 2009;5(4):210-220. doi:10.1038/nrneurol.2009.24.

Lehman C. Confusion in older adults: determining the difference between dementia and delirium. *ARN Network*. 2008;3. http://www.rehabnurse.org/pdf/GeriatricConfusion.pdf

Taylor R. *The Psychological Masquerade.* 3rd ed. New York, NY: Springer Publishing; 2007.

CASE 51 APPENDIX

Cognitive Assessment Tools

TABLE 51-1 Confusion Assessment Method (CAM) Diagnostic Algorithm

Date of assessment: ______________________

Time of assessment: ______________________

	YES	NO
1. Acute onset and fluctuating course? (Acute change in mental status from baseline, fluctuating behaviour through the day)		
2. Inattention? (Difficulty focusing attention, easily distracted, difficulty keeping track of what is being said)		
3. Disorganized thinking? (disorganized or incoherent thinking, rambling or irrelevant conversation, unclear or illogical flow of ideas)		
4. Altered level of consciousness? (This feature is shown by any answer other than "alert", including: hyper-alert, lethargic, stupor, or coma)		

The diagnosis of Delirium by CAM requires the presence of features 1 and 2 *AND EITHER* 3 or 4.

Delirium detected? **YES** **NO**
(Circle)

Reprinted with permission from Inouye SK, Van Dyck CH, Alessi CA, Balkin S, Siegal AP, Horwitz RI. Clarifying confusion: the Confusion Assessment Method. *Ann Int Med.* 1990;113:941-948

TABLE 51-2 Montreal Cognitive Assessment (MoCA)

MONTREAL COGNITIVE ASSESSMENT (MoCA)
Version 7.1 Original Version

NAME :
Education : Date of birth :
Sex : DATE :

		POINTS
VISUOSPATIAL / EXECUTIVE	(E) End, (A), (5), (B), (2), (1) Begin, (D), (4), (3), (C) [ ] ; Copy cube [ ] ; Draw CLOCK (Ten past eleven) (3 points) [ ] Contour [ ] Numbers [ ] Hands	___/5
NAMING	[ ] [ ] [ ]	___/3
MEMORY	Read list of words, subject must repeat them. Do 2 trials, even if 1st trial is successful. Do a recall after 5 minutes.	No points

	FACE	VELVET	CHURCH	DAISY	RED
1st trial					
2nd trial					

		POINTS
ATTENTION	Read list of digits (1 digit/ sec.). Subject has to repeat them in the forward order [ ] 2 1 8 5 4 ; Subject has to repeat them in the backward order [ ] 7 4 2	___/2
	Read list of letters. The subject must tap with his hand at each letter A. No points if ≥ 2 errors [ ] FBACMNAAJKLBAFAKDEAAAJAMOFAAB	___/1
	Serial 7 subtraction starting at 100 [ ] 93 [ ] 86 [ ] 79 [ ] 72 [ ] 65 ; 4 or 5 correct subtractions: **3 pts**, 2 or 3 correct: **2 pts**, 1 correct: **1 pt**, 0 correct: **0 pt**	___/3
LANGUAGE	Repeat : I only know that John is the one to help today. [ ] The cat always hid under the couch when dogs were in the room. [ ]	___/2
	Fluency / Name maximum number of words in one minute that begin with the letter F [ ] ____ (N ≥ 11 words)	___/1
ABSTRACTION	Similarity between e.g. banana - orange = fruit [ ] train – bicycle [ ] watch - ruler	___/2

DELAYED RECALL	Has to recall words	FACE	VELVET	CHURCH	DAISY	RED	Points for UNCUED recall only	___/5
	WITH NO CUE	[ ]	[ ]	[ ]	[ ]	[ ]		
Optional	Category cue							
	Multiple choice cue							

		POINTS
ORIENTATION	[ ] Date [ ] Month [ ] Year [ ] Day [ ] Place [ ] City	___/6

 www.mocatest.org Normal ≥26 / 30 TOTAL ___/30

Administered by: ______________________ Add 1 point if ≤ 12 yr edu

(Reprinted with permission from Z. Nasreddine, MD.)

TABLE 51-3 Montreal Cognitive Assessment (MoCA)

ADMINISTRATION AND SCORING INSTRUCTIONS

The Montreal Cognitive Assessment (MoCA) was designed as a rapid screening instrument for mild cognitive dysfunction. It assesses different cognitive domains: attention and concentration, executive functions, memory, language, visuoconstructional skills, conceptual thinking, calculations, and orientation. Time to administer the MoCA is approximately 10 minutes. The total possible score is 30 points; a score of 26 or above is considered normal.

1. Alternating Trail Making:

   Administration: The examiner instructs the subject: "*Please draw a line, going from a number to a letter in ascending order. Begin here* [point to (1)] *and draw a line from 1 then to A then to 2 and so on. End here* [point to (E)]."

   Scoring: Allocate one point if the subject successfully draws the following pattern: 1- A- 2- B- 3- C- 4- D- 5- E, without drawing any lines that cross. Any error that is not immediately self-corrected earns a score of 0.

2. Visuoconstructional Skills (Cube):

   Administration: The examiner gives the following instructions, pointing to the **cube**: "*Copy this drawing as accurately as you can, in the space below.*"

   Scoring: One point is allocated for a correctly executed drawing.

   - Drawing must be three-dimensional
   - All lines are drawn
   - No line is added
   - Lines are relatively parallel and their length is similar (rectangular prisms are accepted)

   A point is not assigned if any of the above criteria are not met.

3. Visuoconstructional Skills (Clock):

   Administration: Indicate the right third of the space and give the following instructions: "*Draw a* ***clock****. Put in all the numbers and set the time to 10 past 11.*"

   Scoring: One point is allocated for each of the following three criteria:

   - Contour (1 pt.): the clock face must be a circle with only minor distortion acceptable (eg, slight imperfection on closing the circle);
   - Numbers (1 pt.): all clock numbers must be present with no additional numbers; numbers must be in the correct order and placed in the approximate quadrants on the clock face; Roman numerals are acceptable; numbers can be placed outside the circle contour;
   - Hands (1 pt.): there must be two hands jointly indicating the correct time; the hour hand must be clearly shorter than the minute hand; hands must be centered within the clock face with their junction close to the clock center.
   - A point is not assigned for a given element if any of the above criteria are not met.

4. Naming:

   Administration: Beginning on the left, point to each figure and say: "*Tell me the name of this animal.*"

   Scoring: One point each is given for the following responses: (1) lion (2) rhinoceros or rhino (3) camel or dromedary.

5. Memory:

   Administration: The examiner reads a list of 5 words at a rate of one per second, giving the following instructions: "*This is a memory test. I am going to read a list of words that you will have to remember now and later on. Listen carefully. When I am through, tell me as many words as you can remember. It doesn't matter in what order you say them.*" Mark a check in the allocated space for each word the subject produces on this first trial. When the subject indicates that (s)he has finished (has recalled all words), or can recall no more words, read the list a second time with the following instructions: "*I am going to read the same list for a second time. Try to remember and tell me as many words as you can, including words you said the first time.*" Put a check in the allocated space for each word the subject recalls after the second trial.

   At the end of the second trial, inform the subject that (s)he will be asked to recall these words again by saying, "*I will ask you to recall those words again at the end of the test.*"

   Scoring: No points are given for Trials One and Two.

6. Attention:

   Forward Digit Span: Administration: Give the following instruction: "*I am going to say some numbers and when I am through, repeat them to me exactly as I said them.*" Read the five number sequence at a rate of one digit per second.

   Backward Digit Span: Administration: Give the following instruction: "*Now I am going to say some more numbers, but when I am through you must repeat them to me in the backward order.*" Read the three number sequence at a rate of one digit per second.

   Scoring: Allocate one point for each sequence correctly repeated (*N.B.*: the correct response for the backward trial is 2-4-7).

   Vigilance: Administration: The examiner reads the list of letters at a rate of one per second, after giving the following instruction: "*I am going to read a sequence of letters. Every time I say the letter A, tap your hand once. If I say a different letter, do not tap your hand.*"

   Scoring: Give one point if there is zero to one error (an error is a tap on a wrong letter or a failure to tap on letter A).

   Serial 7s: Administration: The examiner gives the following instruction: "*Now, I will ask you to count by subtracting seven from 100, and then, keep subtracting seven from your answer until I tell you to stop.*" Give this instruction twice if necessary.

   Scoring: This item is scored out of 3 points. Give no (0) points for no correct subtractions, 1 point for one correction subtraction, 2 points for two-to-three correct subtractions, and 3 points if the participant successfully makes four or five correct subtractions. Count each correct subtraction of 7 beginning at 100. Each subtraction is evaluated independently; that is, if the participant responds with an incorrect number but continues to correctly subtract 7 from it, give a point for each correct subtraction. For example, a participant may respond "92 – 85 – 78 – 71 – 64" where the "92" is incorrect, but all subsequent numbers are subtracted correctly. This is one error and the item would be given a score of 3.

7. Sentence Repetition:

   Administration: The examiner gives the following instructions: "*I am going to read you a sentence. Repeat it after me, exactly as I say it* [pause]: ***I only know that John is the one to help today.***" Following the response, say: "*Now I am going to read you another sentence. Repeat it after me, exactly as I say it* [pause]: ***The cat always hid under the couch when dogs were in the room.***"

   Scoring: Allocate 1 point for each sentence correctly repeated. Repetition must be exact. Be alert for errors that are omissions (eg, omitting "only," "always") and substitutions/additions (eg, "John is the one who helped today"; substituting "hides" for "hid," altering plurals, etc.).

8. Verbal Fluency:

   Administration: The examiner gives the following instruction: "*Tell me as many words as you can think of that begin with a certain letter of the alphabet that I will tell you in a moment. You can say any kind of word you want, except for proper nouns (like Bob or Boston), numbers, or words that begin with the same sound but have a different suffix, for example, love, love, loving. I will tell you to stop after one minute. Are you ready?* [Pause] *Now, tell me as many words as you can think of that begin with the letter F.* [time for 60 sec]. *Stop.*"

   Scoring: Allocate one point if the subject generates 11 words or more in 60 sec. Record the subject's response in the bottom or side margins.

9. Abstraction:

   Administration: The examiner asks the subject to explain what each pair of words has in common, starting with the example: "*Tell me how an orange and a banana are alike.*" If the subject answers in a concrete manner, then say only one additional time: "*Tell me another way in which those items are alike.*" If the subject does not give the appropriate response *(fruit)*, say, "*Yes, and they are also both fruit.*" Do not give any additional instructions or clarification. After the practice trial, say: "*Now, tell me how a train and a bicycle are alike.*" Following the response, administer the second trial, saying: "*Now tell me how a ruler and a watch are alike.*"

   Do not give any additional instructions or prompts.

   Scoring: Only the last two item pairs are scored. Give 1 point to each item pair correctly answered. The following responses are acceptable:

   Train–bicycle = means of transportation, means of traveling, you take trips in both.

   Ruler–watch = measuring instruments, used to measure.

   The following responses are **not** acceptable: Train–bicycle = they have wheels; Ruler–watch = they have numbers.

10. Delayed Recall:

    Administration: The examiner gives the following instruction: "*I read some words to you earlier, which I asked you to remember. Tell me as many of those words as you can remember.*" Make a check mark (√) for each of the words correctly recalled spontaneously without any cues, in the allocated space.

    Scoring: **Allocate 1 point for each word recalled freely *without any cues*.**

Optional

Following the delayed free recall trial, prompt the subject with the semantic category cue provided below for any word not recalled. Make a check mark (√) in the allocated space if the subject remembered the word with the help of a category or multiple-choice cue. Prompt all nonrecalled words in this manner. If the subject does not recall the word after the category cue, give him/her a multiple choice trial, using the following example instruction, "*Which of the following words do you think it was, NOSE, FACE, or HAND?*"

Use the following category and/or multiple-choice cues for each word, when appropriate:

FACE:	category cue: part of the body	multiple choice: nose, face, hand
VELVET:	category cue: type of fabric	multiple choice: denim, cotton, velvet
CHURCH:	category cue: type of building	multiple choice: church, school, hospital
DAISY:	category cue: type of flower	multiple choice: rose, daisy, tulip
RED:	category cue: a color	multiple choice: red, blue, green

Scoring: **No points are allocated for words recalled with a cue.** A cue is used for clinical information purposes only and can give the test interpreter additional information about the type of memory disorder. For memory deficits due to retrieval failures, performance can be improved with a cue. For memory deficits due to encoding failures, performance does not improve with a cue.

11. Orientation:

Administration: The examiner gives the following instructions: "Tell me the date today." If the subject does not give a complete answer, then prompt accordingly by saying: "*Tell me the [year, month, exact date, and day of the week].*" Then say: "*Now, tell me the name of this place, and which city it is in.*"

Scoring: Give one point for each item correctly answered. The subject must tell the exact date and the exact place (name of hospital, clinic, office). No points are allocated if subject makes an error of one day for the day and date.

TOTAL SCORE: Sum all subscores listed on the right-hand side. Add one point for an individual who has 12 years or fewer of formal education, for a possible maximum of 30 points. A final total score of 26 and above is considered normal.

CASE 52

Agitated and Clapping Hands

IDENTIFICATION: The patient is an 87-year-old Black widowed female currently living in a nursing home for the past 4 years. Her family is not involved with her care. She was referred for a psychiatric consult by the nursing facility staff.

CHIEF COMPLAINT: Nursing facility staff states, "Nothing we do helps the clapping, and it bothers the other residents."

HISTORY OF CHIEF COMPLAINT: The patient has been in the nursing home for 4 years over which time her dementia has progressed to the point of a Montreal Cognitive Assessment equaling zero (see Case 51, Appendix Tables 2 and 3). The behavior leading to this consult is constant clapping. The clapping starts off in a soft pattern, and then escalates at various times during the day and night. The clapping is disturbing to the other residents and has caused other residents to be angry toward her.

PAST PSYCHIATRIC HISTORY: There is no documented psychiatric history prior to the behavioral interventions for her clapping behavior at the nursing home. Assessment of medical conditions that may contribute to the behavior have included a workup for urinary tract infection, urinalysis, culture and sensitivity, complete blood count, chem panel, chest x-ray, kidneys, ureters, and bladder x-ray.

Pain management with acetaminophen to treat potential pain that the patient was not able to express verbally had no effect on modifying the clapping behavior. Behavior modification interventions have included providing items to keep her hands busy, like the busy aprons, offering liquids, limiting time out of bed to prevent fatigue (which may have contributed to the clapping behavior).

Medications that have been tried include selective serotonin reuptake inhibitors (sertraline) to treat anxiety, imipramine to treat anxiety, short-acting benzodiazepine (lorazepam), an atypical antipsychotic (quetiapine), and mood stabilizers (valproic acid and lamotrigine). None of those agents were effective in modifying her behavior.

MEDICAL HISTORY: No known drug allergies, no known food allergies. There is no significant past medical history. The patient is fed by nursing staff and eats 100% of her soft diet.

Medications include acetaminophen 650 mg PRN q8h for pain and discomfort, trazodone 25 mg QHS for sleep.

HISTORY OF DRUG OR ALCOHOL ABUSE: None known.

FAMILY HISTORY: None known.

PERSONAL HISTORY

Perinatal: Information not available.

Childhood: Information not available.

Adolescence: Information not available.

Adulthood: Was married. Currently widowed. Has one niece who visits her in the nursing home.

TRAUMA/ABUSE HISTORY: Not known.

MENTAL STATUS EXAMINATION

Appearance: Sitting in geri chair, not ambulatory. Has a strained, worried, facial expression.

Behavior and psychomotor activity: Agitated, clapping hands constantly.

Consciousness:	Awake, alert.
Orientation:	To person only. She looks up when her name is called.
Memory:	Nonverbal at this time, so unable to assess.
Concentration and attention:	Not able to access.
Visuospatial ability:	Not able to assess.
Abstract thought:	Not able to assess.

Intellectual functioning: Not able to assess.

Speech and language: Nonverbal currently. Six months ago exhibited erratic yelling episodes.

Perceptions: Not able to assess.

Thought processes: Not able to assess.

Thought content: Not able to assess.

Suicidality or homicidality: Not able to assess.

Mood: Labile and more agitated at times, clapping is intermittently louder and more aggressive.

Affect: Blunted.

Impulse control: Poor.

Judgment/insight/reliability: Not able to assess.

FORMULATING THE DIAGNOSIS

Which diagnosis (or diagnoses) should be considered?

799.59 (R41.9) Unspecified Neurocognitive Disorder

This category applies to presentations in which symptoms characteristic of a neurocognitive disorder that cause clinically significant distress or impairment in social, occupational, or other important areas of functioning predominate but do not meet the full criteria for any of the disorders in the neurocognitive disorders diagnostic class. The unspecified neurocognitive disorder category is used in situations in which the precise etiology cannot be determined with sufficient certainty to make an etiologic attribution.

Coding note: For unspecified major or mild neurocognitive disorder, code 799.59 (R41.9). (**Note:** Do *not* use additional codes for any presumed etiologic medical conditions. Behavioral disturbance cannot be coded but may be indicated in writing.)

(Reprinted with permission from the *Diagnostic and Statistical Manual of Mental Disorders*. 5th ed. Arlington, VA: American Psychiatric Publishing; 2013.)

What is the rationale for the diagnosis?

This diagnosis is indicated because the patient presents with major neurocognitive disorder of an unknown etiology. Physical examination and laboratory findings indicate that her neurocognitive disorder is not due to another medical condition. The disorder causes significant impairment as evidenced by her inability to perform any activities of daily living, including feeding herself. She has exhibited persistent behavior disturbances (clapping), which has not responded to any behavioral modification or psychopharmacologic interventions. Therefore, a diagnosis of unspecified neurocognitive disorder is applicable.

What test or tools should be considered to help identify the correct diagnosis?

Neuropsychiatric Inventory Nursing Home Version (Appendix).

Comprehensive Assessment of Psychopathology in Patients with Dementia Residing in Nursing Homes, can be obtained at http://www.dementiamanagementstrategy.com/File.axd?id=c9f7405f-3596-4f5f-9f8d-f322e5188678

What differential diagnosis (or diagnoses) should be considered?

The *DSM-5* does not have a specific code for pseudobulbar affect (PBA); however, the *ICD-10* does.

(F48.2) Pseudobulbar Affect

Applicable to involuntary emotional expression disorder related to neurocognitive disorder.

Code first underlying cause, if known, such as

- amyotrophic lateral sclerosis
- multiple sclerosis
- sequelae of cerebrovascular disease
- sequelae of traumatic intracranial injury

(Reprinted with permission from World Health Organization. *The ICD-10 Classification of Mental and Behavioural Disorders: Clinical Descriptions and Diagnostic Guidelines*. Geneva: World Health Organization; 1992.)

The patient does not exhibit the involuntary emotional expression of crying or laughing, which is considered the standard for the diagnosis of PBA. However, her only means of expression is hand clapping and it fluctuates in intensity and at random. Her hand clapping could be perceived as an involuntary form of emotional expression, but since this is not definitive, the diagnosis of PBA can only be considered as a differential.

FORMULATING THE TREATMENT STRATEGY

What treatment would you prescribe and what is the rationale?

Psychopharmacology: Dextromethorphan-quinidine one capsule daily for 7 days and then one capsule twice daily.

Recent research has indicated that dextromethorphan-quinidine with doses up to 30/10 mg twice daily has been effective as an off-label treatment for agitation in certain patient populations with dementia and has been well tolerated.

Diagnostic Tests: All tests have been completed previously to rule out any medical condition that could be contributing to her agitated clapping behavior.

Referrals: Recreational therapy was ordered to distract the patient and have her focus on other hand-related activities.

Type of Psychotherapy: None indicated.

Psychoeducation: Although this patient's family is not actively involved in her care, information for family caregivers about dementia can be retrieved online at www.caregiver.org/fact-sheets

The nursing staff was educated regarding behavior modification plans for rest, repositioning, and distraction.

What standard guidelines would you use to treat or assess this patient?

Galvin JE. Guidelines for the management of cognitive and behavioral problems in dementia. *J Am Board Fam Med.* 2012;25:350-366. doi:10.3122/jabfm.2012.03.100183.

CLINICAL NOTE

- PBA is defined as a disinhibition of behavior with involuntary crying or laughing resulting from neurologic injury or disorder. It is more commonly associated with Alzheimer's disease. The exact mechanism is not known. Misdiagnosis is common as patients may be thought to be depressed and are treated with antidepressants, which are ineffective. PBA must be identified so that it can be treated appropriately. The recommended treatment is dextromethorphan–quinidine.
- In this specific case, the patient's hand clapping behavior significantly subsided with treatment with dextromethorphan-quinidine.

REFERENCES/RECOMMENDED READINGS

American Psychiatric Association. *Diagnostic and Statistical Manual for Mental Disorder, DSM 5.* 5th ed. Arlington, VA: American Psychiatric Publishing; 2013.

Cummings JL, Lyketsos CG, Peskind ER, et al. Effect of dextromethorphan-quinidine on agitation in patients with Alzheimer disease dementia: a randomized clinical trial. *JAMA.* 2015;314:1242-1254.

Gitlin LN, Kales HC, Lyketsos CG. Managing behavioral symptoms in dementia using non-pharmacologic approaches: an overview. *JAMA*. 2012;308(19):2020-2029. doi:10.1001/jama.2012.36918.

Simmons BB, Hartmann B, Dejoseph D. Evaluation of suspected dementia. *Am Fam Physician*. 2011;84(8):895-902.

Volicer L, Hurley AC. Review article: management of behavioral symptoms in progressive degenerative dementias. *J Gerontol A Biol Sci Med Sci*. 2003;58(9):M837-M845.

World Health Organization. *The ICD-10 Classification of Mental and Behavioural Disorders: Clinical Descriptions and Diagnostic Guidelines*. Geneva: World Health Organization; 1992.

Zarowitz B, O'Shea T. Clinical, behavioral, and treatment differences in nursing facility residents with dementia, with and without pseudobulbar affect symptomatology. *Consult Pharm*. 2013;28(11):713-722.

CASE 52 APPENDIX

Neuropsychiatric Inventory—Nursing Home

TODAY'S DATE ________________ TIME ________________

RESIDENT'S NAME ____________ RATER'S NAME ________________

	√Check appropriate box		O Circle Frequency ×	O Circle Severity	= Score	O Circle Disruption Score
Symptom	No NA	Yes	Frequency 1 2 3 4	Severity 1 2 3	Item Score	Disruption Score 0 1 2 3 4 5
1 Delusions			1 2 3 4	1 2 3		0 1 2 3 4 5
2 Hallucinations			1 2 3 4	1 2 3		0 1 2 3 4 5
3 Agitation			1 2 3 4	1 2 3		0 1 2 3 4 5
4 Depression/Dysphoria			1 2 3 4	1 2 3		0 1 2 3 4 5
5 Anxiety			1 2 3 4	1 2 3		0 1 2 3 4 5
6 Apathy			1 2 3 4	1 2 3		0 1 2 3 4 5
7 Irritability			1 2 3 4	1 2 3		0 1 2 3 4 5
8 Euphoria			1 2 3 4	1 2 3		0 1 2 3 4 5
9 Disinhibition			1 2 3 4	1 2 3		0 1 2 3 4 5
10 Aberrant Motor Behavior			1 2 3 4	1 2 3		0 1 2 3 4 5
11 Nighttime Behavior			1 2 3 4	1 2 3		0 1 2 3 4 5
12 Appetite/Eating Changes			1 2 3 4	1 2 3		0 1 2 3 4 5

Total Neuropsychiatric Inventory Score: ________/144

Total Disruption Score: ________/60

Neuropsychiatric Inventory Raters' Criteria

NEUROPSYCHIATRIC INVENTORY SYMPTOMS

Frequency of behavior:

1. Occasionally, less than once a week
2. Often, about once a week
3. Frequently, several times per week, but less than every day
4. Very frequently, once or more per day

Severity of behavior:

1. Mild (noticeable, but not a significant change)
2. Moderate (significant, but not a dramatic change)
3. Severe (very marked, a dramatic change)
    - For each of the 12 neuropsychiatric inventory (NPI) symptom categories, multiply the frequency score by the severity score
    - If the symptom is not present or not applicable, the score is 0
    - Add the total score for each item, to determine the overall NPI score (maximum is 144 points)
        - Less than 20 points: mild behavioral disturbance
        - 20 to 50 points: moderate behavioral disturbance
        - 50 or more points: severe behavioral disturbance

Caregiver disruption assessment:

0 Points	No distress
1 Point	Minimal (slightly distressing)
2 Points	Mild (not very distressing, generally easy to cope with)
3 Points	Moderate (fairly distressing, difficult to cope with)
4 Points	Severe (very distressing, difficult to cope with)
5 Points	Extreme (extremely distressing, unable to cope with)

- Add each of the 12 NPI symptom caregiver disruption scores to determine the total caregiver disruption score. (Maximum is 60 points.)

Scoring the Neuropsychiatric Inventory

DEFINITION

The NPI is a questionnaire that assesses changes in behavioral and psychological disturbances in a patient for whom a diagnosis of dementia has been made. It also evaluates the impact of these symptoms on the caregiver (eg, family member or professional caregiver). Evaluation is generally performed at 4- or 6-weekly intervals.

THE NEUROPSYCHIATRIC INVENTORY ASSESSMENT TOOL

The NPI assesses 12 neuropsychiatric symptoms exhibited by a patient. (These will be examined in detail along with the scoring.)

1. Delusions (paranoia)
2. Hallucinations
3. Agitation or aggression
4. Dysphoria (depressed mood)
5. Anxiety
6. Apathy
7. Irritability
8. Euphoria
9. Disinhibition
10. Aberrant motor behavior
11. Nighttime behavior disturbances
12. Appetite and eating abnormalities

"NO" indicates that there is no abnormal behavior or the abnormal behavior did not change (eg, the resident is not anxious, or his/her level of anxiety level has not changed). **If the rater checks No/NA, the score for that item is 0.**

YES indicates that symptoms are present or have increased in frequency and severity beyond the resident's baseline. The rater selects a number for the frequency of the abnormal behavior and the severity.

Score	**Frequency**	**Severity**
1	Occasionally, less than once a week	Mild (noticeable, but not a significant change)
2	Often, about once a week	Moderate (significant, but not a dramatic change)
3	Frequently, several times per week but less than every day	Severe (very marked; a dramatic change)
4	Very frequently, once or more per day	

Each neuropsychiatric item score is calculated by multiplying frequency times severity. The total score is obtained by adding the scores for each of the 12 items.

Total score ranges from 1 to 144 (144 is the worst possible score). The higher the total score, the more severe the symptoms:

SCORE RANGE

- Less than 20: symptoms are mild
- 20 to 50: symptoms are moderate
- 50 or over: symptoms are severe

DESCRIPTION OF NEUROPSYCHIATRIC SYMPTOMS

1. *Delusions*. The patient believes that others are planning to harm him or her in some way. He/she believes that others are stealing from him or her. He/she says that family members are not who they say they are or that the spouse is being unfaithful. The patient is not only suspicious, but also convinced these things are happening.
2. *Hallucinations*. The patient acts as if he/she hears voices. He/she talks to people who are not there. He/she seems to see, hear, or experience things that are not present. (This behavior is different from that of believing that a long-dead person is still alive.)
3. *Agitation/Aggression*. The patient has periods of verbal or physical agitation or aggression. Behaviors include screaming, temper outbursts, swearing, repeated calling out, pushing, biting, hitting, scratching, grabbing, throwing objects, spitting, kicking, wandering, pacing, elopement, intrusion into others' rooms, inappropriate voiding. The patient has periods of refusing to cooperate or being resistant to help from others. The patient is hard to handle.
4. *Depression/Dysphoria*.* The patient seems sad or in low spirits. He/she says that he/she feels sad or depressed. He or she cries.
5. *Anxiety*. The patient is very nervous, worried, or frightened for no apparent reason. He/she is very tense or fidgety. The patient becomes upset when separated from an object or person who offers comfort.
6. *Apathy/Indifference*. The patient seems less interested in the world around and in enjoyable daily activities. He/she lacks motivation for starting new activities. He/she is more difficult to engage in conversation.
7. *Irritability/Lability*. The patient gets irritated and easily disturbed. His/her moods are very changeable. He/she is abnormally impatient and cranky.

---

*Dysphoria: Mood disturbance associated with anxiety.

8. *Elation/Euphoria*. The patient has a persistent and abnormally good mood (ie, he/she feels too cheerful or acts excessively happy) for no reason.
9. *Disinhibition*. The patient acts impulsively. He/she does or says things that are not usually done or said in public, that are embarrassing to people, or that may hurt people's feelings. The patient may talk to strangers as if he or she knows them. Inappropriate disrobing or sexual behaviors are also examples of disinhibition.
10. *Aberrant Motor Behavior*. The patient engages in repetitive activities such as pacing, or does things repeatedly such as opening closets or drawers. The patient may constantly pick at clothes or skin, tap fingers, jiggle a leg, or rub an object (eg, "polishing" a piece of furniture).
11. *Sleep*. The patient has difficulty sleeping. He/she wanders at night, gets dressed, awakens during the night, rises too early in the morning, takes excessive naps during the day.
12. *Appetite and Eating Disorders*. He/she has had a change in appetite or eating habits. (Rate N/A if the patient cannot feed himself.) The patient has lost or gained significant weight.

NEUROPSYCHIATRIC INVENTORY—CAREGIVER DISRUPTION ASSESSMENT

Evaluates the impact of these symptoms on caregivers.

Assessment

For each of the 12 neuropsychiatric symptoms, caregivers rate the level of distress they experience on a scale from 0 (none) to 5 (very severe):

0 Points	No distress
1 Point	Minimal (slightly distressing)
2 Points	Mild (not very distressing, generally easy to cope with)
3 Points	Moderate (fairly distressing, not always easy to cope)
4 Points	Severe (very distressing, difficult to cope with)
5 Points	Extreme (extremely distressing, unable to cope)

Total score for caregiver distress ranges from 1 to 60 (60 is the worst possible score).

Stéphane Bastianetto, Ph.D.
August 2005

Ed. ElderAdvocates, Inc. 2006

Grouping Neuropsychiatric Behaviors into Categories for Medication Management

RESIDENT ________________________________ **DATE**__________

HYPERACTIVITY

NPI #	Symptom	Item Score (1–12)
3	Agitation or aggression	
7	Irritability	
8	Euphoria	
9	Disinhibition	
10	Aberrant motor behavior	

AFFECTIVE

NPI #	Symptom	Item Score (1–12)
4	Dysphoria/depressed mood	
5	Anxiety	
11	Nighttime behavior	
12	Appetite/eating abnormalities	

APATHY

NPI #	Symptom	Item Score (1–12)
6	Apathy	
11	Nighttime behavior	
12	Appetite/eating abnormalities	
10	Aberrant motor behavior	

PSYCHOSIS

NPI #	Symptom	Item Score (1–12)
1	Delusions	
2	Hallucinations	
5	Anxiety	

Most effective medication management is based on the category of behavior disturbance, derived from the NPI scores.

INDEX BY DIAGNOSTIC CATEGORY

(Case Number, Diagnosis, and Page Number)

ANXIETY DISORDERS

OBSESSIVE-COMPULSIVE AND RELATED DISORDERS

TRAUMA- AND STRESSOR-RELATED DISORDERS

NEUROCOGNITIVE DISORDERS

PERSONALITY DISORDERS

MEDICATION-INDUCED MOVEMENT DISORDERS AND OTHER ADVERSE EFFECTS OF MEDICATION

CONDITIONS FOR FURTHER STUDY

ALPHABETICAL INDEX OF NON–*DSM-5* DIAGNOSES (*ICD-10* CODES)

LIST OF MEDICATIONS REFERRED TO IN THE CASES

GENERIC NAME	BRAND NAME
acetaminophen/oxycodone	Percocet
alprazolam	Xanax
amitriptyline	Elavil
amphetamine/dextroamphetamine	Adderall
aripiprazole	Abilify
armodafinil	Nuvigil
atomoxetine	Strattera
buproprion	Wellbutrin
buspirone	Buspar
butalbital acetaminophen caffeine	Fioricet
citalopram	Celexa
clonazepam	Klonopin
clonidine	Catapres
clozapine	Clozaril
cyproheptadine	Periactin
dexmethylphenidate	Focalin
dextromethorphan-quinidine	Nuedexta
diazepam	Valium
dicyclomine	Bentyl
diphenoxylate 2.5 mg/atropine 0.24 mg	Lomotil
doxepine	Silenor
duloxetine	Cymbalta
escitalopram	Lexapro
fluoxetine	Prozac
fluvoxamine	Luvox
fluphenazine	Prolixin
gabapentin	Neurontin
guanfacine	Intuniv
haloperidol	Haldol
hydroxyzine	Vistaril
lamotrigine	Lamictal
lisdexamfetamine dimesylate	Vyvanse
lithium ER	Eskalith
lorazepam	Ativan
lurasidone	Latuda
methadone	Dolophine
methylphenidate ER	Concerta
mirtazapine	Remeron

GENERIC NAME	BRAND NAME
naloxone	Narcan
naltrexone	Revia
olanzapine	Zyprexa
paliperidone	Invega
paroxetine	Paxil
prazosin	Minipres
propranolol	Inderal
quetiapine	Seroquel
risperidone	Risperdal
sertraline	Zoloft
trazodone	Desyrel
topriamate	Topamax
valproic acid	Depakote
venlafaxine	Effexor
ziprasidone	Geodon
zolmitriptan	Zolmig
zolpidem	Ambien

CLINICAL PRACTICE TOOLS LIST

INDEX

Note: Page numbers followed by *f* and *t* indicate figures and tables

C

P

T

X

Y

Z